Health Care in Rural South Africa

4

Financial support for the publication of this book has kindly been provided by the Dutch foundation Stichting Dioraphte.

VU University Press is an imprint of
VU Boekhandel/Uitgeverij bv
De Boelelaan 1105
1081 HV Amsterdam
The Netherlands
E-mail: info@vu-uitgeverij.nl

ISBN 90 5383 991 7
NUR 883

Design cover: Titus Schulz, Arnhem

# Contents

# PART III:

## Southern African Catholic Bishops' Conference - AIDS Office (Pretoria)

# Epilogue

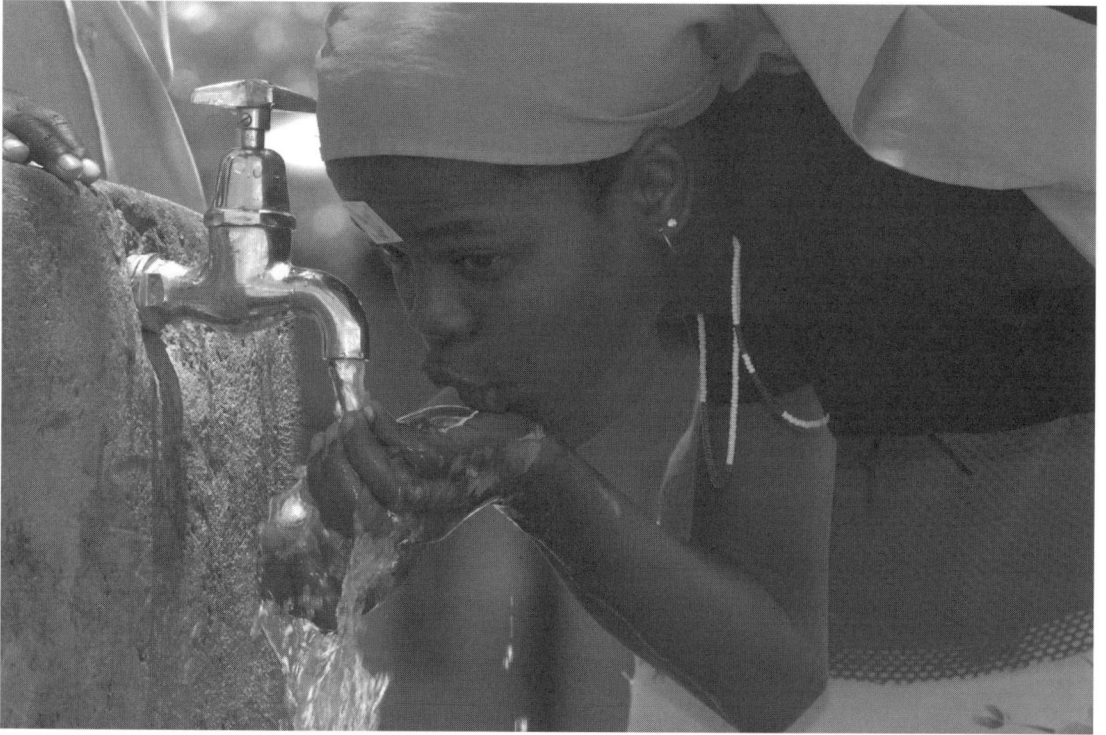

# Preface

It is with great pleasure that I respond to the editors' invitation to write a preface to this book. Since 1993, I have been visiting southern Africa, in particular South Africa, several times a year. I have seen many changes, especially positive developments. As the saying goes, 'you can leave Africa, but Africa never leaves you'. I have learned what this means.

However, we cannot close our eyes for the reality that South Africa is still characterised by great contrasts. Crime and HIV/AIDS dominate the image of the country. These two huge problems go hand in hand with an imposing and almost magic scenery.

I sometimes get the impression that many people in western countries regard southern Africa, in particular South Africa, as a lost continent. Every effort and investment has to be considered as a drop in the ocean. To be clear, I am not of this opinion.

This book testifies to a number of positive developments. The work done by the editors and the people working for the NGOs that have contributed to this book, tell a success story. Set against the background of the huge problems of South Africa, these projects could be perceived as drops in the ocean. However, a waterfall also started with some drops.

The contributions to this book are realistic, but also positive. I hope and trust that the positive message of this book will leave a lasting impression on the reader.

*René Valks*
*Stichting Liberty and Stichting Dioraphte*

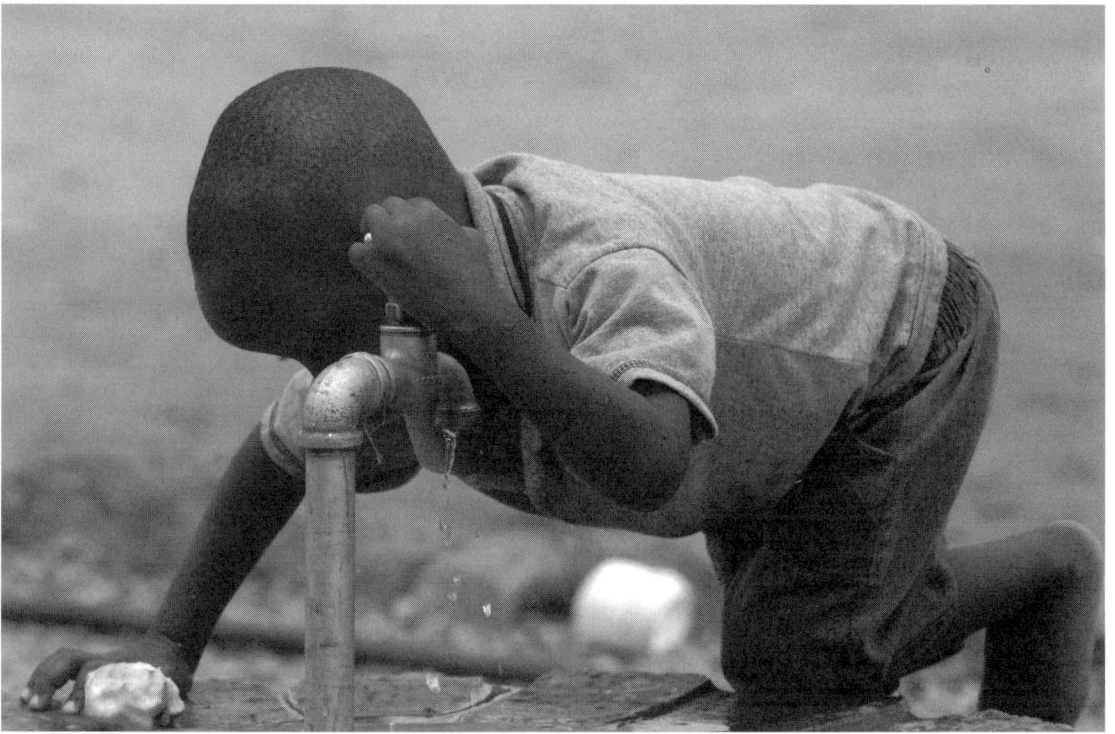

# Introduction

In 2002, co-operation was started between Ndlovu Medical Centre in Elandsdoorn (Mpuma-langa, South Africa) and Sizanani Village in Bronkhorstspruit (Gauteng Province, South Africa) on the one hand, and on the other the Faculty of Social Sciences of the Utrecht University in Utrecht (The Netherlands). This contact was initiated by Mrs. Rita Kok, while the Royal Netherlands Embassy in Pretoria (South Africa) acted as an intermediary. From the start, both sides have felt the relationships developed between them to be quite stimulating and fruitful, which has resulted in several research projects. The common focus of the research described in this book, concerns the evaluation of health care activities carried out by both partners in South Africa, in the meantime joined by a third partner, the Southern African Catholic Bishops' Conference AIDS Office in Pretoria. The planning and realisation of these research projects was facilitated by the substantial financial and managerial support of two Dutch funds, the Stichting Liberty and the Stichting Dioraphte. Out of the mutual connections, a strong co-operation between the various partners has been developed. This book bears witness to this fruitful co-operation.

## Ndlovu Medical Centre

After the development of a great number of health care projects within a period of 5 to 10 years, Ndlovu Medical Centre (NMC) felt a slumbering need to pay attention to the evaluation of these projects, also in view of the fast growing number of activities. As yet, it was chosen to start with the evaluation of the outcome of a nutritional programme for under- and malnourished babies and young children and their mothers, and the evaluation of an AIDS awareness programme for schoolchildren and youth in the Elandsdoorn township area. Furthermore, attention is paid to the development of an antiretroviral treatment programme.

### Evaluation of the Ndlovu Nutritional Unit Programme (NNU)
This programme has been set up for severely under- and malnourished babies and young children. During one year, (grand)mothers receive training in healthy cooking, health behaviour and the starting and maintenance of a vegetable garden. There are presently six nutritional units. The research concerns:
- the programme's effects on the weight, length and general development of the children at discharge, short term and on long term after discharge;
- the identification of factors that determine the participation and completion of the programme by the (grand)mothers;
- the programme's effects on the level of health knowledge of the (grand)mothers.

### Evaluation of the Ndlovu AIDS Awareness Programme (NAAP)
NAAP is conducted by seven young adults, four men and three women. Once a year they visit the senior grades of primary schools and all grades of the high schools in the Elandsdoorn township area and surrounding townships. The programme consists of information about

HIV/AIDS and sex instruction. The performances of the group are a mix of verbal instruction and humoristic sketches. After the performances, the NAAP team 'hangs around' the school for a couple of hours to give students the opportunity to ask questions in an informal setting and to get condoms for free.

The research concerns:
– the programme's effects on safe sex behaviour, in particular condom use;
– the determination of the factors that influence condom use.

## Development of the Highly Active Antiretroviral Treatment (HAART) Programme

One of the most important health care programmes developed by the NMC during the last four years, is the HAART programme. This programme has resulted in an extensive growth of the NMC. In a political context in which even the relationship between HIV and AIDS is under discussion, the NMC has started with a free-of-charge treatment with antiretroviral medicines for HIV patients. The NMC implemented their HAART programme through the start of an Autonomous Treatment Centre (ATC). The Ndlovu HAART programme has three main objectives. NMC would like:
– to become a care provider for the community they work for, firstly in Mpumalanga Province;
– to develop a centre of excellence for integrated TB and HIV/AIDS care in a rural setting, and a model project for others in this field of health care in developing countries;
– to become a capacity builder: health care workers and administrators from both NGOs and public sector are invited to learn from the experiences gained at this project, e.g. by following courses regarding ARV treatment, drug procurement, laboratory- and project management.

This programme is financially supported by the Dutch foundations Stichting Liberty and Stichting Dioraphte and by the PEPFAR programme of the USA.

## Sizanani Village

At the outset, 15 years ago, Sizanani Village primarily offered a home, now called St. Mary's Home, to about 225 disowned, neglected severely disabled children, and children with disabilities whose parents could not take care of them. The situation we encountered in 2002 showed that the children were very well taken care of, that the hygienic circumstances were good, but that despite all this, the amount of treatment, training of elementary daily activities and education to a certain level of independence was minimal. After having assessed the children's needs and the wishes of the childcare workers, it was decided in 2003 to start with the introduction of a development stimulation programme on an experimental basis. A choice was made for a programme called Conductive Education. This is a training and educational programme for children with cerebral palsy or brain injury. The experiment ran until 2005, accompanied by an intervention research with a repeated measurement design. After the successful conclusion of this experiment, it was decided to implement Conductive Education for all children of St. Mary's Home. The introduction and implementation of this programme was supported by the Dutch foundation Stichting Dioraphte.

## The Implementation of Conductive Education in St. Mary's Home

At the moment St. Mary's Home accommodates about 170 children with severe physical and mental disabilities. We feel that Conductive Education (CE), developed in Hungary after the second world war, is an ideal programme for the stimulation of daily independence of children with neurological disorders in particular in developing countries. The starting point of the programme is that children with severe, chronic (that is enduring, unchangeable) motor disorders have to learn to cope with their disabilities and that therapy is not the first thing these children need. The care system itself has to offer these children training situations that teach them to use their potentialities to acquire the skills they directly need in their daily life in order to be as independent as possible.

The research concerns the determination of the CE programme effects on:
- the development of the children's level of independence;
- a change in the intervention style of the childcare workers in their daily interaction with the children, in this case a change from being primarily focused on nursing and caring to being focused on stimulation, training and education;
- the satisfaction of the childcare workers with the new programme.

## Southern African Catholic Bishops' Conference AIDS Office

Over the last years, Sizanani Village has also offered home- and centre-based care for persons with HIV/AIDS. This service is part of a large network of HIV/AIDS care in South Africa under the auspices of the Southern African Catholic Bishops' Conference (SACBC) AIDS Office in Pretoria.

### ARV Treatment Programmes

The SACBC AIDS Office implements ARV programmes on seven locations in South Africa. After a medical screening and selection of HIV/AIDS patients, the patients are supported by local people, some of them also infected with HIV/AIDS, who provide home care. There is regular medical control, but the programme is mainly supported by the social network. The University of Pretoria and the National Research Foundation of South Africa supported the evaluation of these projects by means of qualitative research. The ARV treatment programmes involve mainly adults, but since a few years also children have been participating.

### HIV/AIDS, ARV Treatment and Children's Quality of Life

When children hear that they are HIV/AIDS-infected, this will have a great impact on their perspective of the future, their self-image, their position within the family and their peer relationships. It could be that inclusion in an ARV treatment programme has a positive effect on these aspects of their development. The research executed among children on ARVs took place on four locations: Bronkhorstspruit, Pretoria en two in Johannesburg.

The research question concerns the quality of life of the children involved in the ARV treatment programmes.

This book describes research that has been done in co-operation with the NMC, Sizanani Village and SACBC in South Africa. Not much of this kind of research exists. There is, however, a great need for this type of intervention or evaluative research. Non-governmental organisations (NGOs) are the main subsidisers of health care projects in developing countries. They are highly interested in the results of their- mostly - financial support. Clinical settings, health care centres and health care institutions and organisations, which are responsible for the daily care of their patients, are usually busy day and night, with the organisation and continuation of their activities. There is hardly any time for reflection and systematic evaluation. Feedback by means of effect research proved to be most welcome. The outcomes of these evidence-based research projects would provide starting points for reflection on and - if necessary - readjustment of the programmes described.

All research projects were executed by Master Degree students in Special Education or Developmental Psychology of the Utrecht University in Utrecht (The Netherlands). Also students in Public Health of the Vrije Universiteit in Amsterdam (The Netherlands) were involved in a number of studies. The scientific support and coaching was provided by the departments of these universities. Since last year, also the Department of Psychology of the University of Pretoria has co-operated.

In accordance with the research contacts that have been developed, this book consists of three parts. Descriptions are given of research projects together with:
1. Ndlovu Medical Centre;
2. St. Mary's Home of Sizanani Village;
3. Southern African Catholic Bishop's Conference AIDS Office

In order to place the research projects in the local context, each part of the book starts with an introductory chapter about the aims and activities of the organisation concerned.

The health care activities of the three organisations take place within the context of health care developments in a developing country like South Africa. The research into a number of these activities described here is determined by the investigator's methodological frames of reference. To place these activities in the context of national health care in South Africa, this book opens with a prologue about the developments in this field, in particular with respect to HIV/AIDS. The book closes with an epilogue on how the academia could contribute to health care in developing countries.

All this work is only possible with the help of committed sponsors. The chairman of two of these funds, Stichting Liberty and Stichting Dioraphte, therefore opens this book with his foreword.

Lastly, this book bears a pretentious title: 'An innovative approach'. The fact that the NGOs and NPOs described in this book, allow their activities to be evaluated, attests to a vision. A vision is also expressed in the chapters that offer perspectives for the disaster taking place in South Africa. This disaster is called 'AIDS'. These chapters show an attitude of not accepting, of using all efforts to fight this pandemic. Similarly, a vision is evidenced by the approach of disability: focus on potentials and functionality. The epilogue provides a perspective of the societal importance of the research described in this book.

*Adri Vermeer and Hugo Tempelman,*
*editors*

# Prologue

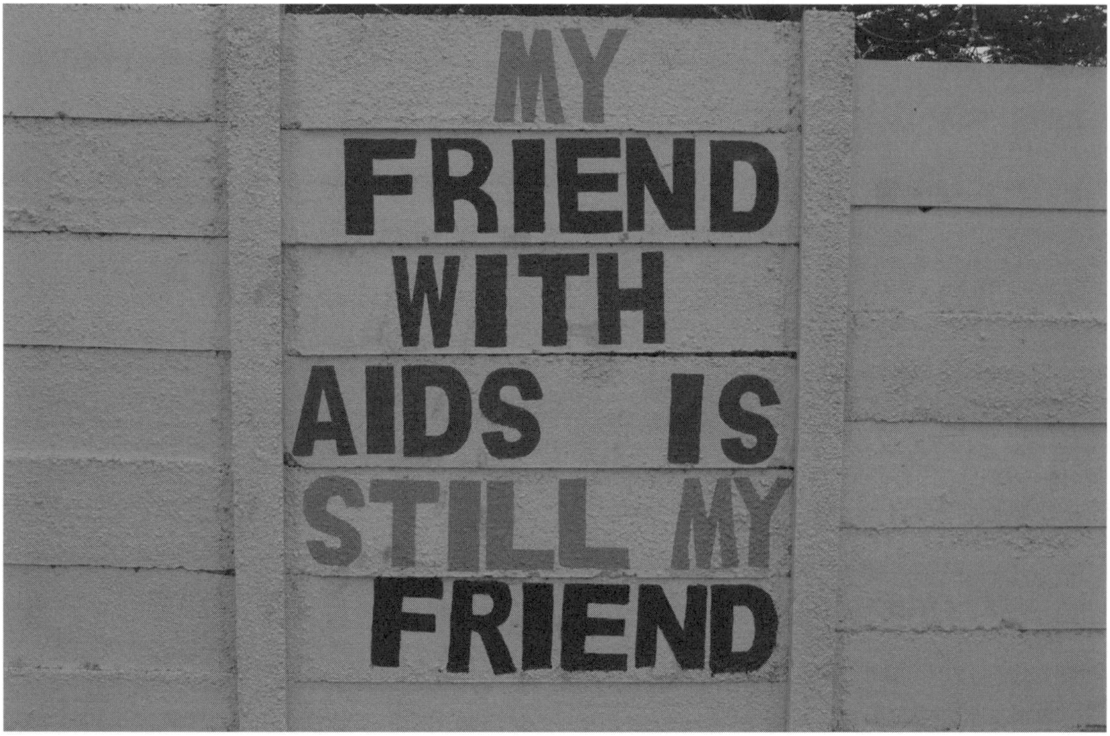
MY
FRIEND
WITH
AIDS IS
STILL MY
FRIEND

# Chapter 1

# Perspectives on HIV Medical Care in South Africa

*Des Martin* [1]

[1] South African HIV Clinicians Society; University of Pretoria, Pretoria, South Africa

## Abstract

South Africa has witnessed an HIV epidemic of catastrophic proportions. The social milieu has provided a fertile ground for this epidemic. Poverty, malnutrition, lack of empowerment of women, an epidemic of sexually transmitted infections and the legacy of apartheid are some of the co-factors that have fuelled the epidemic. Some unique features have included the 'dissident' debacle, the inaction and bungling of successive governments and the role of activism and legal actions in forcing change. Other unique features include various cultural influences, myths and the role of traditional healers and their remedies.

## 1. Introduction

During the 1980s most people were aware of the new disease, AIDS, found mainly amongst injecting drug users and the homosexual community in the United States of America (USA). Many South Africans at the time believed that as South Africa had only very small populations of these societal sub-groups, AIDS would not be a major problem in South Africa. Under the repressive government of mostly religious-conservative members in the 1980s, homosexuality was considered a sin and few gay people had come out of the closet, so numbers were underestimated and the stigma and discrimination associated with HIV and AIDS can only have been heightened by the prevailing attitudes of the time.

Only in the latter years of the 1980s did South Africans become aware of the fact that AIDS was emerging as a heterosexually transmitted disease in central and eastern Africa. Stories began emerging that it was possible that infection could be caused by the preparation and/or ingestion of monkey-meat or as a mode of transmission in countries such as Uganda, Kenya, Burundi, Malawi, Tanzania and other African countries.

The South African public became really conscious of HIV/AIDS as a very real presence in South Africa in 1993, the year after two homosexual South African Airway's employees died from an AIDS-related opportunistic infection. At that time it was thought that the disease was almost exclusively a disease of the gay community, largely due to their practice of anal sex, and also of intravenous drug users. There appeared to be a strong link with the USA, a country frequented by the two SAA employees and where the disease was known to exist in the gay community and among intravenous drug users.

Later, due to 'Slim' disease being prevalent in Uganda and other countries north of South Africa and an outbreak of *Cryptococcal* meningitis in Zaire, another theory was postulated, i. e. that immigrant workers and truckers were bringing the disease into the country. An imported supply of HIV-contaminated blood product (Factor 8) from the USA resulted in many

Johannesburg haemophiliacs becoming infected, alerting healthcare professionals to the risk of untested or 'high risk' donors (or donors in the window period) playing a part in the international spread of the disease. This again confirmed the USA-link. Blood taken from mine workers in the 1970s had been saved and was tested when the HIV-antibody test became available (Abbott's ELISA test; Sher & Reid, 1987). About 5 percent were found to have been HIV-positive, the majority being Malawian mine workers. This resulted in the Malawian government preventing their men from coming to work on South Africa mines. This supported the mineworker-trucker/Northern African countries theory.

In 1983, Ruben Sher and Dennis Sifris (Sher, dos Santod & Lyons, 1985) tested 200 gay males and found that 11 to 12 percent were positive. Locally, studies were carried out in supposed 'high risk' groups, e.g. dental practitioners, intravenous drug users, but HIV was not found in these sections of South African society at that point in time.

South Africa's epidemic came later than in other sub-Saharan African countries because of isolation and limited movement in and out of the country due to the politics of the day, which included sanctions and considerable political 'struggle'. Some epidemiologists also believe that up to 30 percent of political exiles returning to South Africa in 1994, in the wake of the new democratically elected ANC government, were already HIV-positive when they returned home. Also the truckers freighting goods across borders and down the length of the country contributed in no insignificant measure to the spread of disease from more northern countries.

A decade has passed since then, during which time the disease has passed insidiously from gay men to bi-sexual men, from heterosexual men to heterosexual women, from heterosexual women to heterosexual men, and from mother to child. Globally and in South Africa, few health care workers have become infected through 'needle stick' injuries, or from sores and cuts on their hands and the splattering of HIV-infected blood into eyes and open mouths during medical procedures and surgery.

The two governments in power over this period of time were not particularly helpful in mounting a meaningful, powerful attack on the epidemic, which has enabled the small number of infected individuals to spread into an epidemic that is now a pandemic of epic proportions. So in terms of numbers, about 100,000 people may have been HIV-positive by 1990, but it would be seven to ten years before they developed AIDS. Between 1980 and 1990, only a small number of business people spoke with any concern about the possible impact an AIDS epidemic could have on the business sector. The late 1980s were an intense time in the struggle for a democratic government and most white businesses were focusing a lot of energy on supporting change. Much time was spent on labour legislation and later on the incorporation of the Constitutional requirements in labour practice. Only after the change in government and the publishing of the early HIV epidemiology data from prevalence studies did the question of pre-employment screening for HIV infection, provision of benefits for HIV-infected persons by medical schemes, confidentiality in the workplace, training, education and management of HIV-infected employees become issues.

## 2. Challenges and Responses to the HIV Epidemic in South Africa

### 2.1. Impact on the Economy

Over the last fifteen years there has been an evolving attitude by big and medium business to HIV/AIDS largely due to the fact that at first business people did not believe that HIV/AIDS was going to be a major issue and as there was some scepticism in many quarters regarding

the results of early epidemiology studies. The government and a lot of other sections of the community felt that the data were inflated. As time went on, it became clear to almost everyone that the epidemic was growing at an alarming rate. Only then did the business sector start to take note. The AIDS 2000 Conference held in July 2000 in Durban, South Africa (XIIIth International AIDS Conference) was given prominence in the press and big business in particular had to sit up and pay attention to the fact that many people of both sexes, mostly young people in their productive working years, were already infected. The problems foreseen included:
– injuries to AIDS-sick people manning machinery;
– accidents caused by sick truck drivers;
– loss of skilled workers to AIDS;
– absenteeism;
– modes of transmission in the workplace;
– workplace education;
– the role of medical schemes in treatment of HIV and of opportunistic infections and AIDS.

The business response is difficult to define as there are many different companies with very diverse corporate cultures. But the government's questioning of the causal link between HIV and AIDS and related public debates, muddied the field. Adding to the confusion, the Minister of Health repeatedly made reference to the dire toxic side- effects of antiretroviral drugs, and still does. Of course, this still left the key issue faced by the business sector: the (non) employment of HIV-infected persons. Initially, business attempted not to employ HIV-infected by insisting on an HIV test and some employers even tried to dismiss HIV-infected workers or workers who were 'thought' to be infected. Today, HIV testing as a prerequisite to employment is now virtually unheard of in South Africa.

The Employment Equity Act 55 of 1998 regulates workplace medical testing in the context of the workplace: 'Medical testing of an employee is prohibited, unless: legislation permits or requires the testing, or it is justifiable in the light of medical facts, employment conditions, social policy, fair distribution of employee benefits or the inherent requirements of a job or testing of an employee to determine that employee's HIV status is prohibited unless such testing is determined to be justifiable by the Labour Court in terms of Section 50(4) of this Act.' An employer is therefore prohibited from 'testing' or arranging for HIV testing.

## The Effect of HIV/AIDS on the Local Markets
Retail businesses are beginning to have very real concerns regarding the impact of AIDS sickness and AIDS deaths on their consumer markets. Their concern relates to the absolute South African market size and sectors within the market, especially those which market and sell high-priced items mostly paid for on higher purchase agreements. This manner of payment is often used by people in the 20–40 age group which is the group largely affected by the pandemic.

## Response in the Mining Industry
The mining industry has always employed large numbers of migrant labourers now thought to have added to the pandemic (especially Malawians) and although those workers no longer do that, they generally have a higher prevalence than the general population. This is largely due to the social environment in which they live, i.e. single-sex hostels away from their

homes and wives, and the use of groups of prostitutes living in the vicinity of the mines. Due to this situation, mining companies led the way in employee group HIV programmes. Many mines have established clinics and hospitals and some include HIV benefits not just for the employees but also their families. Many studies have been carried out in and around the mining sector, including the treatment of sexually transmitted diseases, education programmes, peer-group counsellors for Voluntary Counselling and Testing (VCT) and antiretroviral treatment (ARVT). Some senior executives have also participated in these programmes to try to increase the uptake of VCT and disclosure to close family members or friends and to form support groups. Anglo American, the second largest gold mining group in the world, began an antiretroviral programme some three years ago. They have now approximately 3,000 thousand patients on the programme.

ARVT regimens do offer businesses an opportunity to keep HIV-infected employees productive for longer periods of time and therefore able to assist children to remain at school and provide income for their families.

*Business Response*
SABCOHA, the South Africa Business Coalition on HIV/AIDS, was launched in February 2000 and is affiliated to the Global Business Council on HIV/AIDS, which was founded in 1997. After several years of stop/start activity, SABCOHA has finally given South Africa a co-ordinated business response to HIV/AIDS. This informal grouping of interested businesses has grown from strength to strength during the last 2–3 years but is still battling for recognition and funding. It also has to compete with AIDS activities in other organised business- or industry-based structures.

The objectives of SABCOHA are to establish a network of expertise and a resource centre to assist the private sector to develop the necessary response to deal with HIV/AIDS in the workplace. There are, however, still many issues and divisions within so-called organised business in South Africa.

A key issue to investigate is what would be best practice for South Africa. HIV should be part of the strategic plan of every organisation and should be matched with a budget and an action plan.

*Life Insurance Industry*
One of the routine tasks undertaken by actuaries is to make long-term projections of expected mortality and disability rates. In most developed countries, actuaries have observed more or less continuous improvements in mortality rates, largely due to improved nutrition, safety and health care. However, early projections of the impact of the HIV/AIDS epidemic showed a significant increase in mortality rates, particularly in the age groups 20-40, which is the most productive age group, paying much of a country's tax, medical aid contributions, life assurance, and retirement fund contributions.

Life assurors have required an HIV test for high insurance cover in line with other similar high-risk and/or chronic diseases, e.g. vascular disease and diabetes which have similar requirements. The Life Officers Association (LOA) has kept abreast of scientific advances and ethics related to HIV, particularly related to counselling and HIV testing with informed consent.

Insurance companies used to include *exclusion clauses* in insurance contracts, which included people suffering from HIV and AIDS. This was a very controversial practice, evolving from the premise that HIV/AIDS could threaten the financial stability of insurance companies. The LOA has, however, discouraged the use of exclusion clauses and, today, they are being relied on less and less by life insurers.

South Africa has also been a leader in responding to the HIV epidemic. The world's first life insurance product for HIV/AIDS patients was developed and marketed in this country.

## 2.2. Impact of HIV/AIDS on the Criminal Justice System

South Africa's criminal justice system is performing abysmally. In 2000 almost 2.6 million crimes were recorded by the police, of which the prosecution service took on 270,000 cases, the remainder being unsolved or withdrawn. Of these, approximately 210,000 cases ended in a conviction of the perpetrators, which reflects that only about 8 percent of the crimes recorded resulted in a conviction.

A number of the prosecutors seeking these convictions are themselves under the age of 30 years and would therefore also fall within a high-risk group for HIV/AIDS. There is a huge 'back log' of cases in the courts that would require a considerable period of time to deal with before any new cases can be accepted. This will be compounded by a prosecution service that may well be losing members to HIV/AIDS or functioning less optimally due to HIV-related illness.

### Police Service

The majority of South Africa's police officers are male and in the younger age group. Police officers stationed in rural areas are also at an increased risk of becoming involved in high-risk behaviour. The impact of HIV/AIDS is therefore likely to have a negative effect on the efficacy of the police force as a whole, which will further aggravate the number of cases submitted to the courts for prosecution.

### Correctional Services

The prison environment is one which is likely to exacerbate factors leading to the transmission of HIV. High-risk sexual behaviour, sexual abuse, rape, sexually transmitted diseases, are all factors which will promote the spread of HIV. The increasing rate of natural deaths among prison inmates is thought to be largely a result of HIV/AIDS. It is estimated that by the year 2010 nearly 45,000 prisoners will die whilst incarcerated, primarily as a result of HIV/AIDS. High rates of HIV infection in the prisons cause an increased burden of work amongst staff and medical services. This leads to a chronic lack of adequate supervision of inmates, thus contributing to a vicious cycle of HIV transmission.

It can thus be seen that the core criminal justice departments (correction services, prosecution and police force) will suffer a dramatic impact as a result of HIV/AIDS. The loss of trained and experienced personnel in the next decade will compound the issues mentioned previously.

### Orphans

The unprecedented number of deaths of young people in South Africa has resulted in an increase in the number of orphans on a scale that was unpredicted. It is estimated that there are close on 1 million South African children under the age of 15 years who have lost one or both parents to AIDS by 2005. This figure is expected to rise to well over 2 million by 2010, according to the National Department of Health.

The deeply rooted kinship systems and extended family networks which previously constituted a social safety net, are unable to cope with the burden of AIDS orphans. This has led to a lack of family support for these unfortunate children and many have become street children. Purely to survive, these children turn to crime which often takes the form of theft of food and clothing, and residential burglary. Street children are both the cause and victims of a range of crimes. Many street children are assaulted, abused, raped and drawn into prostitution rings. They are therefore at risk of becoming HIV-infected themselves.

## 2.3. *Government Response*

One of the results of dissident activities in South Africa and the peculiar fascination that the South African government and the Department of Health has with them, has been that many HIV-positive people taking antiretrovirals (ARVs) have discontinued their ARVs because they fear the 'high toxicity' and question the very nature of the disease. Local politicians have openly expressed and supported the dissident view that HIV infection has multifactorial causes, including poverty and poor nutrition, and is not linked to AIDS.

Formed in 1995, the National AIDS/STD Advisory Committee, with its multi-sectoral members, was dissolved and replaced in 2000 by a new South African National AIDS Council (SANAC). It was highly criticised, as a large number of government officials were listed as members, but none of the internationally and nationally recognised South African medical clinical, laboratory and research HIV experts were included. The government appeared to disregard internationally researched and accepted scientific views regarding the virus, its causation of AIDS and antiretroviral therapy. This further muddied the waters and led to some epidemiological research and much discussion around prevention. Nothing was resolved in the eyes of the government and many South Africans. As a result, a number of HIV-infected South Africans have discontinued ARVs and begun taking non-researched food extracts, herbs, micro- and macro-nutrients and fortified foodstuffs. Few of these have been properly researched in the context of HIV/AIDS and those that have, have proved ineffective and some even hasten the course of the disease process. Many people have died as a result.

Such is the influence of the dissidents on the President and of the President on his staff, that they have remained virtually silent on this issue. It is surmised that they were unwilling to criticise the ANC leadership and former comrades in the struggle. The South African community at large has been confused by the President and the ANC government's stance, so that people simply do not know what to believe or what to do. This attitude has contributed to stigmatisation of the disease and has proved to be a barrier to VCT and disclosure.

The 'Durban Declaration' (2002) emanated from the AIDS Conference held in Durban in 2000, and was a document in support of an evidence-based cause, transmission, testing and treatment of HIV/AIDS. This was signed by approximately 5,000 people (mostly doctors and health care workers) in an attempt to counter the dissidents' influences.

The current views of President Mbeki regarding the causation of HIV/AIDS are not known and he has not commented on the issue for some time. He has largely played a passive role in supporting the HIV/AIDS programmes in the country and as such has influenced senior members of his cabinet and of the ANC. This situation is in stark contrast to other countries in Africa, particularly Uganda and Botswana, where the presidents have championed various AIDS programmes and have acted as shining examples to the rest of the continent.

With a singular lack of conviction an antiretroviral roll-out programme has been endorsed by the government. This programme has been exceedingly slow and inadequate and mainly confined to the larger centres where some infrastructure exists.   This is, once again, in stark contrast to the programmes carried out by large industry, the private sector, faith-based organisations and various non-governmental organisations.

## 2.4. Medical Response

The First International Conference on AIDS was held in Atlanta, Georgia, in the United States of America in 1985. Twenty years ago! It was attended by a well-known South African expert, Ruben Sher, who together with Sue Lyons (Sher, Lyons, dos Santos, Shoub & McGillvray, 1985) developed an indirect fluorescent antibody test, which enabled the first testing of blood to take place in South Africa. The South African Institute of Medical Research commenced routine testing of blood and the South African Blood Transfusion Service (SABTS) introduced HIV-antibody testing for all donors. It was at this time that haemophiliacs were infected by HIV- contaminated Factor 8 infusions, which resulted in the majority of South African haemophiliacs being infected. This prompted the Johannesburg Hospital to open an HIV Clinic in 1985, followed by other Johannesburg hospitals, namely Hillbrow Hospital, JG Strydom Hospital (now Helen Joseph) and the Baragwaneth Hospital (now Chris Hani Baragwaneth Hospital). In these early days, the Johannesburg Hospital Clinic was staffed by part-time doctors, e.g. Steven Miller, Dennis Sifris and Des Martin.

It was also at this time that the South African government, believing that AIDS was confined to certain risk groups, contributed a small amount of money to establish an AIDS Advisory Group headed by Jack Metz, Director of the South African Institute of Medical Research (SAIMR). The government did very little to contain the epidemic and small groups of individuals among the medical professions were left to do their best. It was also at this time that the Treatment Action Campaign (TAC) was formed as an activist group to lobby various stakeholders, including the government, to provide a more meaningful response to the epidemic.

In 1987, Ruben Sher established the first AIDS Training Centre (ATTIC) at the SAIMR, which was to provide a model for the education and training in the field of HIV/AIDS to various health care professionals (Sherr, Christie, Sher & Metz, 1989). The number of ATTICS steadily grew and they provided an excellent service to HIV-infected and affected communities. Unfortunately in early 1993 the Department of Health saw fit to close the ATTIC at the SAIMR, claiming 'a shortage of funds'.

In the early 1990s the Johannesburg City Health Department, under the leadership of the Medical Officer of Health, Hilliard Hurwitz, together with Nicky Padayachee, Clive Evian and Mary Crewe-Brown established an AIDS Information Centre at Hillbrow, Johannesburg. This clinic is still operational and provides expanded services under the expert leadership of Francois Venter, who has attracted support and visits from the rich and famous including the actor Brad Pitt and the billionaire entrepreneur Sir Richard Branson.

But by the early 1990s still only a few medical doctors were really involved in the epidemic and providing diagnosis, treatment and care of the HIV-infected. This group, the AIDS Advisory Group, included Jack Metz, Ruben Sher, B. Schoub, Dennis Sifris, S. Lyons, Steven Miller and Des Martin. Other doctors involved from various other segments of medicine, including those from the Infectious Diseases arena and the Blood Transfusion Service included Shapiro, Richard Crooks, Anton Heynes, Jack Metz and James Gear. It is to be noted that this group was largely male and all were white.

## 2.5. Southern African HIV Clinicians Society

With the growing number of HIV-infected patients in the country the need arose for educational initiatives and networking within the medical professions. 1988 saw the birth of the Southern African HIV Clinicians Society, registered as a South African Medical Association's (SAMA) Special Interest Group (SIG). It is now the largest with approximately 10,000 members, most of whom are general practitioners. The Society's main objective is to support a high standard of health care to populations affected by HIV/AIDS and provide quality clinical care for people living with HIV/AIDS through an increasing number of initiatives.

The Society has witnessed a phenomenal growth since its inception in 1988. The initial membership was 288 and this has grown to over 10,000 members, mainly doctors, mostly within South Africa but also scattered throughout the southern African region. The Society has fostered and supported the growth of branches in Namibia, Botswana, Zimbabwe, Zambia, Swaziland and Lesotho, thus creating a network of active branches within the region. The branches carry out a number of important functions, including monthly meetings, dissemination of information, hosting of continuing medical education courses, and providing faculty for education initiatives. The contact details and other information of every member are maintained on a state-of-art database.

Education of health care professionals remains a prime objective of the Society. To this end, a partnership was formed with the Foundation for Professional Development (FPD), the education division of the South African Medical Association (SAMA). This initiative has flourished and almost 10,000 health care professionals (doctors and nurses) have been trained. The course was launched in September 2001 in order to provide a basic knowledge of 'best practice' standard of care for HIV-infected patients. It was initiated with seed funding from the International AIDS Society (IAS) and a grant from surplus funds from the AIDS 2000 (Durban) Conference. This enables the course to be offered at an affordable price, thus promoting access to all. More recently, sponsorships by mining houses, medical schemes, pharmaceutical companies and other international funders has enabled further courses to be held.

A further educational focus of the Society resides in its widely disseminated publications. These consist of the popular quarterly newsletter *Transcript,* which provides updated information to members regarding meeting dates/venues, current antiretroviral drug prices and an article reflecting on the local HIV milieu. The *Southern African Journal of HIV Medicine,* published quarterly, is the Society's premier publication and is targeted primarily at general practitioners. This journal fills a particular niche because there is a singular lack of a dedicated HIV journal in the region. The editorial board has been strengthened by an international advisory panel, consisting of experts in HIV medicine from other countries. A number of locally relevant management and treatment guidelines have been published within the pages of the journal.

The recognition that an impressive repository of HIV expertise resides within the Society has been provided by a number of bodies. These include the Colleges of Medicine of South Africa (CMSA), for which the Society provides the syllabus and sets the examination in the Diploma of HIV Management (Dip HIV Man SA). The Society also provides consultations to the medical profession, the Department of Health, the pharmaceutical industry, legal access groups, managed healthcare organisations, activist organisations and a variety of NGOs. The Society is affiliated to a number of similar international AIDS Societies.

# 3. The role of Activism

From 1994, when the ANC-led government came to power following a general election, more support was provided by President Mandela's supportive attitude. Sadly, his Minister of Health was influenced by denialists, as was her successor, the present Minister of Health, who believes that garlic, beetroot and other nutrients and micronutrients are helpful in stemming the tide of disease. President Thabo Mbeki is a closet denialist and only the persistence of the Treatment Action Campaign, the AIDS Law Project, the Southern African Clinicians Society, various overseas organisations and disclosure by some very high-profile South Africans (Judge Edwin Cameron, 1999; Zackie Achmat) forced the government into commencing a Public Sector Roll-out of ARVs in 2004. It has been a slow process with hiccoughs in drug supply, inadequately trained medical personnel, and a community afraid to test/disclose due to persistent stigmatisation and probable rejection from partners and family groups.

Despite the denialist attitude, the South African government challenged the patent rights of international pharmaceutical companies in the courts. This action together with Treatment Action Campaign (TAC) activism resulted in significant cost reductions of antiretroviral drugs, which until then had been very highly priced. The TAC then took the government to court for not providing antiretroviral drugs in the public sector. They wanted nevirapine to be made available to HIV-positive mothers to prevent mother-to-child transmission (PMTCT) and a selection (or regimen) of antiretrovirals to be made available to patients with AIDS. This court challenge ended when the Constitutional Court ordered the Department of Health to dispense antiretroviral drugs to pregnant, HIV-infected women.

Various activist organisations have played an enormous role in promoting both human rights and access to antiretroviral treatment in our country. Foremost among these organisations have been the AIDS Law Project (ALP), Treatment Action Campaign (TAC), AIDS Consortium and the National Association of People With AIDS (MAPWA). The AIDS Law Project, started in 1993 by Justice Edwin Cameron, has proved to be an enormous legal resource dealing with various legal and human rights issues in the field of HIV/AIDS. The ALP is now headed by Mark Heywood and one of the defining moments for the organisation was the case against South African Airways, which had a successful outcome in favour of SAA. The ALP was also party to the first judgement in the Constitutional Court in which the precedence of non-discrimination, equality and duty of government was upheld in a case dealing with the employment of an HIV-infected individual. The ALP has been involved in numerous land mark cases since then. In late 1998, the Treatment Action Campaign (TAC) was formed, which has now grown into an extremely powerful local and international activist organisation. Numerous human rights accolades have been awarded to Zackie Achmat, its leader. The TAC has instigated a number of court cases promoting access of standard care for populations living with HIV. Among these are landmark actions brought against the Pharmaceutical Manufacturers Association (PMA), the government and more recently the Rath Foundation, to mention but a few. The Southern African HIV Clinicians Society has been an active partner with various activist organisations in these cases.

# 4. Traditional Healers, Stigma and Myths

Probably one of the most challenging areas in dealing with the epidemic has been the plethora of myths surrounding HIV/AIDS and the number of very destructive beliefs regarding the aetiology, cause(s), mode(s) of transmission and preventative measures. The denialists and the government following have unfortunately done little to dispel any of the myths.

One of the myths is that HIV does not cause AIDS, but poverty and its sequelae do, and that sleeping with a virgin cures HIV/AIDS. The denialists' support of micro- and macronutritional supplementation has rubbed off onto the government with even the Minister of Health frequently exhorting the public to take olive oil, garlic, beetroot etc.

There have been enormous and expensive prevention campaigns which epidemiological statistics and various studies have proved to have been of no positive benefit. Condom usage is still low and not culturally acceptable to many South Africans and women have little bargaining power with their partners. Dry sex, prevalent in South Africa, promotes transmission, as does the high presence of sexually transmitted infections (STIS).

Traditional healers play an important role in the physical and spiritual health of the majority of people in our country. Many patients at some stage during their illnesses, including HIV infection, will consult traditional healers and be given various herbal and other remedies. These have the capacity to cause toxicities in their own right and in some instances to negate the effect of ARV therapies by interacting with ARVs. Our patients are often frightened to tell that they have consulted these healers and clinicians often make incorrect decisions regarding changing therapies due to apparent toxicities of ARVs, whereas the effect is in reality due to the traditional medicines. It is a fallacy to surmise that only the unsophisticated or illiterate members of society consult these healers, as there are well-recorded instances of educated and sophisticated individuals seeking their treatment.

The medical profession has on a number of occasions, with some success, engaged traditional healers in an effort to make them allies in the fight against HIV. The leader and doyen of traditional healers in South Africa, Credo Mutwa was met in an effort to start dialogue at the highest level between our respective organisations. In my opinion this body of individuals and their various cures remain a huge resource in combating HIV, if harnessed and educated.

## 5. Conclusions

South Africa is host to a burgeoning HIV epidemic of catastrophic proportions. The country has the dubious honour of having the most HIV-infected individuals in the world. The roots of the epidemic are complex and lie within a web that embraces poverty, lack of empowerment of women, gender violence and the legacy of the apartheid era. This has led to migrant workers, single-sex hostels and fragmentation of the normal family structures that would be protective in this epidemic. The epidemic in South Africa has further been fuelled by the inaction of both past and present governments and has spawned a society that has discriminated against and stigmatised those who suffer from the disease. The impact of this epidemic on various segments of society may well be disastrous. Is it too late?

## References

Durban Declaration (2002). *Southern African Journal of HIV Medicine, 2.*
Judge Edwin Cameron (1999). *Witness to Aids.* Mail & Guardian. Previous Daily Mail & Report. April, 20.
Sher, R., dos Santos, L. & Lyons, S. (1985). Prevalence of HTLV antibodies in homosexual men in Johannesburg. *South African Medical Journal, 67*, p. 484.

Sher, R., Lyons, S., dos Santos, L., Schoub, B. & McGillvray, G. (1985). An indirect fluorescent antibody test for antibodies against HTLV-111. Letter to the Editor. *South African Medical Journal, 67,* p. 37.

Sher, R. & Reid (Rand Mines) (1987). Seroepidemiology of Human Immunodeficiency Virus in Africa from 1970 – 1974. *New England Journal Medicine,* pp. 450 - 451.

Sherr, L., Christie, G., Sher, R. & Metz, J. (1989). Evaluation of the effectiveness of AIDS training and information courses. *South African Medical Journal, 76,* pp. 358-362.

*Address for correspondence:*
Prof. dr. D. Martin
South African HIV Clinicians Society
Suite 233
PosNet Killarney
Private Bag X2600
Houghton 2041
South Africa
e-mail: des.martin@togalab.co.za

# Part I

# Ndlovu Medical Centre (Elandsdoorn)

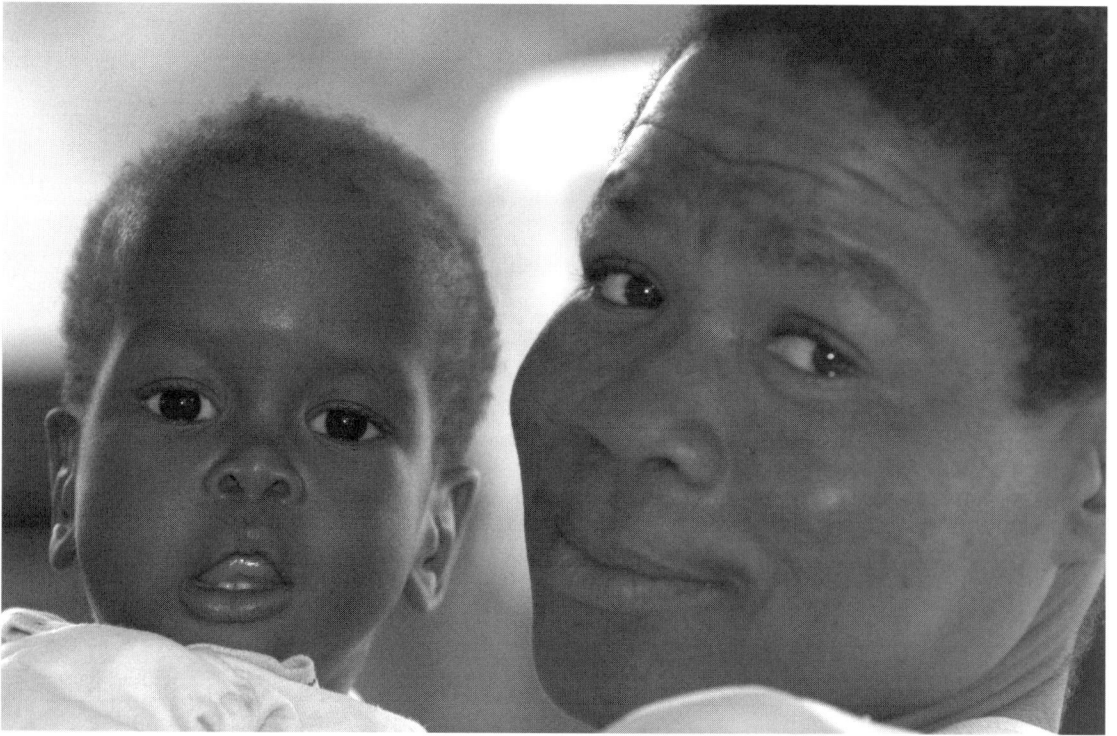

# Chapter 2

# Health Care in Ndlovu Medical Centre

*Hugo Tempelman[1], Liesje Tempelman[1]*

[1] Ndlovu Medical Centre, Elandsdoorn, South Africa

## Abstract

Since 1994, Ndlovu Medical Centre, a private initiative by Liesje and Hugo Tempelman, has functioned in the Moutse area, Mpumalanga, as a private practice and community health care provider. It applies an innovative approach towards public health care, TB care, and HIV/AIDS care. It combines free-of-charge services with private practice and constantly strives for interaction and co-operation with the Department of Health in order to create private-public-partnerships in the provision of health care in resource-poor settings. Recently, the challenge has been to see whether the whole model can be duplicated in the Bushbuckridge area. The emphasis on the health impact of the concept of care provision will only be of greater importance if this initiative will succeed. It might mean the start of a franchise in primary health care facilities in which private and public sector join forces in order to achieve high-quality care for communities that are unable to afford, but do need quality primary care for themselves.

## 1. Introduction

Ndlovu Medical Centre (NMC) combines private and public health care with community development, stimulation of entrepreneurship and self-help projects.

The authors of this chapter, a Dutch medical doctor and a professional nurse, arrived in South Africa in 1990. The first author worked for the Department of Health in KwaNdebele for four years, first as a medical officer and later as the Assistant Superintendent of Philadelphia Hospital in Dennilton. Working at the Department of Health as head of Paramedical Services, he was responsible for the development of primary health care facilities. In 1994, the authors built their own medical clinic, Ndlovu Medical Centre, in Elandsdoorn, Moutse, Mpumalanga. They created a trust for community health projects (Ndlovu Medical Trust, NMT) and a trust for community development projects (Elandsdoorn Development Trust, EDT). The latter will not be discussed in this chapter, but is mentioned to show that a holistic approach to health was chosen. Living and working in a township are makes one aware that health is also closely connected to the availability of primary living conditions. Elandsdoorn Development Trust tries to improve these conditions by initiating water projects, youth employment projects, e.g. a bakery, a fitness centre, a building company, a nappy factory, a car wash, a welding & construction company, a postal agency with 2,000 post-boxes, a waste disposal project, bursaries for promising youth and a library at the secondary school.

Since 1998, the team has been reinforced by a second medical doctor, who previously worked in the former Transkei for a period of seven years. In 2005, the team consisted of six medical doctors and further expansion is expected.

NMT and EDT together have created over 180 sustainable jobs, which makes them a major employer in the area.

## 2. The area

Elandsdoorn is a township in the Moutse district, located on the R25 between Bronkhorst-spruit and Groblersdal, Mpumalanga, South Africa. The population has been estimated at 30,000 – 40,000 people, predominantly Sepedi-, seTswana-, isiZulu- and isiNdebele-speaking. Within a 10-km radius, there are a number of other townships that could benefit from the objectives of the Ndlovu Medical Trust and the Elandsdoorn Development Trust, bringing the total number of potential beneficiaries to 120,000 – 150,000 people.

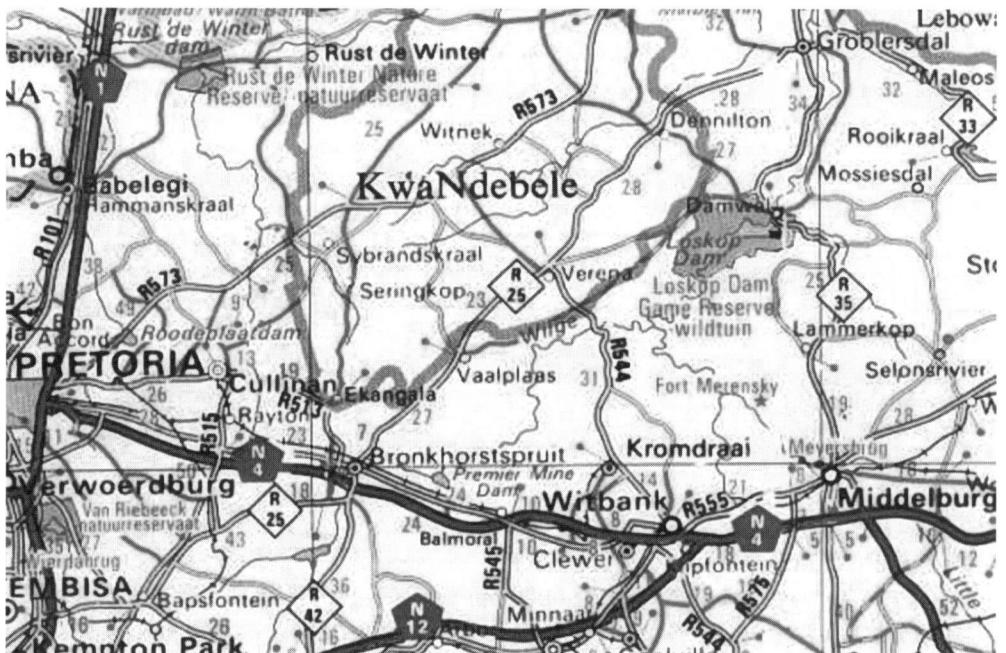

Figure 1: On the map Elandsdoorn is situated next to Dennilton, 30 km from Groblersdal and 30 km from Loskop Dam.

## 3. Health Care Programmes

The NMC operates as a private clinic. It also provides community health care to the area it serves, such as a nutritional programme, an HIV/AIDS awareness programme, a tuberculosis programme, an HIV/AIDS treatment programme, a primary dental care programme, a family planning clinic, a twelve-bed obstetrical hospital with intended beds for AIDS patients and an HIV monitoring laboratory.

The tuberculosis programme provides testing facilities and treatment and arranges home visits to defaulting patients. The HIV/AIDS awareness programme provides awareness programmes to secondary school students, private and group counselling and also distributes information. The nutritional programme treats malnourished children, while their caregivers are taught how to grow vegetables in their own gardens and how to improve the home situation in terms of sanitation, hygiene and health.

The Colombine Maternity Clinic, which offers affordable antenatal, obstetrical and postnatal services, was opened in 1999. Two new programmes were launched in 2003: the Ngwenya Community Dental Care Programme introduces dental health awareness and dental care to primary school children, while the Highly Active Anti-Retroviral Treatment (HAART) project treats AIDS patients with antiretroviral medicines (see for background information, in particular about AIDS in South Africa, Nattrass, 2004).

Although these community health care programmes are provided through the NMC, they are administered by a separate trust, the Ndlovu Medical Trust (NMT).

## 4. Ndlovu Medical Trust

### 4.1. Ndlovu Nutritional Unit Programme (NNU)

The NNU is run in conjunction with the NMC. Mothers or other caregivers often come to the NMC and present their children with chronic diarrhoea or pneumonia. The underlying cause is often malnourishment. Children with acute medical problems that stem from basic malnourishment together with their caregivers are invited to join the programme for treatment. The children are screened for worms, TB, anaemia, HIV, etc. and treated accordingly. During their stay in the programme, they are literally fed until they are back on their normal growth line. All children that are HIV-positive are started on highly active antiretroviral treatment (HAART), together with their siblings and parents.

During the period that the caregiver and the child are in the programme, the caregivers are taught how to start a home vegetable garden (Faber, Phungula, Venter, Dhansay & Benade, 2002) and how to improve the home situation with regard to sanitation, hygiene, etc. The caregivers are provided with seedlings and a garden tool set in order to start their own vegetable gardens. This is done in an effort to structurally improve the nutritional status of the whole family with minimal financial input, using the available human resources of the household instead. Locally trained community health workers (CHWs) carry out regular home visits in order to assist in 'improvements around the home' and to monitor the progress of the home vegetable garden. Besides training in gardening, the caregivers are offered a series of lectures on topics such as diarrhoea and vomiting, burns, immunisation, healthy food and food preparation, caring for children, etc.

In 2000, the first satellite unit was established in Marapong, approximately 12 km from the main unit. This was done in co-operation with the Mpumalanga Department of Health. In 2001, the second satellite unit was established in Ntwane, approximately 5 km from the main unit. The construction of a third unit in Thabakubedu (approximately 15 km from the main unit) was completed in March 2004. The fourth unit has been built in Phooko and has been officially opened in October 2005. Immediately from the start, 34 children with their caregivers were admitted, which proves the tremendous need for services like these in such resource-poor settings. The programme objective is to establish more units in surrounding townships in order to lower the threshold for participating.

With each unit, a pre-school will be established as well. The aim of the pre-schools is twofold:
– to provide good pre-primary education for the community;

– to make all mothers/caregivers aware of the nutritional units and the value those units have regarding good nutrition, good hygiene, home gardening and minor home environment improvements and the health impact all this will have (Steyn, 2000).

At this stage, four schools have been completed and are functioning with an average of 130-150 children per pre-school. Pre-school children's mothers interested in home gardening will also be supplied with knowledge and seedlings, in order to provide a vegetable garden for the family.

Over the years, the amount of children treated, mothers/caregivers educated and households assisted has been growing. A child with its caregiver is approximately 4-6 months in the programme before being discharged and an average of 20-30 children per unit come in every day. With six units, this means that approximately 300 families per annum can be assisted through the Nutritional Unit Programme.

## 4.2. Ndlovu AIDS Awareness Programme for School Children (NAAP)

The Ndlovu AIDS Awareness Programme, started in August 1999, focuses on educating schoolchildren from Moutse and surrounding areas. The idea is to reach them before they become sexually active. The programme consists of a peer education/counselling programme, in which peer educators visit schools and perform a play about HIV/AIDS. After the performance, the peer educators conduct information workshops, in which they go in depth into the problems concerning sexuality, including HIV/AIDS, sexually transmitted diseases (STDs), sexual abuse, child abuse, promiscuity, incest, teacher-pupil relationships, etc. (see also Pavia & Cristenson, 1999). If the schoolchildren want a more private setting, they are referred to the HIV/AIDS advice centre next to the clinic, where well-trained counsellors are available and where they can get condoms (Kingsman, Nakiyingi, Kamali, Carpenter, Quigley, Pool & Whitworth, 2001).

The peer educators are unemployed young adults from Elandsdoorn who are motivated to educate their peers. Professional training has been given to the group in two ways: through courses in crisis debriefing and trauma counselling at the University of South Africa (UNISA) and through drama courses given by various teaching institutions, both from The Netherlands and South Africa.

The programme is not only aimed at young people from the surrounding townships (see Table 1), but tries to create more awareness amongst all South Africans (see also Baldo, 1992; Fawole, Asuzu, Oduntan & Brieger, 1999). Along the R25 between Groblersdal and Bronkhorstspruit, for example, a series of billboards has been erected with slogans to draw people's attention of everyone to this devastating crisis that is disrupting all facets of life in South Africa and will continue to do so in the years to come. These billboards are quite controversial: clear messages like 'Give your jock a jacket' or 'Don't be a fool put a condom on your tool' or 'Women, don't let men dick-tate you', written over a condom of two-meter length are not considered an enrichment for the area by every one. We are pleased with all remarks made about our billboards, however, even negative ones, because we do not care how people speak about this problem as long as they do speak about it. The billboards have been broadcasted all over the world and have even been used in documentaries on CNN and BBC World.

Table 1: Attendance of NAAP events

|  | 2002 | 2003 | 2004 | 2005 |
|---|---|---|---|---|
| N schools visited | 26 | 30 | 34 | 32 |
| N children reached at schools | 7600 | 8600 | 7400 | 8400 |
| N condoms distributed, monthly | 26000 | 22000 | 31000 | 27000 |
| N community events | - | 4 | 20 | 33 |
| N people attending community events | - | 1200 | 6500 | 9100 |
| N centre activities | - | 12 | 12 | 12 |
| N people attending centre activities | - | 1100 | 1800 | 2400 |

## 4.3. An Extended AIDS Awareness Programme

A precondition for initiating treatment is awareness. If the facts around a highly stigmatised disease like HIV/AIDS are not addressed well and the myths and fairytales are not replaced by proper knowledge, the chances of successful treatment are decreasing rapidly.

The awareness programme has a few important tasks:
- provide proper information to the community as a whole;
- address the youth who are not yet sexually active and inform them properly;
- destigmatise HIV/AIDS;
- ensure that people living with HIV/AIDS are accepted in their community and working environment.

This means that interaction at school level only is not sufficient anymore. The AIDS awareness programme for school children is now the start of a much larger concept. The Royal Netherlands Embassy has granted NAAP the funds to form six teams of young adults involving themselves in more aspects of HIV/AIDS education at different interaction levels of the South African communities and to create an HIV/AIDS day care centre. The idea behind this project is to ignore the taboo on HIV/AIDS, to provide proper knowledge about HIV/AIDS and to promote a change in sexual behaviour in order to stop the spread of HIV/AIDS.

The NAAP team will continue to work at school level but also starts programmes in the community, with sex workers, in prisons and in various types of working environment. NAAP will also become a capacity builder for other AIDS awareness groups in order to assist them in building up their knowledge and to pass on the experiences and lessons learnt. A pre-condition for HIV/AIDS treatment programmes is good knowledge about all aspects of HIV/AIDS.

It is our aim to reach as many people as possible, in fact all people from the communities we serve, in order to reach a high rate of VCTs (Voluntary Testing and Counselling) and consequently to supply people who are eligible for HAART with ARVs (see Cohen, Dallabata, Cates & Holmes, 1999).

## 4.4. Ndlovu Tuberculosis Programme (NTP)

Since 1997, the NMC and the provincial Department of Health have been collaborating on a programme to combat tuberculosis. They have formulated a contract for co-operation between the public and private sector for the care of TB patients. The Department of Health has committed itself to provide the NMC with anti-TB drugs and test facilities including sputum tests and micro-cultures, while the NMC has committed itself to provide free TB care for its patients.

In February 2001, the programme introduced a modified version of the directly observed treatment (DOT) principle and a defaulter tracing system. Defaulting patients are visited at home and persuaded to come back to the clinic. Since its implementation, the project has succeeded in reaching a default percentage of 8% of the entire TB patient population over 2001, a default percentage of 10% over 2002, and a default percentage of 8% over 2003. Currently, three TB field workers make home visits and are very successful in reducing the default percentage. The programme is set up in such a way that it can easily be implemented in other townships. It serves as a model of how DOT-TB care can be implemented in rural areas at a relatively low cost.

The growth of this programme is enormous. While we entered 108 patients in the TB programme in 2001, in 2005 until November, there were more than 1,020 confirmed new cases put on treatment. These results are remarkable, more than 80% of the patients completed their six-month treatment and less than 10% defaulted.

About 64% of the TB patients at the NMC are HIV-positive and therefore admitted into the Highly Active Anti-Retroviral Treatment (HAART) programme, after completion of the six-months TB treatment.

It is amazing to see how patients can recover after an initial period of severe illness. Although HAART means lifelong commitment, it also helps people with full-blown AIDS who are adequately treated and educated about lifelong compliancy, to enjoy a good quality of life.

## 4.5. Colombine Maternity Clinic (CMC)

A community maternity clinic was built in 1998 with the help of the Herman van Veen Foundation and the Stichting Colombine, both established in The Netherlands. The clinic has been operational since May 1999. The aim of the clinic is to provide affordable antenatal, obstetrical and postnatal services to the community in the Moutse health district. No other maternity services are available in this district. About 15-30 patients visit the antenatal and postnatal clinic each day. Annually, 300 to 400 deliveries take place at the CMC, and this number increases every year.

Besides antenatal, obstetrical and postnatal services, the clinic also provided a weekly family planning clinic. At this clinic not only contraceptives were distributed, but women were also educated on the subject of sexual hygiene, prevention of sexually transmitted diseases, the danger of HIV/AIDS, sexual abuse, etc. About 180 women visited the family planning clinic each month. It was a great success and a good example of co-operation between a NGO and the Department of Health. Unfortunately, the services had to stop in 2001 because of fraud with government drugs as a consequence of which all supplies to outside institutions were brought to a halt.

Since the start the obstetrical records have been good:
– no maternal losses or major maternal complications;
– two fresh still borns;
– 6 percent of the deliveries started, ended in a Caesarean section.

The CMC is staffed by two midwives, four enrolled nurses, and four auxiliary nurses, which is the absolute practicable minimum for a 24-hour facility. The services are provided far below actual cost. The antenatal services package is provided at R 200 (including the laboratory tests, ultrasounds, and standard medication). A full delivery is provided at R 300. The clinic has its own ambulance, in order to transport patients to a hospital in the event of a Caesarean section being necessary.

Since the introduction of the HAART programme, the CMC is also used to facilitate AIDS patients who started on treatment and do need clinical support. Four beds are reserved for this purpose and the mortality rate of patients with a reconstitution syndrome or low CD4 counts at the start of their treatment has been radically reduced.

## 4.6. Highly Active Anti-Retroviral Treatment (HAART)

In 2003, a project was set up in which HIV-positive patients are treated with antiretroviral (ARV) medicines. A cocktail of three ARVs (triple therapy) is considered to be Highly Active Anti-Retroviral Treatment (HAART). The project had 500 patients on treatment at mid-2005 and will grow to 2,500 patients on treatment in 2008. By treating patients with ARVs, their viral load decreases till undetectable, which gives their immune system a chance to improve, making them less vulnerable to opportunistic infections that would lead to death if no medication is taken. Although ARVs do not cure AIDS, they improve the patients life expectation and quality of life.

With the experience gained, we nearly dare say that HIV/AIDS is a chronic manageable disease not much different from hypertension or diabetes mellitus.

Patients belonging to one of the target groups have to meet clinical, biological, adherence and social criteria. A selection committee verifies whether all selection criteria have been met before a patient is allowed to enter the programme, which is free of charge (see Chapter 8).

## 4.7. Prevention of Mother-to-Child Transmission (PMTCT) Projects

In September 2003, an extensive prevention of mother-to-child transmission (PMTCT) programme was introduced. This programme aims at reducing the HIV transmission from mother to child to less than 1 percent. The programme is run with a very daring protocol in an underprivileged area and might serve as a model to start a new, HIV-free generation in South Africa. Hopefully, this protocol will prove itself so that it can be introduced in the public sector at a later stage, and reduce the rate of HIV transmission from mother to child all over the country (see Chapter 8). PMTCT is also an awareness programme. Awareness is raised by informing the women about the risks, encouraging them to have themselves tested to find out their status, treating the women before and during the delivery to reduce the chances of transmission, and treating the neonate for four weeks after delivery. To prevent HIV transmission through breastfeeding, the women receive formula to feed their babies.

## 4.8. Ngwenya Community Dental Care Project (NCDCP)

Dental care is much neglected in rural black communities. It is considered unnecessary but especially unaffordable, and therefore receives little attention. The old-fashioned way of thinking about dental care - which unfortunately still prevails - is 'painful and loose means extraction'.

In order to start up a dental care awareness programme, NCDCP was developed. It was decided to start with young people. Youngsters can still learn new habits and their dental problems can be treated at an early stage. Ngwenya means 'crocodile' and the programme's name refers to animal's massive jaws and dangerous teeth. The programme consists of two parts: the Dutch part, 'Stichting Ngwenya', and the South African part, NCDCP. The Dutch part seeks funding and volunteer dentists from The Netherlands who would like to work in a rural South African environment for a short while. This is the driving force behind the programme.

In Moutse, the local staff of Ngwenya regularly visits all primary and secondary schools in the area and conducts workshops on dental hygiene and dental care in classrooms. In addition to this, they screen all the children and select those who need dental attention. When the Dutch dentist comes, he/she can be utilised very effectively due to a well-prepared schedule of our local staff. It is a win-win situation for all parties: we get a dentist at no or low cost, while the Dutch dentist will experience South Africa in a way he will never be able to as a tourist and will be exposed to pathology that has been long eradicated in the Western European setting.

This is a low-cost programme with a high impact on the dental health of school children. Approximately 10,000–15,000 school children are screened annually and approximately 1,000 are seen and treated by the dentist.

NPDCP has the approval and assistance of the Department of Dentistry of the University of Pretoria. It is regarded as a pilot project for further research into the question of whether this programme can also be implemented in other areas.

## 5. Future mission

Ndlovu Medical Trust tries to offer a broad spectrum of community health programmes to the community it serves. It is their opinion that this integrated approach of health care is a well functioning and workable system. For all different projects different donors are involved. Each of them has a field of health care supported by them, as the object of their funding possibilities. It is thanks to their commitment that the Trust is able to supply these programmes to the impoverished community as a free-of-charge service. More and more the Department of Health starts to show an interest in their efforts. More and more they start to realise that the health care provided in our area has a positive health impact. The Trust is always striving to improve the relationship with the Department of Health and to encourage them to participate in a public-private partnership with them. If it can prove that this cooperation is possible and valuable, the Trust hopes that their model can finally serve as a delivery system for community health programmes to impoverished and underserved communities and may be of assistance in other parts of South Africa.

## References

Baldo, M. (1992). Lessons learned form pilot projects on school-based AIDS education. *AIDS Health Promotion Exchange, 2,* 14-15.

Cohen, M.S., Dalabatta, G., Cates, W. & Holmes, KK (1999). The global prevention of HIV. In: M. A. Sande & P.A. Volberding (eds.), *The medical management of AIDS (pp. 499-511).* Philadelphia: W.B. Saunders Company.

Faber, M., Phungula, M.A., Ventre, S.L., Dhansay, M.A. & Benade, A.J. (2002). Home gardens focusing on the production of yellow and dark-leafy vegetables increase the serum retinol concentrations of 2-5-y-old children in South Africa. *Journal of Clinical Nutrition, 76,* 1048-1054.

Fawole, I.O., Asuzu, M.C., Oduntan, S.O. & Brieger, W.R. (1999). A school-based AIDS education programme for secundary school students in Nigeria: a review of effectiveness. *Health Education Research, 14,* 675-683.

Kingsman, J., Nakiyingi, J., Kamali, L., Carpenter, L., Quigley, M., Pool, R. & Whitworth, J. (2001). Evaluation of a comprehensive school-based AIDS education programme in rural Masaka, Uganda. *Health Education Research, 16,* 85-100.

Nattrass, N. (2004). *The moral economy of AIDS in South Africa.* Cambridge: Cambridge University Press.

Pavia, A.T. & Christenson, J.C. (1999). Pediatric AIDS. In: M.A. Sande & P.A. Volberding (eds.), *The medical mangement of AIDS (pp. 525-535).* Philadelphia: W.B. Saunders Company.

Steyn, M.P. (2000). A South African perspective on preschool nutrition. *South African Journal of Nutrition, 13,* 9-12.

*Address for correspondence:*
H.A. Tempelman, MD
Ndlovu Medical Centre
P.O. Box 1447
Groblersdal 0470
South Africa
e-mail: tempelman@ndlovumc.org

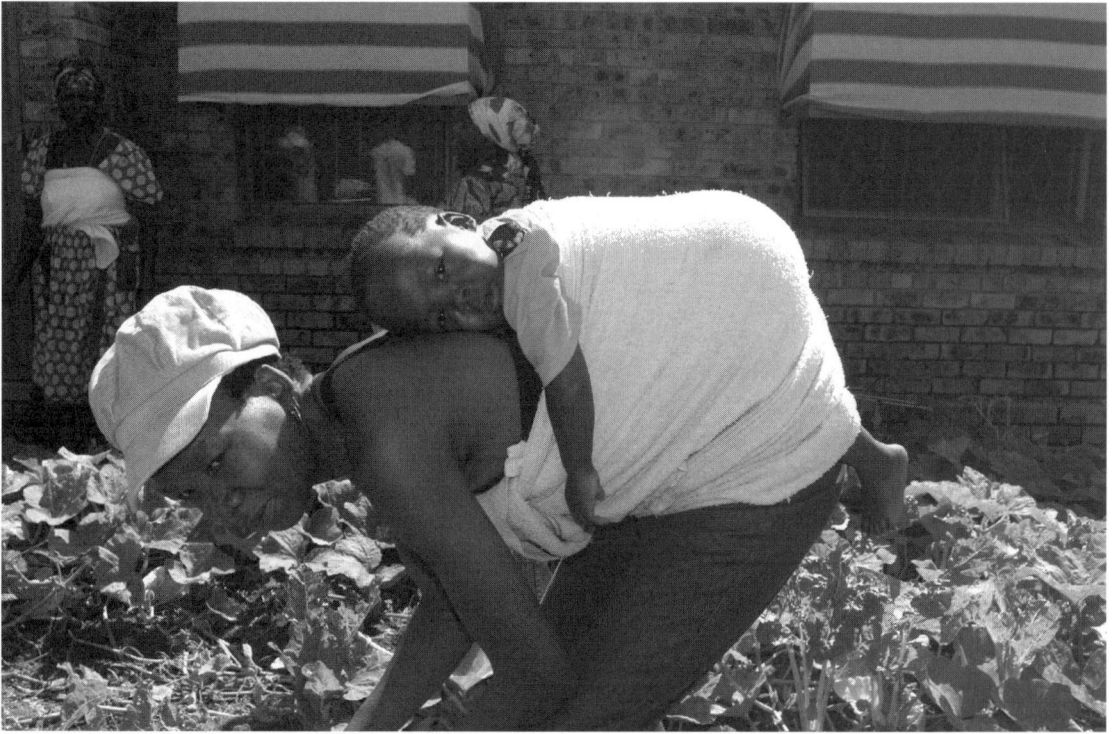

# Chapter 3

# Evaluation of a Nutrition Programme: Participation and Health Effects

*Marieke Westeneng[1], Aukje Okma[1], Janneke Veenstra[1], Hugo Tempelman[2], Adri Vermeer[1]*

[1] Department of Educational Sciences, Utrecht University, The Netherlands
[2] Ndlovu Medical Centre, Elandsdoorn, South Africa

## Abstract

A nutrition programme is conducted in a rural area of South Africa. This study evaluates the factors that determine the participation of the families involved in the educational part of the programme, and the effects of the nutrition part of the programme on the weight, health and developmental condition of the participating children. Interviews were done using a self-constructed questionnaire based on Ajzen's planned behaviour model (1988), kitchen scales to establish the children's weight and two screening checklists – the TQ and the ADLQ – to measure the health and developmental status of the children. The family's attitude towards participation a priori and the perceived ease (or difficulty) of participation in the nutrition programme were found to affect participation. After completion of the programme, 57% of the children had a weight above the 3rd percentile of the age growth curve. Following completion of the programme, the child still appearing backward and slow, speech problems and delayed motor development were the problems most frequently mentioned. Very few functional problems were found to occur after completion of the programme.

## 1. Introduction

### 1.1. Ndlovu Medical Centre

In 1994, Ndlovu Medical Centre (NMC) was established in Elandsdoorn, which is a township in Moutse, Mpumalanga, South Africa. The population of Elandsdoorn has been estimated at between 30,000 and 40,000. Within a 10-km radius of Elandsdoorn, there are many other townships which can benefit from the NMC services, which brings the population reach to about 120,000. The founding of the centre was a private initiative. In addition to the provision of medical care for the surrounding townships, the centre was also established to contribute to the overall development of the area. The NMC provides medical care and community health services. The spacious clinic includes a pharmacy, five consultation rooms, a basic laboratory, an outpatient operating room, an X-ray section, an ultrasound division, a fourteen-bed maternity unit and its own ambulance. The clinic has been registered with the Department of Health, Mpumalanga, as a private hospital with maternity unit attached.

Currently, an AIDS awareness programme, a TB programme and six nutrition units are operating under the auspices of the NMC. Four pre-schools, a bakery, postal services, sports facilities and a day care centre for the elderly have also been built.

## 1.2. Ndlovu Nutritional Unit Programme

Many children with acute medical problems stemming from malnutrition are seen at the NMC. Malnutrition is poor nutritional status due to either an insufficient or poorly balanced diet and/or the inadequate absorption/utilisation of nutrients (Hansen & Bac, 1991). Clearly malnourished children brought to the NMC together with their caregivers were invited to participate in an educational nutrition programme for the feeding of the children. The caregivers followed a training to learn to provide healthy nourishment for their children.

The conduct of the nutrition programme was facilitated with the establishment of six nutrition units. The first nutrition unit was built next to the NMC in Elandsdoorn in 1996. Subsequently, four satellite units were opened in the townships near Elandsdoorn. Each of the nutrition units is equipped with its own water supply to maintain the unit's gardens and provide taps for community use.

The primary aim of the nutrition programme is to rapidly improve the participating children's health status by providing balanced and nutritious meals. The children remain in the programme until they stabilise above the 3rd percentile on the age growth curve. To improve the family's food chain and socio-hygienic status without a major economic investment, the caregivers are trained to establish a home vegetable garden. The caregivers are provided with seeds and a gardening tool set in order to start their own vegetable gardens. Lectures are also presented on the topics of sanitation, hygiene, health and the prevention of disease.

The nutrition units are operated by well-trained community health workers (CHWs). The caregivers and the children visit the unit three times a week for a period of 4-6 six months. On the other two days, the CHWs do home visits in order to assist with around-the-house improvements and monitor the progress being made with respect to the home garden.

After six years of operation, it was decided that the Ndlovu Nutritional Unit (NNU) should be evaluated. Given that this was the first evaluation, it was decided to examine two basic aspects of the programme. First, the factors determining the caregivers participation in the programme were examined. Second, the effects of the programme with respect to the growth and particularly the weight, health and developmental condition of the children participating in the programme were examined. The condition of the home vegetable gardens, the nature of the home environment and the socio-economic status of the families were also examined as part of the evaluation study[1]. All of the information gathered as part of the evaluation study was also supplied to the NNU. Participants discharged by the doctor as well as those participants that had left the programme prematurely were included in the evaluation study. In sum, the following two questions were addressed in this research:

1. Which factors determine participation in the educational part of the nutrition programme?
2. What are the effects of the nutrition part of the programme on the growth and particularly the weight, health and developmental condition of the children following participation?

## 1.3. Nutrition and Growth

'The World Health Organisation estimates that half the world's children are underweight or stunted. In South Africa, the prevalence of children with low weight for age varies from 13 percent in some urban areas to as high as 60 percent in specific rural environments. Children are particularly vulnerable to nutritional inadequacies because of their rapid growth, their dependence on others and their increasing exposure to various environmental hazards' (WHO, 2000; p. 224). More than half of all child deaths are associated with malnutrition, which weakens the body's resistance to illness. Poor diet, frequent illness and inadequate care of young children can lead to malnutrition. In addition, malnutrition during the first two years of life slows down a child's physical and mental growth. And such delays cannot be rectified as the child grows older, which means that the impact of such is likely to be lifelong (Tershakovec & Stallings, 1998).

Examples of the nutrients which children need are vitamin A, iron and iodine. Children need vitamin A to resist illness and prevent visual impairments. Vitamin A can be found in many fruits and vegetables, oils, eggs, dairy products, fortified foods, breast milk and vitamin supplements (Brainbridge & Tsang, 1995; WHO, 2002). Children need iron-rich foods to protect their physical and mental abilities. Iron is found in liver, lean meats, eggs, pulses and green vegetables (Lloyd & Filer, 1995). If a child does not receive sufficient iodine, the child is likely to develop mental, hearing or speech disabilities and may also experience delayed physical or mental development (WHO, 2000).

According to Hansen and Bac (1991), the most common form of malnutrition in childhood is protein energy malnutrition (PEM). The mildest and most prevalent category of PEM is the underweight or stunted child. The only sign of mild PEM is inadequate weight and/or height gain. While the exact effects of infant and child malnutrition have yet to be specified, increased morbidity and compromised development are clearly a consequence of early malnutrition. Early identification enables early intervention and the prevention of more serious complications. For children, a balanced diet with different types of foods containing different nutrients is needed. Children require many nutrients to grow and protect themselves against disease (International College Group, 1999).

## 1.4. The Model of Planned Behaviour

In order to examine those factors which determine the participation of the families in the nutrition programme, use was made of the model of 'planned behaviour' originally put forth by Ajzen (1988) to explain social behaviour. In the model of planned behaviour, the following three factors are assumed to shape the intention towards a particular social behaviour:
– The individual's *attitude* towards the behaviour (i.e. the individual's positive or negative evaluation of participation in the nutrition programme).
– The presence of a *subjective norm* (i.e. the perception of social pressure to either participate or not participate in the nutrition programme).
– *Perceived behavioural control* (i.e. the perceived ease or difficulty of participation in the programme). This determinant is assumed to reflect both past experiences and anticipated impediments or obstacles.

The three aforementioned factors are assumed to influence an individual's *intentions* with regard to a particular *social behaviour*, which is in the present case participation in the nutrition programme. Intentions can predict a variety of action tendencies and thus constitute the antecedents to overt action. Intentions can also change over time, which means that the accuracy of prediction decreases as the interval between measurement of intention and observation of actual behaviour increases. The individual's intention to either perform or not perform a particular behaviour nevertheless remains the immediate determinant of behaviour, as depicted in Figure 1 (Ajzen, 1988; Ajzen & Fishbein, 1980).

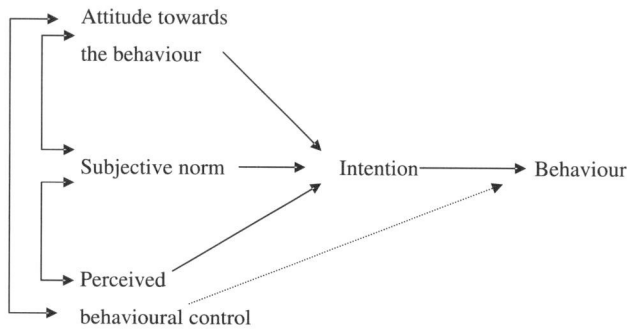

Figure 1: The model of planned behaviour (Ajzen, 1988, p. 133)

## 1.5. *Early Detection of Developmental Disorders in Third World Countries*

Early detection of developmental disorders is secondary prevention. 'It is believed that early intervention of children will help to prevent the occurrence of disabilities and handicaps as well as promote positive outcomes such as sustained parental involvement in their child's development and better future social outcomes' (Thorburn, 1993, p. 4). Early detection involves recognition of the evidence or signs that something is going wrong in a child's development. Early detection involves suspicion of a problem followed by identification of the impairment or disability. E.g. early detection of hearing impairment is important as such an impairment is known to increase the probability of speech and cognitive disabilities. With the early detection of functional disabilities or the emergence of functional disabilities, later developmental delays can be prevented. Early detection can be fostered by the promotion of early recognition on the part of parents, the development of risk registers, the monitoring of selected children, the conduct of community surveys, early referral from key informants and screening. Screening involves all young children as it is aimed at the detection of a condition before it is symptomatic, the identification of cases which have not presented at health facilities and the monitoring of children at-risk for developmental disorders.

In many third world countries, intervention programmes are simply not available and early detection is therefore of little or no use. The relevance of early detection for the present research is to obtain an impression of the health and development of the children who participated in the nutrition programme and then use this information for the improvement of the nutrition programme.

## 2. Methods

### 2.1. *Subjects*

The subject population consists of 166 families participating in the nutrition programme during the period 1996-2002. Those families who participated in 1998 were not included because the names and addresses of these families were not recorded in that year. Each family involved the combination of a caregiver and a child, although a caregiver could have more than one child participating in the programme or participate on two different occasions. In both instances, the different cases of participation were treated separately. A total of 101 families (61%) did not participate in the study. For 52 of these families (31%), only the names and not the addresses were registered. The other 49 families (29%) could not be interviewed because they had moved to another place (N=14), worked many miles away (N=12), could not be found (N=10), were facing difficult family circumstances (N=5), the caregiver(s) had passed away (N=4), or they were not in the programme for a sufficient period of time (N=4). In the end, 65 families (39%) participated in the study.

All of the participating families lived in rural townships around Elandsdoorn. The most pervasive problems in these areas are poverty, lack of water, lack of electricity, unemployment and criminality. The caregivers were the children's mothers in most of the cases (75%), the grandmothers (22%) or the aunts (3%). The children were between the ages of 1 and 9 years, with an average of 5 years; 60% were boys and 40% were girls.

## 2.2. Procedure

The names and addresses of families having completed the nutrition programme during the period 1996-2002 were retrieved from the administrative files of the nutrition units. Those families selected for inclusion in the present study were next visited for an interview in the year 2002 without being informed in advance. People in the township areas of interest do not have telephones and very few have a post office box. All the families agreed to participate despite not being informed in advance.

A structured questionnaire and two screening checklists were administered during the interview, and the child or children participating in the study were then weighed using kitchen scales. Given that the people in this area speak Zulu, Northern-Sotho or Ndebele, a translator was present at all the interviews.

## 2.3. Instruments

The instruments used in this study consisted of a self-developed structured questionnaire and two screening checklists commonly used to establish the health and developmental status of children in developing countries (Thorburn, 1993): the Ten Questions Screen (TQ) and the Activities of Daily Living Questionnaire (ADLQ).

A *structured questionnaire* based on Ajzen's planned behaviour model (1988) was constructed with the help of the NMC professionals, which included a medical doctor and five community health-care workers from the nutrition unit. Six pilot interviews were conducted, and the questionnaire was adjusted as needed. The questionnaire covers the five factors constituting the planned behaviour model:
— twelve questions address the factor 'attitude';
— four questions address 'subjective norm;
— four questions address 'perceived behavioural control';
— three questions address 'intention'; and
— five questions address 'behaviour'. All questions are responded to along a three-point scale ('Yes – I don't know – No').

The TQ is a sensitive and valid tool for the detection of health problems in children between the ages of 2 and 9 years (Thorburn & Marfo, 1994; Thorburn, 1995). The TQ consists of ten questions with a yes-no format and is intended for administration to mothers by community health workers. The questions concern the child's vision, hearing, movement and cognitive abilities. The minimum score is 0, indicating no health problems; the maximum score is 10, indicating multiple health problems.

The ADLQ has been developed to screen children in developing countries from the age of 2 years for developmental (i.e. functional) disabilities. The ADLQ consists of nineteen questions with a 'yes-no-not applicable' response format. 'Not applicable' means that the child is too young to do the daily activity on his own. And if the child is found to have a movement disability, there are two additional questions. The minimum score of 0 indicates no functional disabilities, and the maximum score of 21 indicates functional disabilities in all domains of daily life. The ADLQ has proved to be sensitive to the presence, absence and severity of disability in children in developing countries. The checklist screens for motor, self-help, communication, cognitive and social development problems (Thorburn, Desai & Davidson, 1992; Thorburn, 1995).

The screening checklists were not administered on five occasions: twice because the children were too young; twice because the children had passed away; and once because the child was no longer living with the caregiver.

## 2.4. Statistics

The design of the present research is partly a retrospective survey and partly a retrospective pre-experimental intervention study. The families were interviewed on one occasion as no assessment prior to participation in the nutrition programme occurred.

Structural Equations Modelling (SEM) was used to analyse the questionnaire data (Arbucle, 1997). SEM is a method which uses the paths between the variables in a model to define their relations. SEM calculates the regression weights and covariances between the different variables in a model. The model as a whole is used to calculate the regression weights and covariances (Hox, 1999). The answers to eight of the questions from the questionnaire were re-coded because they were posed in a negative manner. After re-coding, various indices were calculated on the basis of the questions concerned with the same variable. A significance level of 0.05 was used to evaluate the relations between the different variables in the model developed by Ajzen (1988).

The analyses of the TQ and ADLQ data involved calculation of the percentage problems revealed by each screening checklist. Three of the items from the TQ were re-coded as they were posed in a positive direction while the other seven items were posed in a negative direction.

## 3. Results

### 3.1. Factors Determining the Caregivers' Participation in the Educational Part of the Nutrition Programme

The relations between the factors in the planned behaviour model were examined in a regression analysis. The regression weights for the relations between attitude, subjective norm, perceived behavioural control, intention and behaviour are presented in Table 1. As can be seen, the relation between perceived behavioural control and actual behaviour proved significant. Similarly, the relation between attitude towards the behaviour and the behaviour proved significant.

In Table 2, the covariance of the relationships between the independent variables (attitude, subjective norm and perceived behavioural control) are presented. As can be seen, the relation between attitude and perceived behavioural control is significant.

Structural Equation Modelling has been used to evaluate the goodness of fit of the model to the data. The goodness of fit is indicated by the:

a.   $\chi^2$-value, which indicates whether or not the pattern of path coefficients and covariances in the data can be explained by the model, with lower values indicating better fit (N.B. this is not the most informative index, because it is influenced by the sample size);

b. the Normal Fit Index (NFI) which is a measure of complete covariation in the data, with values exceeding 0.90 indicating an acceptable fit; and

c. the Root Mean Square Error of Approximation (RMSEA), which is a measure for assessing models of differing complexity, with values smaller than 0.05 indicating an acceptable fit.

For the model used, the following results were found: $\chi^2$ (1) = 0.139, p = 0.71, NFI = 1.0, RMSEA = 0.00, all indicating that the model fits in with the data very well.

**Table 1: Relations between independent variables (attitude, subjective norm, perceived behavioural control), the intermediate variable (intention) and the dependent variable (behaviour)**

| | | | B | p | Beta |
|---|---|---|---|---|---|
| intention | - | attitude | 1.40 | 0.06 | 0.24 |
| intention | - | subjective norm | 0.37 | 0.11 | 0.19 |
| intention | - | perceived behavioural control | -0.04 | 0.91 | -0.01 |
| behaviour | - | intention | -0.03 | 0.42 | -0.09 |
| behaviour | - | perceived behavioural control | 0.37 | 0.00 | 0.40 |
| behaviour | - | attitude | 0.57 | 0.01 | 0.32 |

B = regression weights or path coefficients
Beta = standardised coefficients

**Table 2: Relations between the independent variables**

| | | | B | p | Beta |
|---|---|---|---|---|---|
| subjective norm | - | perceived behavioural control | 0.02 | 0.31 | 0.13 |
| subjective norm | - | attitude | 0.01 | 0.47 | 0.09 |
| attitude | - | perceived behavioural control | 0.02 | 0.01 | 0.37 |

B = covariances
Beta = correlation coefficients or standardised coefficients

In Figure 2, the data from Tables 1 and 2 have been incorporated into the model of planned behaviour. In contrast to Ajzen's model (1988), attitude towards a particular behaviour was found to significantly influence behaviour.

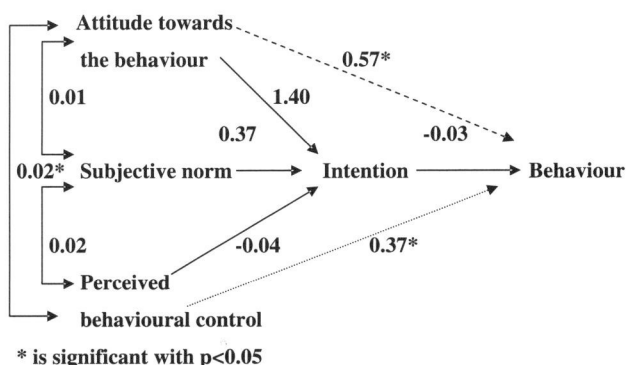

Figure 2: Path coefficients for the factors in the model of planned behaviour

The Squared Multiple Correlations (SMC) indicate what percentage of variation in the dependent variables can be explained by the linear model. For the model used, the following results were found: the SMC for Intention is 0.01, indicating that 1% of the variation in scores on Intention is explained by the model; the SMC for Behaviour is 0.34, indicating that 34% of the variation in scores on Behaviour can be explained by the model. This indicates that the model can better explain Behaviour than Intention.

## 3.2. Effects of the Nutrition Part of the Programme on Weight, Health and Functional Development

The *weight* results, expressed as the children's position on the age growth curves following participation in the nutrition programme, are presented in Table 3. As can be seen, the weight of nine of the children (or 13.8%) could not be established for various reasons. According to Bilo and Voorhoeve (1990), the normal growth figures lie between the 10th and 90th percentiles. For the case of a developing country, the lower weight limit was set at the 3rd percentile and 57.1% of the children were found to weigh between the 3rd and 50th percentiles following participation in the programme, which means that their weight was 'low-to-normal'. The weight of the remaining 42.9% of the children remained 'below normal.'

**Table 3: Position of children on age growth curves for weight following participation in the nutrition part of the programme**

|  | N | % | valid % | cumulative % |
|---|---|---|---|---|
| weight below 3rd percentile | 24 | 36.9 | 42.9 | 42.9 |
| weight between 3rd and 50th percentiles | 32 | 49.2 | 57.1 | 100.0 |
| missing | 9 | 13.8 |  |  |
| total | 65 | 100.0 |  |  |

**Table 4: TQ results regarding health problems following participation in the nutrition part of the programme**

|  |  | yes | no | Total |
|---|---|---|---|---|
| delay motor function | Count | 11 | 49 | 60 |
|  | % | 18,3% | 81,7% | 100,0% |
| diffuculty seeing | Count | 6 | 54 | 60 |
|  | % | 10,0% | 90,0% | 100,0% |
| difficulty hearing | Count | 7 | 53 | 60 |
|  | % | 11,7% | 88,3% | 100,0% |
| does not understand saying | Count | 3 | 57 | 60 |
|  | % | 5,0% | 95,0% | 100,0% |
| weakness in limbs | Count | 8 | 52 | 60 |
|  | % | 13,3% | 86,7% | 100,0% |
| fits or faint | Count | 2 | 58 | 60 |
|  | % | 3,3% | 96,7% | 100,0% |
| does not learn to do things | Count | 4 | 56 | 60 |
|  | % | 6,7% | 93,3% | 100,0% |
| does not speak | Count | 4 | 56 | 60 |
|  | % | 6,7% | 93,3% | 100,0% |
| speech different | Count | 12 | 48 | 60 |
|  | % | 20,0% | 80,0% | 100,0% |
| backward or slow | Count | 16 | 44 | 60 |
|  | % | 26,7% | 73,3% | 100,0% |

In Table 4, the TQ results regarding the children's *health and developmental status* are presented. The most frequently occurring problem was the child still appearing 'backward or slow' when compared to other children of the same age. The second most frequently occurring problem were speech problems. And delayed motor function (i.e. problems in sitting, standing and/or walking) was the third most frequently occurring problem.

In Table 5, the ADLQ results regarding *functional disabilities* are presented. As can be seen, very few problems with respect to the performance of various functional tasks are encountered. The only possible exception is washing and bathing without help.

**Table 5: ADLQ results regarding functional disabilities following participation in the nutrition part of the programme**

| | | yes | no | not applicable | Total |
|---|---|---|---|---|---|
| gets up from lying | Count | 60 | | | 60 |
| | % | 100,0% | | | 100,0% |
| moves both arms | Count | 58 | 2 | | 60 |
| | % | 96,7% | 3,3% | | 100,0% |
| moves both legs | Count | 58 | 2 | | 60 |
| | % | 96,7% | 3,3% | | 100,0% |
| moves round house | Count | 59 | 1 | | 60 |
| | % | 98,3% | 1,7% | | 100,0% |
| eats and drinks | Count | 58 | 1 | 1 | 60 |
| | % | 96,7% | 1,7% | 1,7% | 100,0% |
| washes and bathes | Count | 17 | 14 | 29 | 60 |
| | % | 28,3% | 23,3% | 48,3% | 100,0% |
| cleans teeth | Count | 44 | 4 | 12 | 60 |
| | % | 73,3% | 6,7% | 20,0% | 100,0% |
| uses toilet | Count | 46 | 5 | 9 | 60 |
| | % | 76,7% | 8,3% | 15,0% | 100,0% |
| dresses | Count | 38 | 2 | 20 | 60 |
| | % | 63,3% | 3,3% | 33,3% | 100,0% |
| understands speech | Count | 57 | 3 | | 60 |
| | % | 95,0% | 5,0% | | 100,0% |
| expresses thoughts | Count | 58 | 2 | | 60 |
| | % | 96,7% | 3,3% | | 100,0% |
| others understand | Count | 54 | 2 | 4 | 60 |
| | % | 90,0% | 3,3% | 6,7% | 100,0% |
| plays | Count | 58 | 2 | | 60 |
| | % | 96,7% | 3,3% | | 100,0% |
| school | Count | 11 | 2 | 47 | 60 |
| | % | 18,3% | 3,3% | 78,3% | 100,0% |
| familie activities | Count | 51 | 4 | 5 | 60 |
| | % | 85,0% | 6,7% | 8,3% | 100,0% |
| moves in community | Count | 48 | 1 | 11 | 60 |
| | % | 80,0% | 1,7% | 18,3% | 100,0% |
| community activities | Count | 38 | | 22 | 60 |
| | % | 63,3% | | 36,7% | 100,0% |
| household tasks | Count | 21 | | 39 | 60 |
| | % | 35,0% | | 65,0% | 100,0% |
| works | Count | | | 60 | 60 |
| | % | | | 100,0% | 100,0% |

# 4. Conclusions and Discussion

## 4.1. Methodological Issues

It has to be realised that the research took place in a township area in a developing country. All kind of methodological difficulties in carrying out the planned evaluation research have been met and practical solutions had to be found. This could affect the validity of the results and the applicability of the findings to other settings. It has been tried to cope with these constraints and to carry out the research optimally in a situation where no research has been done up till now.

Of the participants, 39% were surveyed. 61% did not participate in the study for all kind of external reasons, e.g. had moved to another place, could not be found, caregivers had passed away. There are no indications that these persons differ meaningfully from those who were interviewed. At the time they took part in the nutrition programme, they lived in the same area, were in similar socio-economic situations, had the same difficult family circumstances and similar numbers of caregivers passed away compared to those who took part in the study.

A retrospective survey of participants up to six years after they have completed the nutrition programme may affect the reliability of the outcomes. To this end, correlations were calculated between the first cohorts (1996+1997) and the last cohorts (2001+2002). An effect of time could not be established.

The assessment of the programme's effects on growth, health and development were established by means of a pre-experimental design, viz. without a meaningful comparison group. The status of current nutrition and development could have changed during or after participation in the programme as a result of changes in food supply or other extraneous factors. Based on descriptions of the family and environmental circumstances in the medical files of the NMC, it could be stated that no big changes in these circumstances took place over time.

A final limitation on this study may have been the need to use a translator. The use of a translator for the questions asked and the answers given may have influenced the reliability of the present results. We tried to minimise the problem of interpretation to the greatest extent possible by training the translators before the interview and providing strict instructions.

## 4.2. Factors Determining Participation in the Educational Part of the Nutrition Programme

The first aim of this study was to examine the factors which appear to determine the participation of families in the educational part of a nutrition programme (i.e. behaviour). The factors 'attitude' and 'perceived behavioural control' were indeed found to significantly influence participation. In contrast, 'subjective norm' and 'intention' did not appear to influence the participation of the families in the programme. Stated differently, the decisions of the families to participate in the programme (or not) were not influenced by other people in their environment. Similarly, the factor 'intention' did not influence their participation. However, the a priori positive or negative family evaluations of participation in the programme and the perceived ease (or difficulty) of participation did affect their actual participation.

According to Ajzen's model of planned behaviour, 'intention' should have been the main predictor of 'behaviour'. However, this was not found to be the case in this study. One possible explanation may lie in the length of time between the measurement of intention and the measurement of actual behaviour. As already noted, the longer the interval between the measurement of intention and the performance of the target behaviour, the lower the predictive value of intention. When the correlations between intention and behaviour for the first cohorts (1996+1997) and the last cohorts (2001+2002) were compared, however, an effect of time on the relations between 'intention' and 'actual behaviour' was not detected. An explanation for the discrepancy between the suppositions of the model and the results of this study may lie in the fact that Ajzen's model is a typically Western model in which people basically 'do what they intend to do'. It could be that in the African situation other factors, such as personal and cultural characteristics, determine behaviour to a higher extent.

## 4.3. Effects of the Nutrition Part of the Programme on Weight, Health and Functional Development

The second aim of this study was to evaluate the growth, health and developmental condition of the children following participation in the nutrition part of the programme. As already noted, 57% of the children had gained weight to above the 3rd percentile of the age growth curves, while 43% of the children remained below the 3rd percentile and were therefore still underweight.

The TQ results showed the child appearing to be backward or slow to be the main health problem following participation in the nutrition programme. This may be due to a lack of iron-rich foods and iodine (WHO, 2000; Lloyd & Filer, 1995). Speech problems were also mentioned fairly frequently, which may be due to a lack of iodine (WHO, 2000). Delayed motor function is probably due to a shortage of iron and iodine (WHO, 2000; Lloyd & Filer, 1995). Further research into the composition of the food in the area of the research is needed to verify this supposition. The established health problems may also be a result of a lack of environmental stimulation. For instance, there is a lack of any stimulation of play and movement activities in the township area.

The results of the present study show growth delays still to prevail - despite the operation of a nutrition programme - and to influence the health of children in a negative manner. Just how long the children were malnourished prior to participation in the programme is unknown. As already pointed out, severe undernourishment during the first years of life can damage the development of children irreparably (Tershakovec & Stallings, 1998). A poor nutrition regime and the presence of disease *after* completion of the programme may also have influenced the present results, and further research is therefore needed to separate the influences of various factors.

The ADLQ results showed no severe problems with respect to the functional development of the children. The washing and bathing of oneself constituted the only exception but actually appeared to depend on the socio-economic circumstances of the families and the pervasive lack of water in the area.

In closing, it should be recalled that early detection without intervention is of little or no use. Further research should also be undertaken to compare the results for malnourished children participating in a nutrition programme with the results for malnourished children not participating in such a programme. And the specific effects of the nutrition programme on the various delays in the growth and development of children should be more carefully investigated as well.

# References

Ajzen, I. (1988). *Attitudes, personality and behaviour.* Chicago: The Dorsey Press.

Ajzen, I. & Fishbein, M. (1980). *Understanding attitudes and predicting social behaviour.* New Jersey: Prentice-Hall, Englewood Cliffs.

Arbucle, J. (1977). *Amos user's guide.* Chicago: Smallwaters.

Bainbridge, R, Tsang R.(1995). Optimal nutrition in low birth weight infants. In: F. Lifshitz (ed), *Childhood Nutrition (pp. 33-42).* Boca Raton: CRC Press.

Bilo, R.A.C. & Voorhoeve, H.W.A. (1990). *Kind in ontwikkeling. Een handreiking bij de observatie van jonge kinderen [Children in development. A guide for the observation of young children].* Lochem: De Tijdstroom.

Davidson, L.(1995) The development of the Ten Questions: A tool to screen for serious disability in children in countries with few professional resources. In: M.I.M. Schuurman (ed.), *Assessment of childhood disabilities in developing countries (pp 11-20).* Utrecht: Bisschop Beckers Institute.

Hansen, J.D.L. & Bac, M. Malnutrition. In: M.A. Kibel & L.A. Wagstaff (eds.), *Child health for all. A manual for Southern Africa (pp 221-232).* Cape Town: Oxford University Press.

Hox J.J. (1999). Principes en toepassing van structurele modellen [Principles and application of structural models]. *Kind en Adolescent, 20,* 200-217.

International Colleges Group. *Home Health Care. The human body, nutrition and children.* International Colleges Group; 1999.

Lloyd, J. & Filer, J.R. (1995). Iron deficiency. In: F. Lifshitz (ed.), *Childhood Nutrition( pp. 53-60).* Boca Raton: CRC Press.

Tershakovec, A.M. & Stallings, V.A. (1998). Paediatric nutrition and nutritional disorders. In: R. Behrman & R. Kliegman (eds.), *Essentials of paediatrics (pp.56-92).* Philadelphia: W.B Saunders Company.

Thorburn, M.J. (1993). *Early detection of children with disabilities in third world countries* Jamaica: Unpublished paper.

Thorburn, M.J. & Marfo, K. (1994). *Practical approaches to childhood disability in* developing countries. *Tampa (Fl): Global Age Publishing.*

Thorburn, M.J. (1995). Achievements of the Ten Questions and possibilities for its practical use. In: M.I.M. Schuurman (ed.). *Assessment of childhood disabilities in developing countries (pp. 78-86).* Utrecht: Bisschop Beckers Institute.

Thorburn, M.J., Desai, P. & Davidson L. (1992). Categories, classes and criteria in childhood disabilities. Experiences from a survey in Jamaica. *Disability and Rehabilitation, 14,* 122-133.

WHO. (2002). Nutrition and growth. In: *Facts for life.* Genova: World Health Organization..

## Address for correspondence:
H.A. Tempelman, MD
Ndlovu Medical Centre
P.O. Box 1447
Groblersdal 0470
South Africa

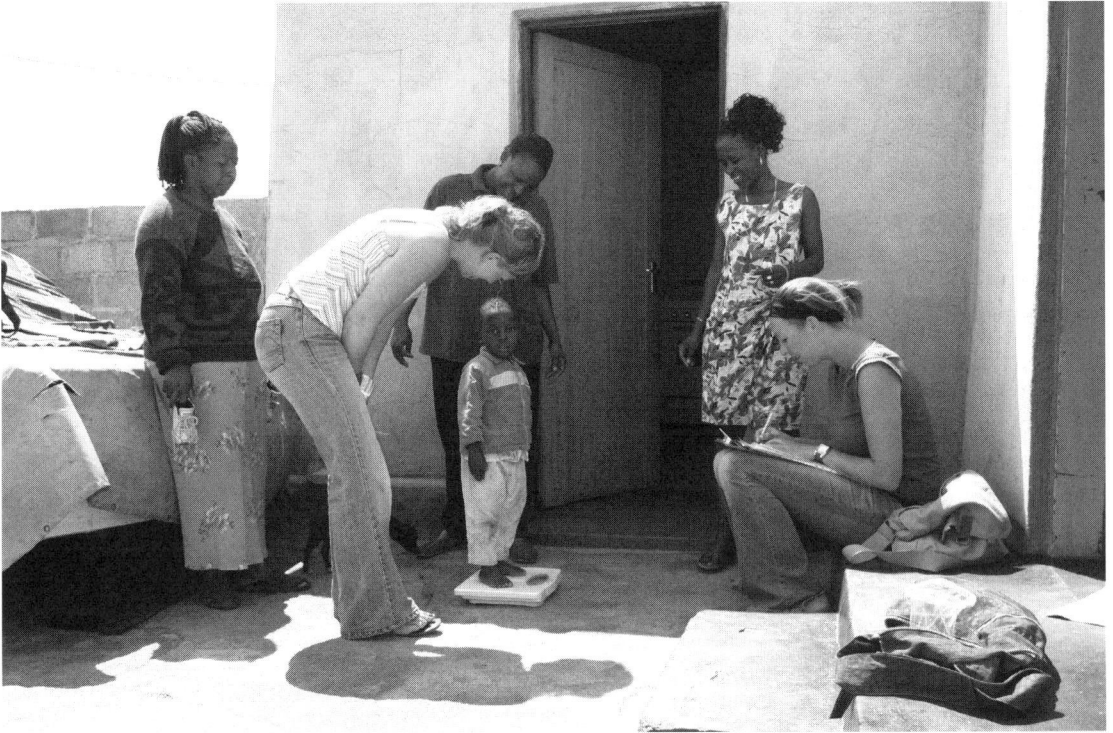

# Chapter 4

# Effects of a Nutrition Programme on the Health and Development of Undernourished Children

*Florieke Stofmeel[1], Florence Wehmeijer[1], Hugo Tempelman[2], Marcel van Aken[1], Adri Vermeer[3]*

[1] Department of Developmental Psychology, Utrecht University, Utrecht, The Netherlands
[2] Ndlovu Medical Centre, Elandsdoorn, South Africa
[3] Department of Educational Sciences, Utrecht University, Utrecht, The Netherlands

## Abstract

The objective of this follow-up study was to establish the effects of a nutrition programme conducted in a rural area of South Africa on the health and development of undernourished children. Forty children who participated in the programme were compared with a matched control group of 35 children who did not participate in the programme. Kitchen scales were used to establish the weight of the children and a tape measure to establish the children's length and head circumference. Three screening checklists – the TQ, ADLQ and SDQ – were used to measure the children's actual health and functional and behavioural development. Weight (in kg) and length (in cm) were higher in the treatment group than in the control group. No differences were found in length and weight on the growth chart. No differences were found in head circumference both in cm and on the growth chart. No differences in actual health on the TQ, except for the question 'difficulty in hearing', were found between the treatment and the control group. No differences in functional development on the ADLQ were found between the two groups. On behavioural development on the SDQ, two differences were found between treatment and control group. There were more emotional problems in the treatment group, while the control group showed more hyperactivity problems. Of the treatment group, 30% showed a relapse in health after finishing the programme. No factors related to this relapse were found. Aspects of the programme to be improved in the future are longer aftercare, better record keeping, more stimulation and activities for both children and mothers and improvement of the home visits.

## 1. Introduction

### 1.1. Nutritional Units at Ndlovu Medical Centre

At the Ndlovu Medical Centre (NMC) in Elandsdoorn, Mpumalanga, many children are seen with acute medical problems, originating from underlying malnutrition. Malnutrition is a poor nutritional status because of an insufficient or poorly balanced diet or results from inadequate absorption or impaired utilisation of nutrients (Hansen & Bac, 1991).

The undernourished children seen at the medical centre together with their caregivers are invited to a nutrition programme for treatment and training. The primary aim of the Nutritional Unit Programme is to quickly improve the child's health status, particularly, to return children to a normal weight, as determined by the appropriate growth curve. This is done by close monitoring of the children's health during their participation in the programme and by providing the children with balanced and nutritious meals. Children are discharged by a medical doctor when they are stable for at least three months above or a little below the 3rd percentile on the growth curve for weight and show now signs of undernourishment.

A second aim is to improve the family's food chain and socio-hygienic status with a minor economic investment. This is done by training the caregivers how to establish a home vegetable garden. Also, lectures are offered on how to improve the home situation concerning sanitation, hygiene, health and prevention of diseases. The caregivers are provided with seeds and a gardening tool set in order to start their own vegetable gardens.

The first nutritional unit was built next to the NMC in Elandsdoorn in 1996. Four satellite units opened in townships near Elandsdoorn. Each unit is equipped with its own water supply, used to maintain the unit's gardens and to provide taps for community use.

Local women are extensively trained as community health workers (CHWs) and work at the nutritional units. The caregivers and the children come to the unit on Mondays, Wednesdays and Fridays. On Tuesdays and Thursdays the CHWs do home visits in order to assist in 'around-the-house' improvements and to monitor the progress of the home gardening. The programme lasts about one year.

## 1.2. Results of the Previous Study

In 2002, an evaluation study has been performed on the Nutritional Unit Programme (see chapter 3). The research questions were: 'Which factors determine the participation of the families who have been involved in the nutrition programme?', and, 'How is the growth and particularly the weight, health and developmental condition of the children after participation in the nutrition programme?'

For the first research question, a questionnaire was used which was based on the model of planned behaviour (Ajzen, 1988). This model explains social behaviour and distinguishes three factors that determine the intention towards a social behaviour. These three factors are the individual's attitude, the subjective norm and the perceived behavioural control. These three factors or determinants influence the intention towards participation in the nutrition programme. The results of this part of the study show that participation of a family was influenced by the family's attitude towards participation and their perceived ease or difficulty of participation (perceived behavioural control).

For the second research question, kitchen scales and two screening checklists were used. The results show that after the programme, 57% of the children had gained weight to above the 3rd percentile of the age growth chart, while 43% of the children remained below the 3rd percentile and were therefore still underweight. Two screening checklists, the Ten Questions Screen (TQ) and the Activities of Daily Living Questionnaire (ADLQ), were used to establish the health and developmental status of the children. Results of the TQ show that the problem occurring most frequently in the sample is that the child appears to be 'mentally backward or slow' compared to other children of this age. Secondly, there were speech problems. Delay in motor function, i.e. sitting, standing and/or walking, is the third most frequently occurring problem. The ADLQ shows no severe problems, except for washing and bathing. This appears to be a socio-economic problem, because there is a severe lack of water in the area. It is not clear to what extent these problems occur in children who have not been involved in the programme. The expectation is that the problems mentioned above are more severe and more frequently occurring in children who have not followed the programme.

## 1.3. Present Study

In this research, a follow-up study of the evaluation of the Ndlovu Medical Centre nutrition programme was carried out. Because in the previous study no control group was used, it was not possible to draw conclusions about the programme's effect on children's health and development. Without a control group, the role of external influences cannot be ruled out. In this study, besides a new treatment group, a control group was used. The treatment group consisted of 40 children with caregivers who participated in the nutrition programme in the period of September 2002 until September 2004. The control group consisted of 35 children with caregivers who did not participate in the programme during this period. These children were on the waiting list in October/November 2004 and planned to follow the programme. The general question of this research was whether the nutrition programme has an effect on the health and development of undernourished children. Health and development of these groups were established. Health was defined as weight, length, head circumference and actual health score. Development was defined in terms of functional and behavioural development. It was also examined whether children of the treatment group showed a relapse in their health and which variables had a possible effect on this relapse. In this study, a relapse was defined as a weight loss of more than 10% of the expected weight on the growth curve at the moment of measuring, and/or a child showing clinical signs of undernourishment, e.g. kwashiorkor, marasmus. Kwashiorkor is defined as severe malnutrition in infants and children that is characterised by failure to grow and develop, changes in the pigmentation of the skin and hair, edema, fatty degeneration of the liver, anaemia, and apathy, and is caused by a diet excessively high in carbohydrate and extremely low in protein. Marasmus is defined as a condition of chronic undernourishment occurring especially in children and usually caused by a diet deficient in calories and proteins but sometimes by disease or parasitic infection.

Specific research questions for this study were:
1. What is the weight, length and head circumference of the children who have and of the children who have not participated in the nutrition programme?
2. How is the actual health and the functional and behavioural development of the children who have and of the children who have not participated in the nutrition programme?
3a. How many children who participated in the nutrition programme remain healthy after completing the programme?
3b. When children show a relapse in their health, which variables are related to this relapse?

The expectation in this study was that the health and development of the children who have followed the programme is improved, compared to the health and development of those who have not followed the programme.

## 2. Methods

### 2.1. Subjects

During the period of September 2002 until September 2004, 113 children were involved in the nutrition programme. A child participates in the programme with his or her caregiver. If a caregiver had brought more than one child to the programme, this was counted separately. 61 children finished the programme, and 52 children did not. The reasons for not finishing the programme were: the family moved to another place, the caregiver started working, the caregiver became pregnant or ill. In many cases the reasons were unknown (48%). Of all 61 discharged children, 40 children (65.6%) could be retraced and participated in our study. 21 children could not be found. 5 children of the 40 participants were discharged in 2002, 16 children in 2003 and 19 children in 2004. 7 of these children followed the programme in Elandsdoorn, 15 in Ntwane, 14 in Marapong and 4 in Thabakubedu.

The control group consists of 35 children who have not participated in the programme. These children were on the waiting list in October/November 2004 and planned to follow the programme. It was tried to find a control group matching the treatment group as much as possible in age and sex at the moment of registration at the nutrition unit.

All participating families were living in rural townships around Elandsdoorn. Common problems in these areas are poverty, lack of water and electricity and unemployment. The interviewed persons were the mothers (54.7%), grandmothers (21.3%), aunt/uncle (13.3%), sister/brother (5.3%) or CHW (5.3%). 50.7% of the children were boys, 49.3% were girls. The total group of children (N=75) was between 1 and 7 years old. The average age of this group of children was 2.69 years.

The initial treatment group (N=40) and the initial control group (N=35) were compared for age and gender. The groups matched in gender (p>0,05), but were different in age (p<0,05). To match the groups, the four eldest children of the treatment group and the four youngest children of the control group were removed. After this, the age for the treatment group varied from 0 to 5 years (M=2.89; SD=1.3, whereas the age for the control group varied from 1 to 6 years (M=2.35; SD=1.4). The new treatment group consisted of 19 boys (52.8%) and 17 girls (47.2%). The new control group consisted of 15 boys (48.4%) and 16 girls (51.6%). No significant differences in age and gender remained between the new treatment and control group.

## 2.2. Instruments

### Weight

In this study, weight is expressed both in kilograms and as the child's position on the age growth chart. Kitchen scales were used to establish the children's weight. A growth chart from the NMC with weight-for-age curves was used to compare the weights of the children with the weights of healthy children of the same age. On this growth chart, the 3rd percentile curve, the 50th percentile curve and the 97th percentile curve are shown. For each child the weight is determined as below 3rd percentile, between 3rd and 50th percentile or above 50th percentile. In this study, a child is labelled as undernourished when it is under the 3rd percentile on the growth chart for weight and/or shows clinical signs of undernourishment.

### Length

Length is an indication of the child's rate of growth over a long period of time. Significant variations in length cannot be attributed to adverse events (i.e. malnutrition) restricted to the recent past (Pollitt, William & Leibel,1982). In this study, length is expressed both in centimetres and as the child's position on the age growth chart. A tape measure was used to establish the length. To compare the lengths of the children with the lengths of healthy children of the same age, a growth chart with length-for-age curves was used from the Centres for Disease Control and Prevention (CDC) (National Centre for Health Statistics, 2000). Seven percentile curves are shown: the 5th, 10th, 25th, 50th, 75th and 90th. For each child, the length is determined to be below the 5th percentile, between 5th and 50th percentile, or above the 50th percentile. A child whose length is below the 3rd percentile for his/her age is defined as stunted (King & Burgess, 1993).

## Head Circumference
Head circumference is a presumed physical correlate of brain growth, which is particularly important during infancy and the early pre-school years (Pollitt et al., 1982). In this research, a tape measure was used to measure the head circumference. A growth chart with head circumference-for-age curves was used from the CDC. This growth chart is available for children up to 36 months. The 5th, 10th, 25th, 50th, 75th, 90th and 97th percentile curves are shown. For each child up to 36 months the head circumference is determined as below 5th percentile, between 5th and 50th percentile or above 50th percentile (National Centre for Health Statistics, 2000). Head circumference below the 5th percentile is called microcephal. Microcephaly is a condition of abnormal smallness of the head, usually associated with mental retardation.

## Actual Health, Functional Development and Behavioural Development
To establish the children's actual health and the functional and behavioural development, three screening checklists were used: the Ten Questions Screen (TQ), the Activities of Daily Living Questionnaire (ADLQ) and the Strengths and Difficulties Questionnaire (SDQ). The TQ and ADLQ are screening checklists to establish the health and developmental status of children in developing countries (Thorburn & Marfo, 1994). The SDQ is a behavioural screening checklist (Goodman, 1997).

## Actual Health
The TQ is a sensitive and valid tool for detecting health problems in children from 2 to 9 years old (Davidson, 1995; Thorburn, 1995). The TQ consists of ten questions concerning the child's vision, hearing, movement and cognitive abilities. The questions are asked in a 'yes-no' format, where 'yes' indicates a disability. Three questions were re-coded, because these were asked in the other direction. The total score is the sum of problems appearing in the checklist. The minimum score is 0, indicating no problems and the maximum score is 10, which means problems on all domains of the TQ. The TQ was designed to be administered to mothers by a community health worker and does not take more than ten minutes.

## Functional Development
The ADLQ was developed to screen children in developing countries from the age of 2 years on development, viz. functional disabilities. The ADLQ consists of nineteen questions, divided over five scales: a motor scale, self-help scale, communication scale, cognitive scale and social scale. The questions are asked in a 'yes-no-not applicable' format. 'Not applicable' means that the child is too young to do the daily activity on his own. If the child has a movement problem, two more questions are asked. A total score of 0 indicates that the child has no functional problems and a score of 21 means that the child has problems with all activities of daily life. A scale score can also be calculated. The ADLQ has proved to be sensitive to identify the presence, absence and severity of a disability in children in developing countries (Thorburn, Desai & Davidson 1992; Thorburn & Marfo, 1994).

*Behavioural Development*

The SDQ is a behavioural screening questionnaire for 3-16 year olds. In this study, the SDQ was used for children from 2 years up. The SDQ asks questions about 25 attributes, some positive and others negative. These 25 items are divided over five scales: an emotional symptoms scale, a conduct problems scale, a hyperactivity scale, a peer problems scale and a pro-social scale. Answering possibilities are 'not true', 'somewhat true' and 'certainly true'. Five of the questions of the SDQ were re-coded, because these were asked in a positive direction and the other twenty in a negative direction. For each scale, the score can be divided in 'normal', 'borderline' and 'abnormal'. Summing the scores from all scales except the pro-social scale generates a total difficulties score. This screening questionnaire can be completed in five minutes. The SDQ is a very promising screening checklist for measuring behavioural problems in young children in different cultural populations (Mullick & Goodman, 2001).

## 2.3. Procedure

The community health workers were taught how to use the questionnaires. Then two screening checklists were tried out in a pilot study. Subsequently, problems and difficulties were discussed until all questions were clear to the CHWs.

The names and the addresses of the children who had participated were found in the administrative files of the nutrition units. These files contained child information such as admission date, date of discharge, length, weight, medical diagnosis, vaccination status, medical history of the child/family and allergies. For the children on the waiting list, files had already been made with most of the above-mentioned information.

With help from the CHWs, the families were visited at home where the screening checklists were gone through by means of an interview. After each interview, the child's weight, length and head circumference was established. In some cases the interviewing and measuring of the children was done in the nutritional unit, after the children visited the medical doctor with their caregiver. Because people in this area speak Zulu, Northern-Sotho or Ndebele, the CHWs also acted as translators. In general, the families were visited without informing them in advance. It was not possible to do so, because people in the areas concerned do not have telephone and hardly anyone has a post office box. However, because the CHWs lived in these townships too, they sometimes could inform the families about the visits. It seemed to be no problem when they had not been informed in advance.

## 2.4. Statistics

A pre-experimental design with one measurement has been used in this research (Campbell & Stanley, 1963). Children who had followed the programme (treatment group) and children who did not follow the programme (control group) were compared. The first question concerned the weight, length and head circumference of the children who did and the children who did not participate in the nutrition programme. To answer this, t-tests and chi-square tests were used. T-tests were used for the continuous variables weight in kilograms and length and head circumference in centimetres. Chi-square tests were used for the group variables weight, length and head circumference expressed as the position on the growth chart. To answer the second question about the actual health and functional and behavioural development of the children who did and the children who did not participate in the nutrition programme, t-tests were used. These tests were used because the TQ questions, ADLQ scales, the SDQ scales, the total TQ score, the total ADLQ score and the total SDQ score are continuous variables.

The third question, 'how many children who participated in the nutrition programme remain healthy?', was answered by calculating the total amount of relapse and non-relapse children in the treatment group. After answering the third question, it was tried to find variables possibly related to relapse. To answer this fourth question, the relapse and the non-relapse group were compared for the variables of the first two questions and for extra information on the files. T-tests were used for the variables length and head circumference in centimetres, age, possibility of gardening, water distance, vaccination status and total TQ score, ADLQ score and SDQ score. For the variables length and head circumference on the growth chart, gender, water available and medical history of the child, chi-square tests were used. Because weight had already been included in measuring relapse, this was not mentioned separately.

## 3. Results

### 3.1. Weight, Length and Head Circumference

Table 1 shows that length in centimetres and weight in kilograms were higher in the treatment group than in the control group ($p<0.01$). No difference between the groups was found on head circumference in centimetres.

**Table 1: Means and standard deviations on length (cm), weight (kg) and head circumference (cm) of treatment and control group**

|  | Treatment group (SD) | Control group (SD) | t |
|---|---|---|---|
| Length in cm | 90.43 (10.40) | 83.77 (11,80) | 2.40 ** |
| Weight in kg | 12.50 (2.43) | 11,02 (2.87) | 2.25 ** |
| Head circumference in cm | 48.54 (2.08) | 47.67 (2,27) | 1.17 |

* p< 0. 05; ** p<0.01

As can be seen from Table 2, the differences in weight, length and head circumference ($p>0.05$) between the treatment and the control group are not significant when expressed as the position on the age growth chart.

**Table 2: Length, weight and head circumference on the growth chart of treatment and control group**

| Difference between treatment and control group | chi-square | df | p |
|---|---|---|---|
| Length growth chart | 0.82 | 2 | 0.66 |
| Weight growth chart | 2.16 | 2 | 0.34 |
| Head circumference Growth chart | 1.87 | 2 | 0.39 |

* p< 0.05; ** p<0.01

### 3.2. Health, Functional and Behavioural Development

The treatment and control group were compared for the results of the three screening checklists: the TQ, the ADLQ and the SDQ. Results can be found in Table 3.

For the TQ, the control group showed a higher score on two of the ten questions. However, these differences were not significant. The only significant difference was found in 'difficulty in hearing' ($p<0.05$). The treatment group showed more problems in this area than the control group. The total problem score on the TQ was higher for the treatment group than for the control group. However, this difference is not significant.

The control group showed higher scores than the treatment group on two scales of the ADLQ (motor function problems and communication problems) and a higher total score. However, these differences were not significant either.

When groups were compared for the SDQ, differences are found on the emotional symptoms scale (p<0.05) and the hyperactivity scale (p<0.01). The treatment group showed more emotional problems than the control group and the control group showed more problems on the hyperactivity scale. The treatment group had a higher total difficulties score than the control group, but again not significantly so.

**Table 3: Means and standard deviations of the TQ questions, ADLQ and SDQ scales and their total problem scores**

|  |  | Treatment (SD) | Control (SD) | t |
|---|---|---|---|---|
| *TQ* | delay motor function | 0.50 (0.51) | 0.45 (0.51) | 0.34 |
|  | difficulty seeing | 0.10 (0.31) | 0.05 (0.22) | 0.72 |
|  | difficulty hearing | 0.13 (0.35) | 0.00 (0.00) | 2.11* |
|  | does not understand saying | 0.07 (0.25) | 0.05 (0.22\|) | 0.29 |
|  | weakness in limbs | 0.00 (0.00) | 0.05 (0.22) | -1.00 |
|  | fits or faint | 0.10 (0.31) | 0.00 (0.00) | 1.80 |
|  | does not learn to do things like others | 0.00 (0.00) | 0.05 (0.22) | -1.00 |
|  | does not speak | 0.13 (0.35) | 0.29 (0.46) | -1.28 |
|  | speech different | 0.17 (0.38) | 0.10 (0.30) | 0.75 |
|  | backward or slow | 0.13 (0.35) | 0.05 (0.22) | 1.08 |
|  | *total problem score TQ* | *1.33 (1.58)* | *1.10 (1.74)* | *0.66* |
| *ADLQ* | motor function problems | 0.00 (0.00) | 0.19 (0.87) | -1.00 |
|  | Self help problems | 0.47 (0.73) | 0.29 (0.56) | 1.00 |
|  | communication problems | 0.23 (0.50) | 0.52 (0.81) | -1.45 |
|  | cognitive problems | 0.07 (0.25) | 0.05 (0.22) | 0.29 |
|  | social problems | 0.03 (0.18) | 0.00 (0.00) | 1.00 |
|  | *total score on ADLQ* | *0.80 (0.89)* | *1.05 (1.72)* | *-0.61* |
| *SDQ* | emotional symptoms | 1.00 (0.85) | 0.52 (0.75) | 2.10 * |
|  | conduct problems | 0.96 (0.92) | 0.52 (0.75) | 1.84 |
|  | hyperactivity | 1.33 (0.88) | 1.90 (0.30) | -3.28 ** |
|  | peer problems | 0.37 (0.72) | 0.52 (0.87) | -0.68 |
|  | pro-social behaviour | 0.47 (0.82) | 0.76 (0.94) | -1.16 |
|  | *total difficulties score SDQ* | *1.15 (0.82)* | *1.00 (0.84)* | *0.61* |

* p< 0.05; **p<0.01

## 3.3. Relapse

At the moment of measuring, twelve children of the treatment group (30%) showed a relapse in weight after completion of the programme. This means that 27 children (67.5%) of the treatment group showed no relapse and remained healthy after following the programme. For one child (2.5%) no data were available.

## 3.4. Factors related to relapse

To determine which factors were possibly related to relapse, a comparison is made for relevant dependent and independent variables between the relapse group (N=12) and the

non-relapse group (N= 27). As can be seen from Table 4 and 5, no significant differences were found between the relapse group and the non-relapse group. The results for the t-tests are shown in Table 4 and the results for the chi-square tests in Table 5.

**Table 4: Differences between relapse group and non-relapse group for relevant variables**

| Variables | Relapse (SD) | Non-relapse (SD) | t |
|---|---|---|---|
| Length in cm | 93.67 (10.50) | 90.96 (11.46) | -0.72 |
| Head circumference in cm | 49.00 (1.00) | 48.41 (2.31) | -0.65 |
| Age | 3.58 (1.51) | 3.11 (1.58) | -0.89 |
| Possibility of gardening | 2.08 (1.00) | 2.26 (1.20) | 0.48 |
| Water distance | 1.67 (0.52) | 1.50 (0.51) | -0.69 |
| Vaccination status | 1.64 (1.80) | 2.38 (1.79) | 1.13 |
| Total TQ score | 1.58 (1.62) | 1.41 (2.24) | -0.26 |
| Total ADLQ score | 0.42 (0.67) | 0.91 (0.92) | 1.79 |
| Total SDQ score | 0.91 (0.94) | 1.10 (0.79) | 0.57 |

* p< 0.05; **p<0.01

**Table 5: Differences between relapse group and non-relapse group for several variables**

| Difference between relapse and no-relapse group | chi-square | df | p |
|---|---|---|---|
| Length on growth chart | 4.58 | 2 | 0.10 |
| Head circumference on growth chart | 1.59 | 1 | 0.21 |
| Gender | 0.14 | 1 | 0.71 |
| Water available | 7.71 | 5 | 0.17 |
| Medical history child | 12.08 | 10 | 0.28 |

* p< 0.05; **p<0.01

# 4. Discussion

## 4.1. Results

The results of this study show that length in centimetres and weight in kilograms were higher in the treatment group than in the control group. This means that children who followed the programme were heavier and taller than children who did not follow the programme. As expected, their growth had improved. These differences were not found for weight, length and head circumference expressed as the child's position on the age growth chart. This could be explained by the less detailed level of measuring that was used when determining the position on the growth chart (only three categories could be formed). This may have led to a loss of information.

No differences were found between children who did and who did not participate in the programme in head circumference in centimetres and on the growth chart. Effects of undernourishment on a child's head circumference can probably only be found after a long period of undernourishment.

Results show that, except for one question, the treatment and control group show no differences for the outcome of the TQ. This means no differences were found for health problems between children who did and who did not participate in the programme. The only difference between the two groups was found for the question 'difficulty in hearing', in which the treatment group showed more problems than the control group. Reasons for this difference are unclear.

There were no differences on the ADLQ scales among the treatment and the control group. This means that no differences in functional disabilities were found between children who did and who did not participate in the programme.

Differences were found between the treatment group and the control group for two scales of the SDQ. The treatment group showed more emotional problems than the control group. The control group showed more hyperactivity problems.

A possible reason for the small differences between the scores of the treatment and the control group for the three screening lists could be that malnutrition had not yet visibly affected the actual health, functional development and behavioural development. If malnutrition did already have an effect, the small differences could be explained by the programme's incapacity improve the health and development of the children. Another reason could be that the screening lists used did not show the differences between the groups.

Of the treatment group, 30% showed a relapse. This means that the majority of the children who participated in the programme showed no relapse after an average of 10.5 months after being discharged.

In this study, no variables related to relapse were found. However, some of the findings can provide useful information for improvement of the programme. Results for 'water distance' show that many families have access to water at the nutritional units. Of the non-relapse group 45.8% gets water at the nutritional units, versus 16.7% of the relapse group. This shows the great importance of the water supply at the nutritional units for the health of families in the townships. The gardens of the non-relapse group are of better quality than those of the relapse group. Of the non-relapse group, 14.8% scored 'good' and 3.7% 'excellent' for 'possibility of gardening', in contrast to the relapse group, in which 8.3% scored 'good' and 0% 'excellent'.

In general, it can be concluded that the question whether the Nutritional Unit Programme has an effect on the health and development of undernourished children cannot be answered affirmatively in this study.

## 4.2. Limitations of the Study

It has to be realised that this study took place in a township area in a developing country. All kind of methodological difficulties in carrying out the planned research were met and practical solutions had to be found. This could affect the validity of the results and the applicability of the findings to other settings. It has been tried to cope with these constraints and to conduct the research as optimally as possible.

Of the 61 participants who finished the programme, 40 children (65.6%) were surveyed. The other 21 children could not be found. There are no indications that these children differ significantly from those who were interviewed. At the time they took part in the nutrition programme, they lived in the same area, were in similar socio-economic situations and had the same family circumstances, compared with those who took part in the study.

To investigate whether the nutrition programme has an effect, ideally children should be randomly assigned to a treatment and a control group. However, it is ethically impossible to exclude a child from the nutrition programme. In this study, we tried to have the treatment and control group in matching in on sex and age as well as possible. Minor differences in age appeared to remain, although these were not significant. Also, the treatment and the control group should be measured twice. The treatment group should be tested before and after participation in the nutrition programme, the control group should be tested at the same time. Unfortunately, this was not possible due to the short period of time given to conduct the research.

This research was performed up to 22 months after the treatment group completed the nutrition programme. The status of current nutrition and development could have changed during or after participation in the programme as a result of changes in food supply or other extraneous factors. Based on descriptions of the family and environmental circumstances in the medical files of the NMC, it can be expected that no significant changes in these circumstances have taken place over time.

The use of a translator for the questions asked and the answers provided may have influenced the reliability of the present results. It was tried to minimise the problem of interpretation to the greatest extent possible by training the translators before the interview and providing strict instructions.

Information about the child's behaviour was gathered by interviewing the caregivers. A consequence of this is that answers concerning the caregivers behaviour are coloured by the caregiver's ideas of normal and abnormal behaviour. Culture-specific concepts of what is normal or abnormal can also affect the way in which a child's behaviour is perceived (Hackett & Hackett, 1999).

## 4.3. Further Improvement
After studying the results and observations gained during this research, several suggestions for the improvement of the programme can be made. It is advised that longer aftercare should be provided for children and their caregivers, up to two years after following the programme. Maintaining contact with the children and observing their health can prevent relapse. Long- term monitoring also allows more research to be conducted, which makes it possible to establish the long-term effects of the nutrition programme.

More precision is needed in the records. This is necessary for monitoring children during the programme and for the evaluation of the home situation.

On the basis of observations during the research, more stimulation and activities for the children and their caregivers are advised. Examples of activities for caregivers are knitting and sewing. Co-operation with pre-schools is advised for new ideas for educational activities for the children.

The lectures the community health workers give to the caregivers should be checked and brought up-to-date. While giving the lectures, the caregivers should be asked to participate.. This creates more interaction and the opportunity to ask questions and have discussions. In this way, important information can be passed on effectively by the CHW to the caregivers.

It is important that the home visits should be improved. Solutions should be found for the participants who have no gardens. Also, more attention should be given to drop-outs. They should be motivated to rejoin the programme.

Of the treatment group, 44.7% of the children and 20% of the children of the control group did not show signs of undernourishment on the date of admission. This could have influenced the measured effect of the nutrition programme. In the future, CHWs and medical doctors should pay more attention to weight and health status of the children before admitting them to the programme.

Hopefully, the results of this study will be useful for the improvement of the Nutritional Unit Programme. Improvement of the programme can help the families living in and around Elandsdoorn to have a better quality of life.

## References

Ajzen, I. (1988). *Attitudes, personality and behaviour*. Chicago: The Dorsey Press.

Bilo, R.A.C. & Voorhoeve, H.W.A. (1990). *Kind in ontwikkeling: Algemene aspecten van de ontwikkeling en groei bij het jonge kind*. Lochem: Uitgeversmaatschappij de Tijdstroom.

Campbell, D.T. & Stanley, J. (1963). *Experimental and quasi-experimental designs for research*. Boston, Massachusetts: Houghton Mifflin Company.

Davidson, L. (1995). The development of the Ten Questions: A tool to screen for serious disability in children in countries with few professional resources. In: M.I.M. Schuurman (ed.), *Assessment of childhood disabilities in developing countries (pp. 11-20)*. Utrecht: Bisschop Beckers Institute.

Goodman, R. (1997). The Strengths and Difficulties Questionnaire: A Research Note. *Journal of Child Psychology and Psychiatry, 38*, 581-586.

Hackett & Hackett, (1999). Child psychiatry across cultures. *International Review of Psychiatry, 11*, 225-235.

Hansen J.D.L. & Bac, M. (1991). Malnutrition. In: M.A. Kibel & L.A. Wagstaff, (eds.), *Child Health for all. A manual for Southern Africa (pp. 221-232)*. Cape Town: Oxford University Press.

King, F.S. & Burgess, A. (1993). *Nutrition for developing countries*. Oxford University Press.

Mullick M.S.I. & Goodman, R. (2001). Questionnaire screening for mental health problems in Bangladeshi children: a preliminary study. *Social Psychiatry and Psychiatric Epidemiology, 36*, 94-99.

National Centre for Health Statistics. CDC Growth Charts: United States. Advance Data No. 314, Vital and Health Statistics of the Centres for Disease Control and Prevention, May 30, 2000.

Pollitt, E., William, W. & Leibel, R.L. (1982). The relation of growth to cognition in a well-nourished pre-school population. *Child Development, 53*, 1157-1163.

Thorburn, M. J. (1995). Achievements of the Ten Questions and possibilities for its practical use. In: M.I.M. Schuurman (ed.), *Assessment of childhood disabilities in developing countries (pp. 78-86)*. Utrecht: Bisschop Beckers Institute.

Thorburn, M. J., Desai, P. & Davidson, L. (1992). Categories, classes and criteria in childhood disabilities. Experiences from a survey in Jamaica. *Disability and Rehabilitation, 14*,122-133.

Thorburn, M.J. & Marfo, K. (1994). *Practical approaches to childhood disability in developing countries*. Tampa: Global Age Publishing.

## Website

*Medline Plus. A service of the U.S. national library of medicine and the national institutes of health. Medical dictionary. http://www.nlm.nih.gov/medlineplus/mplusdictionary.html*

*Address for correspondence:*
H.A. Tempelman, MD
Ndlovu Medical Centre
P.O. Box 1447
Groblersdal 0470
South Africa
e-mail: hltemp@ndlovumc.org

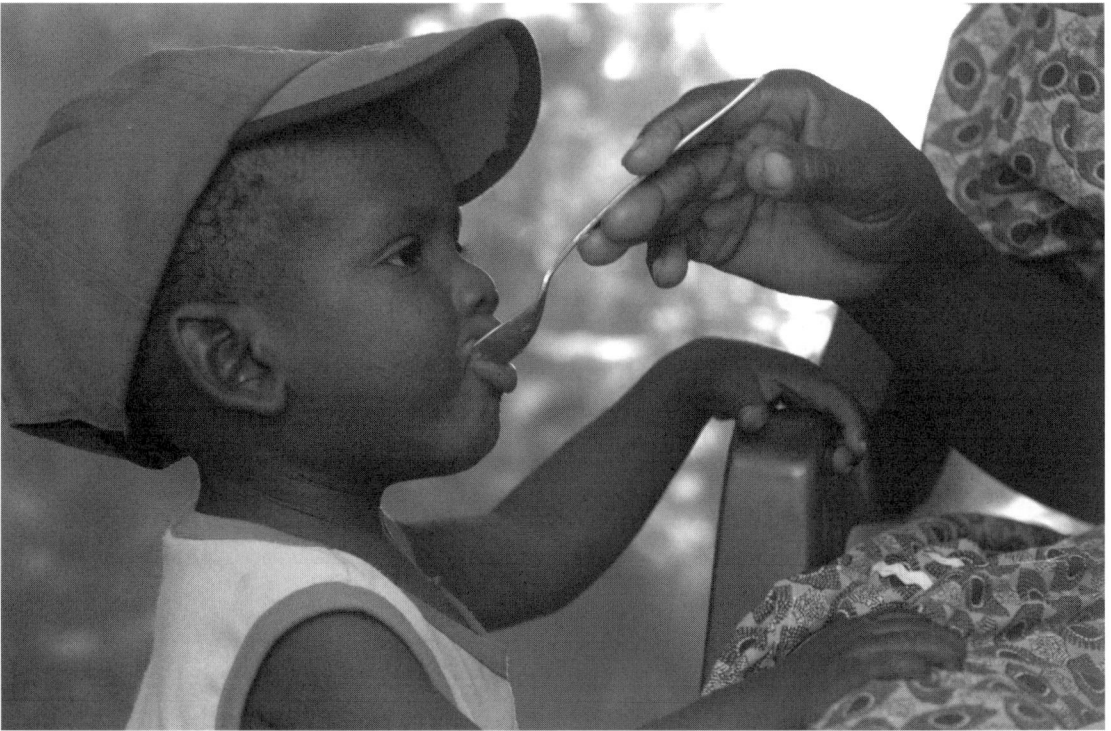

# Chapter 5

# Effects of a Nutritional Training Programme on Nutritional Knowledge in a Rural Area of South Africa.

*Elsbeth Klop[1], Anke Gardeniers[2], Hugo Tempelman[2], Adri Vermeer[3]*

[1] Akkermans & Partners, Utrecht, The Netherlands
[2] Ndlovu Medical Centre Elandsdoorn, South Africa
[3] Department of Educational Sciences, Utrecht University, Utrecht, The Netherlands

## Abstract

The objective of this study was to evaluate the effectiveness of the Ndlovu Nutritional Unit Programme with regard to the level of nutritional knowledge in a population-based study in South Africa. This study is a community-based, cross-sectional, case-controlled survey in the Elandsdoorn area, Mpumalanga, South Africa. Chi-square and t-tests were used to compare the level of nutritional knowledge of participants who have been exposed to the programme with participants who have never been exposed to the programme using a self-developed questionnaire. The study sample consisted of 82 participants pairs. A case pair (N=47) was defined as a caregiver and child who have participated in the programme. A control pair (N=35) was defined as a caregiver and child who have never been exposed to the programme. Participants in the programme score approximately one point higher on the knowledge scale of 1-10 than non-participants. These data show an increase in nutritional knowledge of the caregivers after joining the programme, compared to caretakers who have never followed the programme. Further studies are needed to examine the actual nutritional behaviour of the caregivers. In particularly, pre- and post-surveys are advised to evaluate the real effect of the programme on the level of nutritional knowledge.

## 1. Introduction

### 1.1. Malnutrition

Malnutrition is a major health problem all over the world, especially in developing countries. More than a third of child deaths have malnutrition as underlying cause (Chopra, 1999). South Africa is a country with mortality rates of 45.2 deaths per 1,000 live births and 61 per 1,000 for children younger than 5 years old (Labadarios, Steyn, Mgijima, & Daldla, 2005). Recently, the National Food Consumption Survey in children aged 1-9 years in South Africa has shown that 10.3% of the children is underweight for age and 21.6% of the children are stunted (Labadarios et al., 2003; Steyn, Labadarios, Maunder, Nel, & Lombard, 2005). The prevalence of stunting was 25.5% in children aged 1-3 years (Labadarios et al., 2003).

Many studies have consistently observed different determinants related to stunting. For instance, building material of the house, type of toilet in the household, presence of a television in the house, educational level of the caregiver of the child, and maternal educational level (Steyn, Labadarios, Maunder, Nel, & Lombard, 2005). Other determinants for malnutrition, the education level of the mother, whether the last child was breastfed and the duration of breast-feeding, the presence of a toilet, were found to be significantly related to under-weight-for-age (Chopra, 2003). Poor hygienic practices and a low educational level of the mother or caregiver of the child were found to be the most influencing factors for developing malnutrition (Chopra, 2003). It is known that parental education level improves the nutrition status of the child (Lomperis, 1991; Vella et al., 1992). Education about different health topics is needed to fight child malnutrition, especially in developing countries.

In South Africa many children die as a result of undernutrition. Even when the child survives, undernutrition will have a great impact on the resistance to illness, on growth, and on intellectual development of the child (Chopra, 1999). Poverty and lack of knowledge about different health topics are for instance major basic causes of malnutrition, as well as intermediate causes such as poor hygienic environments and caring practices, diseases or lack of food (Chopra, 1999). Lack of awareness and knowledge about these basic and intermediate causes of malnutrition significantly contributes to a poor nutritional status of children, even in households where adults have enough daily food requirements (Kilaru, Griffiths, Ganapathy, & Ghosh, 2005). The caregivers of the malnourished children might not handle the available sources of food well enough because of cultural beliefs and lack of knowledge about healthy food. Large-scale educational interventions have previously shown to be effective in changing the way caregivers use the available sources, such as offering healthy food, increasing dietary intake, thereby improving child growth (Penny et al., 2005). This shows there is a need for good nutritional programmes to educate caregivers about the different causes of child malnutrition. Here, we evaluate the effects of the Ndlovu nutrition programme on the level of nutritional knowledge in the Elandsdoorn area of South Africa.

## 1.2. Ndlovu Nutritional Unit Programme

The Ndlovu Nutritional Unit Programme (NNUP) is a large community development project in the area of Elandsdoorn, a township in Moutse, South Africa. Ndlovu Medical Centre (NMC), functioning since 1994, is a private health clinic, which also provides community health care to the Elandsdoorn population. The NNUP is a programme working in connection with the NMC. At the clinic children are seen with acute medical problems based on underlying malnourishment. These children and their caregivers are invited to join the programme for treatment. The children are screened and accordingly treated for worms, TB, anaemia, HIV, and other diseases. All children who are found to be HIV-positive are started on highly active antiretroviral treatment (HAART), together with their siblings and parents. During the treatment period, the caregivers of the children are trained how to establish their own vegetable garden and how to improve the home situation concerning sanitation, hygiene and preparing healthy food. The caregivers are provided with seedlings and a garden tool set to start a vegetable garden. This is done in an attempt to provide structural improvement of the feeding status of the whole family. The caregivers are offered different lectures on several important health topics, such as TB, diarrhoea, immunisation, hygienic food preparation and healthy food. During the days at the unit the children get their daily meals until they are back on their normal growth line. The community healthcare workers (CHWs), locally trained staff, are doing regular home visits in order to assist in the home improvements and to monitor the progress of the home gardening.

## 1.3. The Area and Units

Elandsdoorn is a township in Moutse, located between Bronkhorstspruit and Groblersdal, Mpumalanga, South Africa. The population has been estimated at 30,000 to 40,000 people and mainly speaks North Soto, Tswane, Zulu and Ndebele. The population is exclusively black and lives largely in the surrounding rural townships (Kocken, 2000).

The main unit of the NNUP is located in Elandsdoorn, next to the NMC. Four satellite units are opened in the meantime. The objective of the programme is to establish more units in surrounding townships to lower the threshold for participation (Kocken, 2000).

# 2. Methods

## 2.1. Study Sample

This study is a population-based, cross-sectional, case-controlled survey with 82 participant pairs in the townships around Elandsdoorn area, which aims to evaluate the effects of the programme on nutritional knowledge. A participant pair is a combination of a caregiver and one child. If the caregiver has taken more than one child to the programme, this is considered as more than one participant. The case group consists of participant pairs who have followed the programme (N=47) and had or still have children who were/are underweight. The control group consists of participant pairs who have never participated in the programme (N=35) and have children that are not underweight. To reach the goal of this survey, there are a number of questions focusing on the level of nutritional knowledge included in the questionnaire.

In this study sample, 47 cases and 35 controls were interviewed. The median age of the children was 48.5 months (range 13.0⊠88.0). All the participating caregivers were female with a median age of 36 years old (range 16.0⊠75.0). In the case group, 46.8% of the children were male and 53.2% of the children were female. The control group consisted of 60.0% male children and 40.0% female children. One case pair was excluded from the study because it did not meet the selection criteria. The caregiver joined the NNU programme, but her child was not malnourished according to the WAZ-scores. To prevent confounding, this caregiver was excluded from the analysis.

## 2.2. Indicator of Nutritional Status

In order to measure the nutritional status of children aged between 1-8 years, the Weight-for-Age Z-score (WAZ) was used. Epi info 2000, a database and statistical programme, is used to calculate the WAZ-scores, a programme recommended by the World Health Organisation (Dean, 1999; Dean, Sangam, Sunki, Friedman, Lanting, et al., 2000). The US National Centre for Health Statistics (NHCS) population was used as reference population. The children who are below 2 SD (3rd percentile) from the median weight for age of the WHO/NCHS reference population are underweight (Chopra, 2003; Dean, 1999; Dean, Sangam, Sunki, Friedman, Lanting, et al., 2000).

The nutritional programme uses weight-for-age Z-scores to determine the nutritional status. Children under the third percentile of their weight curve are admitted to the programme.

## 2.3. Level of Nutritional Knowledge

Respondents were questioned about different health topics, the three food groups, malnutrition, tuberculosis, diarrhoea, how to prepare food in a hygienic way, and how to prepare baby formula. The questions used for the different health topics are based on the lectures given during the programme. These questions were put into a ten-point scale. Within this scale, higher scores are associated with a better knowledge level of the caregiver. We compared the level of nutritional knowledge of the caregivers who have been taught according to the lectures in the programme about these health topics (case group) with the nutritional knowledge of caretakers who have never been exposed to these lectures (control group).

## 2.4. Statistical Analyses

SPSS software was used for data-entry and statistical analyses. Prevalence and means were calculated to compare the nutritional knowledge level between the cases and controls. Chi-square and t-tests were used to test the significance of the comparisons. The significance level used in this study was p=0.05. P-values above this level (p=0.05) were reported as not statistically significant.

# 3. Results

## 3.1. Baseline Socio-economic Characteristics of the Study Sample

Table 1 shows the socio-economic characteristics of the study sample at baseline. The majority of this study population has electricity and sanitation in the household. All toilets in the households are pit latrines. In this study population, the main source of water is a borehole. There is a statistically significant difference in the median age of the caregivers for both groups. The median age of the caregivers was higher in the case group in comparison with the control group. The study sample depended on two main sources of income, pension and paid jobs. In the case group, 43.0% have a person in the household with a paid job, 60.0% of the income in the household is obtained from a pension and 19.0% have neither. In the control group, 59.0% have a person with a paid job in the household, 44.0% of the income is obtained from a pension, and 9.0% have neither. Approximately an average of 1.9 people in the case group share a room, against an average of 1.7 people in the control group. An average of R 56.6 per person is spent on food by the cases and R 69.7 by the controls. The case group on average lives closer to a health clinic (4.97 km) compared to the control group (6.84 km). There is a statistically significant difference in the division of the relationship between mother and child. In the control group, 62.9% of the caregivers is the mother of the child, against 48.9% in the case group. In the case group, 46.8% of the caregivers are grandmothers. There is also a statistically significant difference in the marital status of the caregivers. In the case group, 55% of the caregivers are married, compared to 29.0% in the control group.

## 3.2. Nutritional Status of the Children

The cases and controls were selected on participation in the programme and the child's nutritional status. Weight-for-Age Z-scores (WAZ) were calculated to determine the nutritional status of the child. The case group has a mean WAZ-score of -2.80 with a standard deviation of 0.64, and the mean Z-score for the control group is 0.69 with a standard deviation of 0.58.

**Table 1: Distribution of socio-economical factors among the samples**

|  | Case sample N = 47 | Control sample N = 35 |
|---|---|---|
| Age child in months (median; range) | 42.0 (13-88) | 60.0 (24-72) |
| Gender child (%) |  |  |
| - boy | 46.8 | 60.0 |
| girl | 53.2 | 40.0 |
| Age caregiver in years (median; range)* | 43.0 (18.0-75.0) | 26.0 (16.0-67.0) |
| Income (%) |  |  |
| - paid job | 42.6 | 58.8 |
| - pension | 59.6 | 44.1 |
| - neither | 19.1 | 8.80 |
| Number of people per room (mean; range) | 1.88 (0.60-6.50) | 1.67 (0.26-4.50) |
| Total amount Rand spent on food per person (mean; range) | 56.55 (20.00-183.33) | 69.69 (18.75-200.00) |
| Distance to the health clinic in km (mean; range) | 4.97 (0.50-20.0) | 6.84 (1.00-15.0) |
| Electricity in the household (%) |  |  |
| - yes | 97.9 | 94.3 |
| - no | 2.10 | 5.70 |
| Sanitation in the household (%) |  |  |
| - yes | 89.4 | 85.7 |
| - no | 10.6 | 14.3 |
| Relationship caregiver – child (%)* |  |  |
| - mother | 48.9 | 62.9 |
| - grandmother | 46.8 | 17.1 |
| - other | 4.30 | 20.0 |
| Marital status caretaker (%)* |  |  |
| - married | 55.3 | 29.4 |
| - widow | 8.50 | 2.90 |
| - other | 36.2 | 66.7 |
| Source of water (%) |  |  |
| - tap | 27.7 | 11.4 |
| - well | 10.6 | 14.3 |
| - borehole | 40.4 | 54.3 |
| - buy | 21.3 | 20.0 |

* Significant group differences within p<0.05

## 3.3. Nutritional Knowledge Level of the Caregiver

Table 2 shows the results for the distribution of different knowledge questions. The majority of the children in the study sample were immunised. When the child is ill and does not want to eat most of the caregivers in this study population still fed their child. Only half of the caregivers in both groups knew that fat food is bad for a sick child. In the case group, 94.0% of the caregivers has breastfed their child, compared to 88.0% of the caregivers in the control group. In the case group, statistically significantly more caregivers (89.5%) knew what healthy food was, compared to the control group (70.0%). In the control group, 91.0% knew how to prepare food in a hygienic way and could give examples, compared to 81.0% of the cases who knew how to prepare food in a hygienic way and could give some examples too. In the case group, 89.0% of the caregivers knew that when the child has diarrhoea, it still needs to eat, compared to 69.0% of the caregivers in the control group. When questioned what the symptoms of TB are, 77.0% of the cases and only 54.0% of the controls could tell. In the case group, 77.0% knew how to recognise a malnourished child, in comparison to 63.0% of the control group. The results show that the case group scores statistically significantly one point higher on the scale of knowledge (0-10) in comparison to the control group.

**Table 2: Distribution of knowledge among the samples**

|  | Case sample N = 47 | Control sample N = 35 | p |
|---|---|---|---|
| Breastfed the child (%) |  |  | 0.371 |
| - yes | 93.6 | 87.9 |  |
| - no | 6.40 | 12.1 |  |
| Know what healthy food is (%)* |  |  | 0.005 |
| - yes | 89.5 | 70.0 |  |
| - no | 10.5 | 30.0 |  |
| Know how to prepare food in a hygienic way (%)* |  |  | 0.047 |
| - yes | 80.9 | 90.9 |  |
| - no | 19.1 | 9.10 |  |
| If the child is ill and does not want to eat, do you feed your child (%) |  |  | 0.148 |
| - yes | 87.2 | 74.3 |  |
| - no | 12.7 | 25.7 |  |
| Do you think that if the child has diarrhoea, the child needs to stop eating (%) |  |  | 0.072 |
| - yes | 10.6 | 31.3 |  |
| - no | 89.4 | 68.7 |  |
| Do you think that fat food is bad for a sick child (%) |  |  | 0.416 |
| - yes | 51.1 | 52.9 |  |
| - no | 48.9 | 47.1 |  |
| Child is immunised (%) |  |  | 0.136 |
| - yes | 85.1 | 96.3 |  |
| - no | 14.9 | 3.70 |  |
| Recognise a child with TB (%)* |  |  | 0.008 |
| - yes | 77.2 | 54.3 |  |
| - no | 12.8 | 45.7 |  |
| Recognise a malnourished child (%) |  |  | 0.231 |
| - yes | 76.6 | 62.9 |  |
| - no | 23.4 | 37.1 |  |
| *Knowledge level of caretaker in a scale of 1 – 10 (mean; range)** | 5.36 (3.00 – 7.00) | 4.51 ( 2.00 – 8.00) | 0.002 |

* Significant group differences within p<0.05

# 4. Discussion

This study evaluated the effects of the Ndlovu Nutritional Unit Programme with regard to the level of nutritional knowledge among caregivers in the rural area of Elandsdoorn. These data show that NNUP participants (case group) on average score one point higher on the ten-point scale of knowledge in comparison to non-participants of the NNUP (control group). Some limitations need to be discussed.

The cross-sectional data limits to test the real effect of the programme. No systematic measurements were taken on the level of nutritional knowledge of the caregivers before being admitted to the programme, so the difference in nutritional knowledge before and after being exposed to the programme cannot be determined. To evaluate the real effect of the programme on the level of nutritional knowledge, pre- and post-surveys would be advised.

The control group limits to be an excellent comparable group to the case group. Controls only have well-nourished children and the cases who joined the programme all have under-nourished children. Therefore, besides measuring the effect of (not)following the programme on the level of nutritional knowledge of both groups, the effect of having well-nourished or undernourished children is measured too. There is also a statistically significant difference in some baseline characteristics for both groups. There is found to be a difference in the age of the caregiver, the relationship caregiver-child, and the marital status of the caregiver. These determinants could be possible confounders in the differences between the two groups for nutritional knowledge of the caregiver.

This study is based on education of the caregivers about different health topics to prevent malnutrition among children in a rural area of South Africa. Only the level of knowledge is measured, but the actual behaviour of the caretakers is not known. For instance, the food intake of the children, the handling and storage of water, the cleaning of the house and environment, daily food choices for meals, and action after recognition of different diseases, are all examples of actual behaviours needed to prevent child undernutrition. The first step, gaining knowledge about the different health topics, is tested, but the important step of acting accordingly needs to be looked at as well. In conclusion, this population-based study shows an increase in the caregivers' nutritional knowledge after following the lectures about different health topics, compared to caregivers who have never followed the programme. Further studies are needed to examine the actual nutritional behaviour of the caregivers. In particularly, pre- and post-surveys are advised, in order to evaluate the real effect of the programme on the level of nutritional knowledge.

# References

Chopra, M. (1999). Under-nutrition in South Africa. *Up Date* (47), 3-4.
Chopra, M. (2003). Risk factors for undernutrition of young children in a rural area of South Africa. *Public Health Nutrition, 6*(7), 645-652.
Dean, A.G. (1999). Epi Info and Epi Map: current status and plans for Epi Info 2000. *J Public Health Management Practise, 5*(4), 54-57.
Dean, A.G., Sangam, S., Sunki, G.G., Friedman, R., Lanting, M., et al. (2000). *Epi Info 2000, A database and statistical programme for public health professionals for use on Windows 95, 98, NT and 2000 computers.* Atlanta.
Kilaru, A., Griffiths, P.L., Ganapathy, S., & Ghosh, S. (2005). Community-based Nutrition Education for Improving Infant Growth in Rural Karnataka. *Indian Pediatrics, 42*(5), 425-432.

Kocken, T. (2000). *Het Umlazi Initiatief*. Utrecht: Utrecht University.

Labadarios, D., Maunder, E., Steyn, N., MacIntyre, U., Swart, R., Gericke, G., et al. (2003). National food consumption survey in children aged 1-9 years: South Africa 1999. *Forum Nutrition, 56*, 106-109.

Labadarios, D., Steyn, N. P., Mgijima, C., & Daldla, N. (2005). Review of the South African nutrition policy 1994-2002 and targets for 2007: achievements and challenges. *Nutrition, 21*(1), 100-108.

Lomperis, A. M. (1991). Teaching mothers to read: evidence from Colombia on the key role of maternal education in preschool child nutritional health. *Journal of Developping Areas, 26*(1), 25-52.

Penny, M.E., Creed-Kanashiro, H.M., Robert, R.C., Narro, M.R., Caulfield, L.E., & Black, R. E. (2005). Effectiveness of an educational intervention delivered through the health services to improve nutrition in young children: a cluster-randomised controlled trial. *Lancet, 365*(9474), 1863-1872.

Steyn, N.P., Labadarios, D., Maunder, E., Nel, J., & Lombard, C. (2005). Secondary anthropometric data analysis of the National Food Consumption Survey in South Africa: the double burden. *Nutrition, 21*(1), 4-13.

Vella, V., Tomkins, A., Borghesi, A., Migliori, G.B., Adriko, B.C., & Crevatin, E. (1992). Determinants of child nutrition and mortality in north-west Uganda. *Bulletin World Health Organisation, 70*(5), 637-643.

*Address for correspondence:*
Mrs. A.C. Gardeniers, MSc
Ndlovu Medical Centre
PO Box 1447
Groblersdal 0470
South Africa

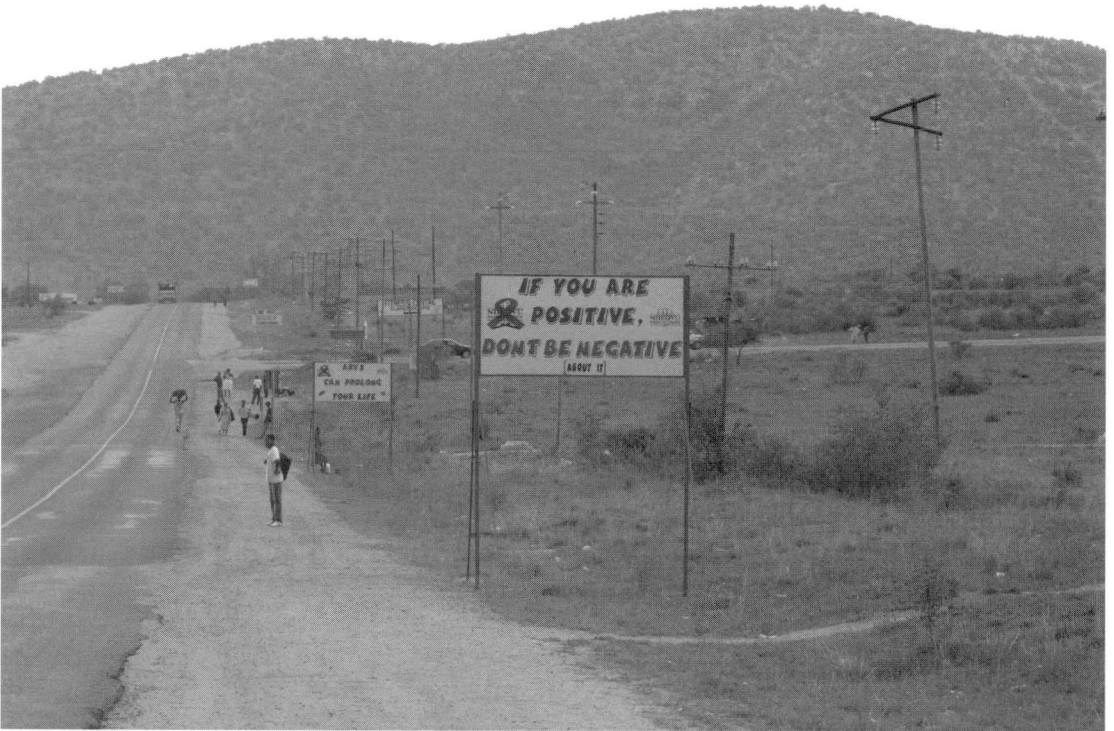

# Chapter 6

# Evaluation of an AIDS Awareness Programme

*Koen van der Lubbe[1,2], Marloes Schinnij[1], Hugo Tempelman[2],*
*Adri Vermeer[1]*

[1] Department of Educational Sciences, Utrecht University, Utrecht, The Netherlands
[2] Ndlovu Medical Centre, Elandsdoorn, South Africa

## Abstract

The evaluation of an AIDS awareness programme was conducted in a township in a rural area in South Africa. The effects of the programme were measured through a self-constructed questionnaire. First, the increase of knowledge about HIV/AIDS was measured and participants were questioned about cultural and personal beliefs. The second part of the questionnaire consisted of questions regarding sexual behaviour. The third and last part was based on the theory of planned behaviour (TPB) (Ajzen, 1991) and tried to verify the predicted influence of the factors of the TPB on condom use. The questionnaire has been completed by 349 children between the ages of 12 and 25, who have attended the programme never, once or more than once. The knowledge increase appeared not to be significant after attending the programme once, but after attending the programme more than once it was. The questions about cultural beliefs showed a great lack of knowledge and the presence of culturally influenced beliefs. The results of the second part, about behaviour, showed a fairly high percentage of sexually active children before seeing the programme (26.6%). After following the programme once, 70.5% of the children said they were willing to change their behaviour. The last part of the questionnaire showed that the model of the TPB has a good fit to the data, that condom use is influenced for boys through intention and for girls through intention and perceived behavioural control.

## 1. Introduction

### 1.1. Ndlovu AIDS Awareness Programme (NAAP)

Ndlovu Medical Centre is a centre that combines private and public health care with community development, stimulation of entrepreneurship and self-help projects. The NMC was established in 1994 as a private initiative and is situated in the Elandsdoorn township, Mpumalanga.

NAAP started as an initiative of Ndlovu Medical Centre in 1999. The goal of the NAAP is to make children aware of the HIV/AIDS problems in their community and to inform and educate them about HIV/AIDS prevention. In order to provide the students with factual information and to promote healthy sexual behaviour, the NAAP performances are focused on these issues. The NAAP team consists of six young adults from Elandsdoorn, who were selected and trained by UN Peace Corps Volunteers and a Dutch drama teacher to do the performances. The NAAP reaches about 25,000 children every year, of which almost 80% through school visits, the remainder has been reached through community events and an unspecified number of people have been counselled at the Aids Awareness Centre in Elandsdoorn. The programme is aimed at children between the ages of 12 (last grade of primary school) and 18 (secondary schools). The NAAP team visits schools in Elandsdoorn and the surrounding area once a year. Visiting one or two grades at a time, each performance is attended by 50 to 100 children. The performances are given in the classroom or at the playground. When not performing in schools, the team is available at the Aids Awareness Information Centre, next to Ndlovu Medical Centre, where they counsel both individuals and groups and where condoms are available for free.

The programme is a combination of information, drama and discussion. To promote healthy sexual behaviour and to provide the children with information on the subject, different dramas are performed. There are six different dramas:

1. AIDS and available help;
2. AIDS and tests, counselling;
3. AIDS and opportunistic infections;
4. AIDS and its implications on South African households and the economy;
5. AIDS and poverty;
6. AIDS and traditional beliefs.

There is one new drama 'AIDS and youth' which has not been performed yet. The choice of the dramas that are performed, can be made by the school or by the NAAP team itself depending, on the main problems of a particular area. Sometimes more than one drama is done. The performances always have the same structure: it starts off with general information about HIV/AIDS, how it is transmitted, how the disease develops and how it can be prevented. After that, there is a drama and a discussion about a specific subject. A performance usually takes about 90 minutes, depending on the children's participation in the discussion.

The NAAP team works with the so-called ABCD of prevention. 'Abstaining', 'Being faithful', 'Condom use' and 'Delay' are the four strategies one can use to prevent getting infected with HIV/AIDS. Condom use is the strategy most emphasised by the NAAP team. The distribution of condoms is one of the most important elements of the NAAP, besides providing knowledge and trying to change behaviour. In their pursuit of changing behaviour, the availability of condoms is the first step in achieving the desired behaviour.

The goals of the Ndlovu AIDS Awareness Programme are:

– Providing factual information on HIV/AIDS and sexual health education to secondary school students and community groups; sexual health education includes information on sexually transmitted infections (STIs), sexual abuse, child abuse, incest and teacher-student relationships.
– Promoting change in sexual behaviour and moral behaviour in order to reduce new transmissions of the HIV virus.
– Promoting the use of condoms and raising awareness of the risks of promiscuity.
– Promoting sexual health for the entire population in the Moutse area, in co-operation with the existing community structures (Tempelman & Botha-Standaert, 2002).

## 1.2. Research questions

After five years, the opportunity was there to get insight into the effectiveness of the NAAP, and to see whether the programme reaches its goals. Besides, it is good to know which factors influence sexual behaviour: understanding the behaviours that put individuals at risk of HIV infection, and identifying ways to change these behaviours are important strategies to help halt the spread of HIV in Africa (Kebaabtswe & Norr, 2002). Therefore, the two research questions are:

1. *Does the Ndlovu AIDS Awareness Programme increase knowledge about HIV/AIDS and does it result in a change of sexual behaviour?*
2. *Which factors influence condom use in the NAAP target group?*

## 1.3. HIV/AIDS in Africa

South Africa is one of the countries with the highest number of HIV-infected persons. Approximately 5.5 million South Africans in the age of 15-49 years are currently HIV-positive. According to Booysen, Geldenhuys and Markinov (2003), the adult prevalence amongst 20-65 year olds will be 24.1%. Every day, 1,700 persons are infected and 600 persons die as a result of AIDS.

The Philadelphia district, where Elandsdoorn is situated, has a population of almost 500,000 people. 14.7% of them are reported HIV-positive, i.e. 73,500 people. 54.5% of the population have not been tested yet. Most new HIV infections occur in people between the ages of 15 and 49 years (Stadler & Hlongwa, 2002).

Male condoms have remained central to HIV prevention campaigns due to their proven efficiency in protecting sexual partners against HIV. As in many parts of the world, condom use in Africa tends to be low in many populations. There are significant barriers to male condom use in South Africa; such barriers include lack of female control over condom use, costs of condoms, limited availability of condoms, lack of knowledge about the effectiveness of condoms, fear of embarrassment associated with using condoms, lack of knowledge about HIV, perceived lack of HIV risk, decreased condom use in sexual acts following alcohol consumption, and culturally specific stigmas associated with condom use (Shapiro & Kapiga, 2002). Although condom use remains low, many people see it as the way to prevent oneself from getting infected with HIV/AIDS. In research done with mineworkers in 2003, 94% responded by saying condom use was the way to protect oneself from HIV/AIDS (Day, Miyamura & Rant et al., 2003).

## 1.4. Theoretical Background

The theory of planned behaviour (TPB) is a model used for explaining social behaviour.

The model focuses on theoretical constructs that are concerned with individual motivational factors as determinants of the likelihood of performing a specific behaviour (Montano & Kasprzyk, 1990). The theory of planned behaviour posits that a person's behaviour is a result of his/her intention to perform the particular action (Ajzen, 1991). The individual's intention to engage in a particular behaviour is supposed to be influenced by three factors: the attitude towards the behaviour, the perceived attitudes of important others (subjective norm) and the perceived behavioural control.

*Attitudes* towards a particular behaviour are a result of beliefs about the consequences of engaging in the specific behaviour and subjective evaluations of those consequences. For example, an individual who believes that a condom is likely to prevent HIV transmission and that HIV transmission is undesirable, may be more likely to use a condom (Bogart, Cecel & Pinkerton, 2000).

*Subjective norms* are defined as the individual's perception of social pressure to perform or not to perform the specific behaviour. Hence, subjective norms are a result of the likelihood that important others think that an individual should engage in a particular behaviour and the individual's motivation to comply with the desires of important others. For example, if a man believes that his sex partner and his friends would like him to use a condom and he values their opinion, he would be more likely to use a condom (Bogart et al., 2000).

*Perceived behavioural control* reflects the control an individual thinks to have over his/her own behaviour. This factor reflects past experience as well as external factors, such as anticipated impediments, obstacles, resources and opportunities that may influence the performance of the specific behaviour. It consists of two sub-factors: the perceived likelihood of encountering factors that will facilitate or inhibit the successful performance of the behaviour, weighted by their perceived power to facilitate or inhibit performance. Perceived behavioural control has affinity with the social cognitive theory construct of self-efficacy, but is not synonymous (Bennet & Bozionelos, 2000).

The model (see Figure 1) proposes that attitudes and subjective norms exert their influence towards a specific behaviour through their impact upon intentions, while perceived behavioural control may influence both intention to perform the specific behaviour and actual behaviour. Other factors as personality, demographics, and other variables external to the model operate through the model constructs, and do not independently contribute to explaining the likelihood of performing a behaviour (Fisher & Fisher, 2000).

## 2. Methods

### 2.1. Subjects

The participants in this research (N=349) are all children attending primary and secondary schools in Marapong in the Elandsdoorn area. The choice of schools and grades depended mostly on the schedule of the NAAP team and on the co-operation of the schools. The NAAP team visits almost every school in the area once or twice a year. Within their schedule, a random choice of schools and grades was made. The schools chosen are not different from other schools in the area. All schools in this township area are government schools. They all have to cope with similar poor conditions. The co-operation of the schools was good, although one school did not want HIV/AIDS education for religious reasons and a few schools had no time to co-operate due to exams.

Five grades from three different schools were chosen. All teachers and almost all children were willing to co-operate. The children could leave the classroom if they did not want to fill in the questionnaire. On one school, a few did leave, saying that they did not feel well. The children were all between the ages of 12 and 25. The group of respondents consisted of 187 boys and 162 girls. The groups of children differ in the number of times they have attended the Ndlovu Aids Awareness Programme (see Table 1).

**Table 1: Subject statistics**

| Gender | Number of times seen the programme | N | Mean Age |
|--------|-----------------------------------|-----|----------|
| Boys | 0 | 57 | 14.88 |
| | 1 | 57 | 14.96 |
| | ≥2 | 72 | 18.20 |
| Girls | 0 | 52 | 13.93 |
| | 1 | 52 | 13.96 |
| | ≥2 | 59 | 16.68 |
| Total | 0 | 109 | 14.40 |
| | 1 | 109 | 14.49 |
| | ≥2 | 131 | 17.58 |

The amount of non-response is low (N=18 is 5%). The eighteen non-response questionnaires were taken out of the data-set. Some questionnaires only had a non-response in one or two parts, but had a useful third part. The N for partial non-response is 10 and was found in the group who had attended the programme more than once. Non-response is mostly a result of a poor level of understanding English or due to a misunderstanding about how to fill in the questionnaire.

## 2.2. Instruments

The data of this research are gathered through a self-developed questionnaire, because there was no suitable questionnaire for the particular circumstances. The questionnaire was con-structed with the help of staff at the NMC. To answer the first research question the respon-dents' knowledge had to be measured and insight had to be gained into the sexual behaviour of the respondents. Furthermore, a theory-based part was needed to answer the second re-search question. Therefore, the questionnaire was set up in three different parts.

*Part A* is partly based on the HIV-Knowledge Questionnaire-18 (Carey & Schroder, 2002) and partly on the information presented by the NAAP team. The first section of part A (1-22) is about HIV/AIDS, ways of infection, prevention and possible cure. The second section (23-33) is about beliefs. Part A consists of 33 questions, with the answering possibilities 'true', 'false' and 'don't know'. All questions of part A are based on the content of the NAAP and its goals.

*Part B* has 17 multiple choice questions and yields insight into the actual sexual behaviour of the children. The results of this part are used to find out if a change in behaviour is established after attending the programme.

*Part C* is based on the theory of planned behaviour (Ajzen, 1991) and consists of 48 ques-tions divided over the factors attitude, subjective norm, perceived behavioural control, inten-tion and actual behaviour. These questions are answered through answers on a 3-point scale.

A try-out (N=10, 5 boys and 5 girls) showed that the initial version of the questionnaire, particularly part C, was too long and the answering possibilities too difficult. As a result of these findings, the questionnaire was revised. Part C was narrowed down to condom use only (instead of abstaining, being faithful, condom use and delay) and the answering possibilities were brought back from a 5- to a 3-point scale. Also a language problem emerged in the try-out. The translation of some English words into Sotho and Zulu proved to be necessary. The children had the possibility of asking questions whilst filling in the questionnaire, if they did not understand a question. The people from the NAAP team speak fluent Zulu and Sotho and were able to answer all questions. The assistance given, though, was only a clarification of the questions asked. Because of the differences in languages and the level of some of the ques-tions, this kind of assistance was inevitable. Doing research in an underdeveloped country may implicate that certain adjustments need to be made in order to achieve the objective, viz. gaining information about knowledge, beliefs and actual behaviour, but that does not mean that this interferes with the reliability and validity of the research.

## 2.3. Procedure

The NAAP team made prior arrangements with schools to do the programme. Some schools did not want the NAAP team to perform at their schools for several reasons. At the time of the research, some schools could not find time in their busy schedule because of the exams. Other schools did not want any AIDS education because of their religion or beliefs. A random selection had to be made out of the schools visited by the NAAP team. As many of the arrangements were made at short notice, it was not possible to make before measurements at all grades/ schools. The permission to execute the research was easily obtained. Most principals and teachers were enthusiastic about the research and willing to co-operate. A copy of the questionnaire was given to all teachers and principals. At the schools the children were first given a brief introduction about the questionnaire, explaining how to fill it in. The explaining was done either by somebody of the NAAP team or by one of the researchers. There were at least three people per class ready to answer any questions. The children needed between 30 minutes and 1.5 hours to fill in the questionnaire. The children were given enough time to do this, so there was no time pressure.

## 2.4. Design

There are differences in the number of times the children have attended the Ndlovu Aids Awareness Programme. There is a group that had never been exposed to the NAAP and a group that had attended the NAAP once. These measurements were done at a grade 7 (never N=109, once N=109). There was also a group that had seen the programme twice or more. These measurements were done at grade 9, 10 and 11 (N=131). This research could be considered as a cross-sectional research. The group of children that had attended the programme twice or more, consists of children who saw the programme twice (N=69), three times (N=24) and four times (N= 8). These categories were rather small and it was decided to combine these groups. The choice of schools, grades and classes mostly depended on where the NAAP team was going and whether schools were co-operative.

## 2.5. Statistics

A total score over the 22 questions of Part A was calculated and means were established for grades, gender and the number of times the children had attended the programme. No means were calculated for the questions of Part B. Percentages were given to these questions to describe the kind of behaviour the children were engaged in. Structural Equations Modeling (SEM) was used to analyse the questionnaire data of Part C (Arbucle, 1997). SEM is a method that uses the paths between the variables in a model to define their relations. SEM calculates the regression weights and covariances between the different factors of a model. The model as a whole is used to calculate the regression weights and covariances (Hox, 1999). The answers to six of the questions of Part C of the questionnaire were recoded because they were posed in a negative manner. Questions concerning the same variable were given one value for further calculation. A significance level of .05 was used to evaluate the relations between the different variables in the model of planned behaviour (Azjen, 1991).

## 3. Results

The results of this research can be divided into three parts. In the line with the questionnaire, there are results for knowledge and beliefs, for behaviour and for the theoretical part based on the TPB. The results for knowledge, beliefs and behaviour show whether the NAAP is effective or not. The results for the third part tell us which factors influence the desired behaviour. Concerning the increase of knowledge about HIV/AIDS, it has to be mentioned that it is difficult to attribute a knowledge increase to the NAAP alone. In between performances, children are exposed to different kinds of media, educators and other influences that may increase their knowledge about HIV/AIDS.

## 3.1. Knowledge about HIV/AIDS

The first part of Part A consisted of 22 'true/false' questions about facts of HIV/AIDS. A reliability analysis showed a Cronbach's alpha of Part A of 0.70. A one-way ANOVA shows, as can be seen from Table 2, that for all groups the percentages of correct answers do increase after attending the programme more often. The increase itself is small though. For ten children there is no score over the 22 questions. Although these children have unusable scores in Part A, they are included in Part B and C of the research.

Table 2: Percentages of correct answers for the first section of part A, per gender and number of times attended the programme

| Gender | Number of times attended the programme | % answers correct | N |
|---|---|---|---|
| Male | 0 | 47.5 % | 57 |
| | 1 | 54.0 % | 57 |
| | ≥2 | 57.7 % | 72 |
| Female | 0 | 45.4 % | 52 |
| | 1 | 47.2 % | 52 |
| | ≥2 | 55.6 % | 59 |
| Total | 0 | 46.5 % | 109 |
| | 1 | 50.8 % | 109 |
| | ≥2 | 56.7 % | 131 |

As can be seen from Table 3, there is a non-significant knowledge increase for the whole group of 4.3% after attending the programme once, and a significant 5.9% increase after attending the programme twice or more than twice. The increase in questions that was answered correctly by boys and girls separately is different. The number of questions answered correctly increases non-significantly after attending the programme once, with 6.5% for boys and 2.8% for girls. After having attended the programme twice or more, the knowledge increases with a non-significant 3.7% for boys, but significantly with 8.4% for girls. There is a significant overall knowledge increase for both boys and girls (the increase being the difference in the percentages of correct answers between children who had never seen the programme and those who had seen it twice or more).

Table 3: Increase of percentages of correct answers after attending the programme once and twice or more than twice and its significance.

| Planned comparison | | Increase of percentage correct answers | p |
|---|---|---|---|
| Male | 0 - 1 | 6.5 % | 0.051 |
| | 1 - ≥2 | 3.7 % | 0.509 |
| | 0 - ≥2 | 10.2 % | 0.000*** |
| Female | 0 - 1 | 2.8 % | 1.000 |
| | 1 - ≥2 | 8.4 % | 0.006** |
| | 0 - ≥2 | 11.2 % | 0.001** |
| Total | 0 - 1 | 4.3 % | 0.083 |
| | 1 - ≥2 | 5.9 % | 0.006** |
| | 0 - ≥2 | 10.2 % | 0.000*** |

* = $p < .05$; ** = $p < .01$; *** = $p < .001$

86

The questions about the beliefs concerning HIV/AIDS will not be discussed in the same way as the knowledge questions, as it is more difficult to discuss beliefs in terms of wrong or right answers. What can be said though, is that the percentages of pupils who give the answer 'don't know' were high before and after attending the programme once and twice or more. Especially the questions about antiretrovirals (ARVs) resulted in high percentages of children who answered 'don't know', even after following the programme once or more times. Only three of the eleven belief questions: 'Having more girlfriends proves that you are a man' (N (1)=107, N (≥2) = 19), 'Sex with a virgin cures AIDS' (N (1)=103, N (≥2)=119), and ARV's can cure AIDS' (N (1)=106, N (≥2)=117), had significant (p< .05) decreases after attending the programme twice or more. All the other percentages of 'don't know' remained high (or were even higher) after attending the programme once or more, but did not change significantly (see Table 4).

**Table 4: Percentages of 'don't know' per number of times attending the programme**

| | 0 | 1 | ≥2 |
|---|---|---|---|
| 23. When you are circumcised (uma ubuya engomeni/ ge o bolotse) you are a man and you are ready to have sex | 15.1 % | 14.8 % | 11.6 % |
| 24. When you have a STI you can show your friends that you have had sex | 25.2 % | 23.2 % | 27.7 % |
| 25. Having more girlfriends proofs that you are a man | 20.9 % | 15.8 % | 2.5 % *** |
| 26. A traditional healer is always right | 31.1 % | 30.8 % | 28.0 % |
| 27. A traditional healer can cure STIs | 26.3 % | 33.6 % | 28.4 % |
| 28. Aids does not exist | 21.5 % | 29.0 % | 19.8 % |
| 29. Sex with a virgin cures AIDS | 22.3 % | 28.2 % | 6.7 % *** |
| 30. ARVs (AIDS treatment) are poisonous drugs | 34.9 % | 44.7 % | 31.0 % |
| 31. ARVs (AIDS treatment) can cure AIDS | 32.4 % | 35.0 % | 18.8 % *** |
| 32. ARVs (AIDS treatment) will only prolong your life a bit | 35.6 % | 36.4 % | 35.3 % |
| 33. ARVs (AIDS treatment) are not worth taking | 34.6 % | 40.2 % | 46.2 % |

*** = p <.05

## 3.2. Changes of Sexual Behaviour

Part B was about actual sexual behaviour. Seventeen multiple choice questions were asked. Four questions of Part B of the questionnaire were used to determine if a change in behaviour was found. The other questions were used to get more insight into the behaviour of the children and can be used for research in the near future. The difference in the number of respondents who answered the questions is due to the fact that not all of the 109 children have filled in every question. This goes for all groups and for all questions discussed in this part.

The answers given to the first of these four questions 'How often do you use a condom?' show that before attending the programme 9.7% of the pupils who are sexually active (42.7%) always use condoms. Therefore, 22.7% of the sexually active children always use condoms. After attending the programme once, 9.5% of the pupils who are sexually active (26.7%) say that they always use condoms, which means 35.7% of the children who are sexually active always use condoms. This means that there is an increase of 13% for always using condoms. This is not totally true, however. If we look at Table 3, the percentage of children who say they always use condoms is 9.7% before and 9.5% after attending the programme. The difference in percentages as stated before (22.7% and 35.7%) is due to the fact that the group of children who say they are not sexually active is larger in the second group. The increase of 13% should therefore rather be interpreted as a decrease in sexual activity.

**Table 5: Degree of condom use per number of times attending the programme (Question 7: How often, when you have sex, do you use a condom?)**

| Number of times attending the programme | Always | Almost every time | Sometimes | Never | Not sexually active | N |
|---|---|---|---|---|---|---|
| 0 | 9.7% | 12.6% | 4.8% | 15.5% | 57.3% | 103 |
| 1 | 9.5% | 3.8% | 8.5% | 4.7% | 73.3% | 105 |
| ≥2 | 27.4% | 11.1 % | 14.5 % | 3.4 % | 43.6% | 117 |

What can be seen in Table 5 for the children who saw the programme twice or more is that there is a small group of children that 'never use condoms' (3.4%), a fairly large group of children who say they are 'not sexually active' (43.6%) and a group of 27.4% that says they 'always use condoms'. The remaining groups, which use condoms 'almost every time' or 'sometimes' together constitute of 25.6%.

A second question asks 'if a person can avoid HIV/AIDS by changing his/her behaviour'. To this question, 34.6% of the children (N=104) before attending the programme answered 'yes'. After attending the programme once, 30.8% (N=104) thought a person could avoid HIV/AIDS by changing his/her behaviour. This decrease was not significant (p=1.000). Of the children who saw the programme twice or more, 64.7% (N=119) said they thought someone could avoid HIV/AIDS by changing his/her behaviour.

Of the children who had never seen the programme, 21.5% (N=107) answered the third question that, 'yes', 'they felt to be at personal risk of getting HIV/AIDS'. This percentage increased to 23.4% (N=107) after attending the programme once. This increase was not significant (p=1.000). The children who saw the programme twice or more (N=116) were feeling more at risk of getting HIV/AIDS (45.7%).

The children who had seen the programme before were asked at the fourth question 'if they had made any changes after following the programme'. 69.1% (N=97) said they did. After attending the programme twice or more, 78% (N=109) said they had made changes after seeing the programme.

## 3.3. Factors Influencing Condom Use

Part C consisted of 48 questions and is based on the theory of planned behaviour (Ajzen, 1991). The theoretical model describes several factors which are supposed to influence a certain behaviour, in this case condom use. A reliability analysis showed a Cronbach's alpha of part C of 0.70.

The data collected in the research has a good fit to the model. Through the statistical programme AMOS (Arbucle, 1997), statistical equation modelling (SEM) was used to evaluate the goodness of fit of the model to the data. The following indices were examined:

a.  the $\chi^2$ statistic that indicates whether or not the pattern of covariation in the data can be explained by the postulated factor structure (although it is not the most informative index, as it is highly sensitive to sample size, it gives some information when comparing models, with lower values indicating better fit);

88

b. the ratio of $\chi^2$ to degrees of freedom ($\chi^2$/df) which decreases and approaches zero as the fit of the model improves;

c. the Normed Fit Index (NFI), which provides a measure of complete covariation in the data, with values > 0.90 indicating an acceptable fit; and

d. the Root Mean Square Error of Approximation (RMSEA) an evaluative statistic suitable for assessing models of differing complexity, with values < 0.05 indicating an acceptable fit.

As can be seen from Table 6, the NFI and RMSEA indicate an acceptable fit for the whole group and for boys.

Table 6: Goodness of fit of the model to the data through Structural Equation Modeling (SEM)

| | $\chi^2$ | Df | $\chi^2$/df | NFI | RMSEA |
|---|---|---|---|---|---|
| Total Group | .099 | 2 | .0495 | .998 | .000 |
| Boys | 1.197 | 2 | .5985 | .948 | .000 |
| Girls | 7.121 | 2 | 3.5605 | .879 | .126 |

Note: NFI = Normed Fit Index; RMSEA = Root Mean Square Error of Approximation

The path coefficients and covariances found for the factors in the model are presented in Table 7.

Table 7: Path coefficients and covariances of TPB for total group

| Path coefficients | B | p | Beta |
|---|---|---|---|
| Attitude ————> Intention | .355 | .054 | .13 |
| Sub. norm ————> Intention | .323 | .038* | .14 |
| PBC ————> Intention | .368 | .027* | .14 |
| Intention ————> Behaviour | .483 | .000*** | .23 |
| PBC ————> Behaviour | .471 | .110 | .09 |
| *Covariances* | | | |
| Sub. norm <————> Attitude | .017 | .000*** | .20 |
| PBC <————> Sub. Norm | .010 | .044* | .11 |
| PBC <————> Attitude | .002 | .664 | .02 |

* = p < .05; *** = p < .001
Note: B = Unstandardised coefficients, Beta = Standardised coefficients

As can be seen in Figure 1 the standardised path coefficients indicate that the relation between perceived behavioural control and the actual behaviour is not significant (p= 0.110) neither is the relation between attitude and intention (p=0.054). The covariance between attitude and perceived behavioural control is also not significant (p=0.664). The other factors do influence the behaviour as expected by the model.

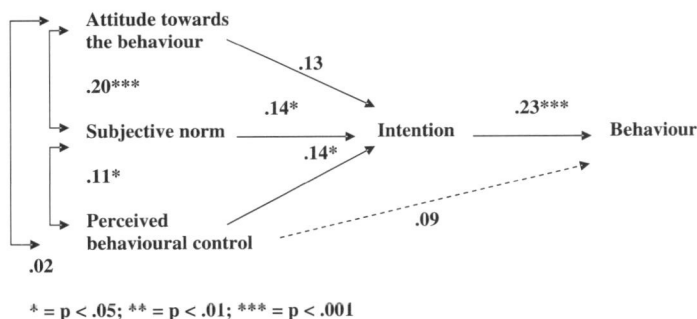

Figure 1: Theory of planned behaviour with standardised path coefficients and standardised covariances for the total group

When the respondents are divided into two groups based on gender, some interesting differences are found. As can be seen from Table 8, the path coefficients and covariances differ between boys and girls. This means that behaviour for boys is influenced in a different way than for girls. As can be seen, the behaviour of boys is only significantly influenced through intention. Furthermore, subjective norm and perceived behavioural control influence each other.

Table 8: Path coefficients and co-variances of TPB per gender

| | Boys | | | Girls | | |
|---|---|---|---|---|---|---|
| Path coefficients | B | p | Beta | B | p | Beta |
| Attitude ———————> Intention | .137 | .495 | .060 | .874 | .007* | .262 |
| Sub. norm ———————> Intention | .176 | .317 | .090 | .462 | .077 | .171 |
| PBC ———————> Intention | .266 | .153 | .128 | .316 | .264 | .106 |
| Intention ———————-> Behaviour | .491 | .036* | .192 | .408 | .010* | .244 |
| PBC ———————> Behaviour | -.155 | .704 | -.029 | .120 | .004** | .224 |
| *Co-variances* | | | | | | |
| Sub. norm < ———————> Attitude | .013 | .052 | .144 | .021 | .001** | .265 |
| PBC < ———————> Sub. Norm | .019 | .011* | .191 | .019 | .933 | .007* |
| PBC < ———————> Attitude | -.001 | .831 | -.016 | -.001 | .200 | .102 |

* = p < .05; ** = p < .01; *** = p < .001
Note: B = Unstandardised coefficients, Beta = Standardised coefficients

The behaviour of girls is influenced by intention (just like boys) and the intention of girls is significantly influenced by their attitude. Furthermore, the perceived behavioural control also significantly influences the behaviour of girls. Girls also show a significant mutual influence between subjective norm and attitude.

## 4. Conclusions and discussion

### 4.1. Knowledge about HIV/AIDS

Looking at the first research question, '*Does the Ndlovu AIDS Awareness Programme increase knowledge about HIV/AIDS and does it result in a change of sexual behaviour?*', a slight non-significant increase in knowledge is found, in comparison to children who have never attended the programme, for children who have attended the programme once, and a larger

90

significant increase after attending the programme twice or more. Distinguished by gender, there is a significant increase for boys after following the programme once, but not for girls. The knowledge increase after attending the programme twice or more, compared to attending it once, is significant for girls, but not for boys.

Although there seems to be some significant increases in knowledge, it has to be realised that these are not necessarily due to the Ndlovu AIDS Awareness Programme. In an area like this, where there is much information and education about HIV/AIDS, it is hard to find out whether an increase in knowledge can be specifically attributed to the NAAP, and not to other factors like maturation or other forms of education and media.

The results of the second section of Part A, about beliefs, show high percentages of children who answer the questions with 'don't know'. Attending the programme once or more than once has hardly any influence on the percentage of children who answer these questions with 'don't know'. This could be because not enough attention is paid to these beliefs in the NAAP or because the children find it hard to decide whether a belief is true or false.

A remark has to be made about these results. The children who never saw the programme before were the youngest children in this research and had the most difficulties filling in the questionnaires. It took them the longest, and they had the most questions. The children who attended the programme twice or more, were older than the children from the other two groups (as can be seen in Table 1) and had the least problems with all three parts of the questionnaire.

## 4.2. Changes of Sexual Behaviour

The question whether the Ndlovu AIDS awareness programme does entail a change in sexual behaviour is difficult to answer. Again, we must consider the possibility that other factors may have influenced the children and their behaviour. We can see that among the children who have attended the programme once, a group of 69.1% say they have changed their way of life after attending the programme. Of the children who followed the programme twice or more 78% say they made changes in their lives as a result of the information they received in the Ndlovu AIDS Awareness Programme. This percentage shows that children do change their behaviour. Exactly how and what they changed, should be further investigated. What is also important to know, is that after seeing the programme once 23.4% of the children feel at personal risk, while only 17% of the children engage in dangerous sexual activities (using condoms almost every time, sometimes and never, see Table 3).

We also found a slight increase in the number of not sexually active children, which could mean that one of the effects of the programme is actually a decrease in sexual activity.

## 4.3. Factors Influencing Condom Use

For the second research question, '*Which factors influence condom use in the NAAP target group?*' we found that not all the factors presumed by Ajzen (1991) to influence behaviour (in this case condom use), significantly do so. After looking at the group as a whole, we considered which factors of the model influenced condom use for boys and girls separately, and found that the behaviour (condom use) was influenced in a different way for boys and girls. The behaviour of boys was influenced through intention and there was a significant correlation between perceived behavioural control and subjective norm. The behaviour for girls was also influenced through intention, and intention was influenced through attitude. Behaviour was also directly influenced through perceived behavioural control. The attitude towards condom use and the subjective norm of girls influenced each other.

## 4.4. Final Conclusions

The results of this evaluation study enable a number of conclusions to be drawn.

In the first place, more attention has to be paid to the transfer of knowledge. The actual knowledge increase proved to be small and not always significant. Also the high percentages of pupils answering 'don't know' to questions about beliefs are a point of concern. The children who answer 'don't know' do not necessarily mean that they do not know the answer to the question. Their answer could also imply that somebody does not want to give an answer. Torn between cultural and western truths, they might find it difficult to choose. Whether this is the case or not, more attention has to be paid in the NAAP to discussing beliefs.

Secondly, it has to be said that the NAAP seems to establish behavioural change. Not only do the respondents say they have changed their behaviour, some of them have also 'stopped being sexually active'.

Furthermore, if the goal is to change behaviour, one should be fully aware of the factors through which such behavioural change can be realised. A different approach of boys and girls seems to be preferable, but this does not mean different education is necessary. Splitting up groups by gender during education removes the factors of discussion and the possibility of integrating one's own point of view with that of the other gender. Because sexual behaviour should be a matter of mutual consent, boys and girls should have the opportunity to discuss the issues and to make the first steps in reaching such consent in the presence of the opposite sex. What might be possible is to start the programme with a basic informative introduction for everybody, followed by two gender-separate discussion groups.

Future research has to provide more information about the influence of the cultural background and the perceptions and beliefs of black South African children in Elandsdoorn and also which aspects influence the significant factors found in this research. This can only be achieved through in-depth-interviews.

## References

Ajzen, I. (1991): The Theory of Planned Behaviour. *Organizational Behaviour and Human Decision Processes, 50,* 179-211.

Arbucle, J. (1997). *Amos user's guide.* Chicago: Smallwaters

Bennett, P. & Bozionelos, G. (2000). The theory of planned behaviour as predictor of condom use: A narrative review. *Psychology Health & Medicine, 5,* 307-326.

Bogart, L.M., Cecel, H. & Pinkerton, S.D. (2000). Hispanic Adult's Beliefs, Attitudes, and Intentions Regarding the Female Condom. *Journal of Behavioural Medicine, 23* (2), 181-206.

Booysen, F. Le R., Geldenhuys, J.P. & Markinov, M. (2003). *The impact of HIV/AIDS on the South African Economy: Review of Current Evidence.* Department of Economics, University of the Free State.

Carey, M.P.& Schroder, K.E.E. (2002). Development and psychometric evaluation of the brief HIV knowledge questionnaire. *AIDS Education and Prevention, 14* (2), 172-182.

Day, J.H., Miyamura, K., Grant, A.D., Leeuw, A., Munsamy, J., Baggaley,T. & Churchyard, G.J. (2003). Attitudes to HIV voluntary counselling and testing among  mineworkers in South Africa: will availability of antiretroviral therapy encourage testing? *AIDS CARE, 15,* (5), 665-672

Fisher, J. D., & Fisher, W. A. (2000). Theoretical approaches to individual- level change in HIV risk behaviour. In: J. L. Peterson & R. J. DiClemente (eds.), *Handbook of HIV prevention AIDS prevention and mental health (pp. 3-55).* New York, NY: Kluwer Academic/Plenum Publishers.

Hox, J.J. (1999). Principes en toepassing van structurele modellen. *Kind en Adolescent, 20,* 200-217.

Kebaabtswe, P. & Norr, K.F. (2002). Behavioural change: Goals and Means. In: M. Essex, S. Mboub, P.J. Kanki, R.G. Marlink & S.D. Tlou (eds.), *Aids in Africa (pp. 415-426)*. Academic, New York.

Montano, D.E.& Kasprzyk, D. (1990). The theory of reasoned action and the theory of planned behaviour. *Health Behaviour and Health Education*, 4, 67-95.

Shapiro, R.L.& Kapiga, S.H. (2002). Male condom and Circumcision. In: M. Essex, S. Mboub, P.J. Kanki, R.G. Marlink & S.D. Tlou (Eds.), *Aids in Africa (pp. 498-506)*. Academic, New York.

Stadler, J,& Hlongwa, L. (2002). *Monitoring and evaluation of LoveLife's AIDS prevention and advocacy activities in South Africa 1999-2001*. Reproductive Health Research Unit, Chris Hani Baragwanath Hospital.

Tempelman, H.A., Botha-Standaert, E.J.A. (2002). *Report on Project Activities 2002 Government of South Tyrol, Italy*. Ndlovu Medical Centre, Groblersdal

*Address for correspondence:*
Koen van der Lubbe, MSc
Ndlovu Medical Centre
P.O. Box 1447
Groblersdal 0470
South Africa

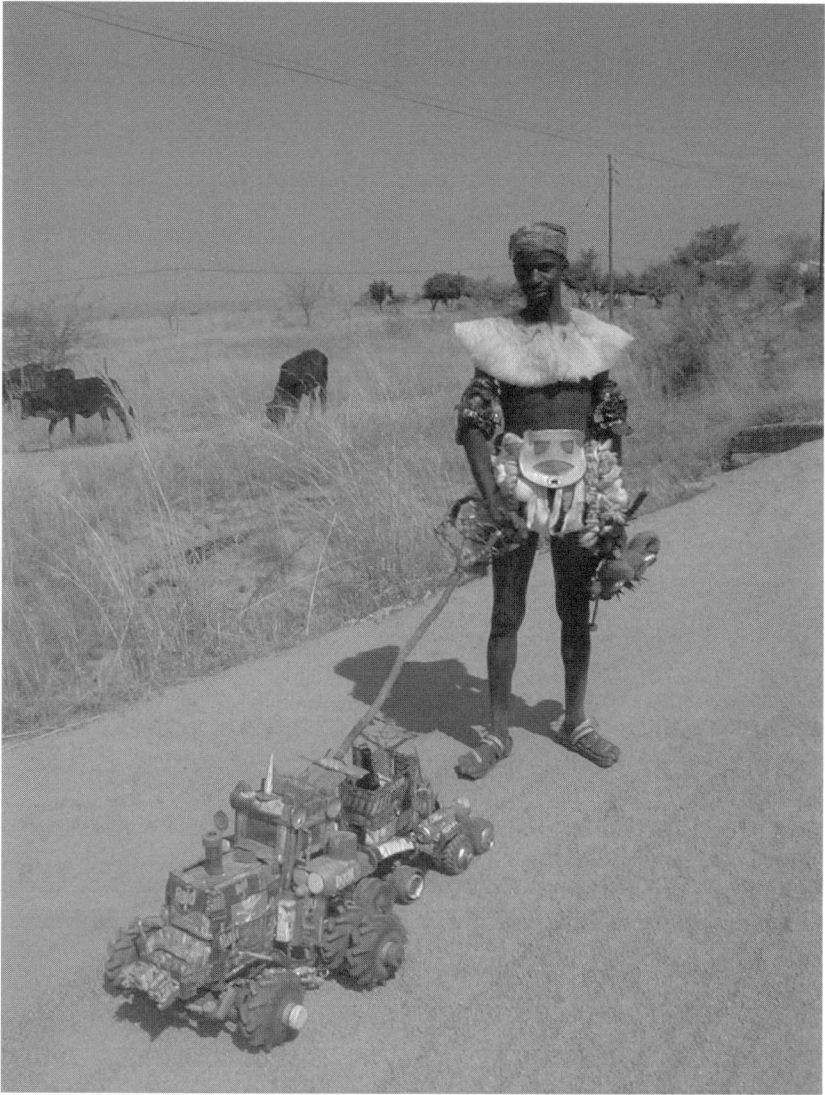

# Chapter 7

# Cultural Influences on Sexual Behaviour of Participants in an AIDS Awareness Programme

*Anneke van Dijk[1], Hanna van den Dries[1], Hugo Tempelman [2], Adri Vermeer[1]*

[1] Department of Educational Sciences, Utrecht University, Utrecht, The Netherlands
[2] Ndlovu Medical Centre, Elandsdoorn, South Africa

## Abstract

In 2003, research was done to evaluate the Ndlovu AIDS Awareness Programme (NAAP). The goal of the NAAP is to make children aware of the HIV/AIDS problems in their community and to inform and educate them on HIV/AIDS prevention. Sexual and moral behaviour changes are promoted in order to reduce new transmissions of HIV. Condom use is the main strategy used by the NAAP. Besides measuring newly acquired knowledge about HIV/AIDS and actual sexual behaviour, also determinants of sexual behaviour were established among school children by means of a self-constructed questionnaire, based on the theory of planned behaviour of Ajzen (1985). Results of this research showed that attitude and perceived behavioural control significantly influenced behaviour in a direct way and not through intention as supposed by Ajzen's model.

Hereafter, a new research was done, focusing on the question to which extent cultural factors influence sexual behaviour and its determining factors. Again the knowledge about HIV/AIDS among school children who had attended the NAAP performances was established. Questions about cultural determinants were added to the questionnaire already used in the earlier study. The questionnaire was based on a combined model of the theory of planned behaviour (Ajzen, 1985) and a model by Eaton, Flisher & Aorø (2003) in which determinants of behaviour are described in three different contexts: the personal, proximal and distal context. 62 school children between the ages of 14 and 18 completed the questionnaires. Almost all of the respondents witnessed one or more NAAP performances. Knowledge about HIV/AIDS was measured through eleven true/false questions. The knowledge questions were followed by questions about cultural beliefs, behaviour, and determinants of behaviour according to the Ajzen model. Afterwards, a structured interview was designed to get in-depth information from the school children. Results show that the level of knowledge of the respondents was insufficient. A significant relationship between knowledge and behaviour was not found. Most of the respondents showed the intention to abstain until marriage. When these intentions were compared with the actual sexual behaviour reported by the respondents, it was found that only 27% of the respondents abstained and 78% of those who were sexually active did not practice safe sex. There was a significant relationship between intention and behaviour. There also was a significant relationship between perceived behavioural control and sexual behaviour. Surprisingly, answers to the questionnaire differed from the answers given during the interviews. The respondents did not show very strong cultural beliefs in their questionnaire answers, but they did admit to believing in certain myths and traditions in the interviews. Belief in ancestors and myths about being able to cure AIDS was common among the respondents. The results of this research lead to a number of recommendations for the NAAP.

# 1. Introduction

## 1.1. Ndlovu AIDS Awareness Programme (NAAP)

The NAAP started in 1999 as an initiative of the Ndlovu Medical Centre. Its goal is to make children aware of the HIV/AIDS problems in their community and to inform and educate them in preventing HIV/AIDS. The members of the NAAP team are six young adults from Elandsdoorn. The NAAP reaches about 25.000 children every year, of which almost 80% through school visits (For a further description see Chapter 2 and 6).

The NAAP works with the so-called ABCD of prevention. 'Abstaining', 'Being faithful', ' Condom-use' and 'Delay' are the four strategies one can use to prevent infection with HIV/ AIDS. Condom use is the strategy mostly used by the NAAP. The distribution of condoms is one of the most important things the NAAP does, besides providing information and trying to change sexual behaviour.

Apart from factual information on HIV/AIDS, the NAAP offers health education to secondary school students and community groups. Sexual health education includes information on sexually transmitted infections (STIs), sexual abuse, child abuse, incest and teacher-student relationships. Changes in sexual and moral behaviour are promoted in order to reduce new transmissions of HIV. This is done by promoting the use of condoms and raising awareness of the risks of promiscuity. Last, but not least, sexual health is promoted for the entire population in the Moutse area, in co-operation with the existing community structures.

## 1.2. HIV/AIDS in Africa

South Africa is one of the countries with the highest number of HIV-infected persons. Approximately 5.5 million South Africans in the age group of 15-49 years are now HIV-positive. Every day 1,700 people are infected, and 600 people die as a result of AIDS. The Philadelphia district, where Elandsdoorn is situated, has a population of almost 500,000 people. 14.7% of them are reported HIV-positive, which amounts to 73,500 people. Most new HIV infections occur in people between the ages of 15 and 49 years (Stadler & Hlongwa, 2002).

There are several factors that contribute to the high prevalence of HIV infections in Africa, compared to the rest of the world. One important factor is poverty. The health conditions in South Africa, like malnutrition, the quality of water and access to health care, determine the susceptibility to diseases (Stillwagon, 2001). Poverty not only creates biological conditions that increase the susceptibility to diseases, it also limits the possibilities of treatment. In spite of the fact that poor populations are more susceptible to disease, AIDS (in contrast to other diseases) is almost entirely preventable (Elder, 2001). This is only possible if sexual behaviour is changed. However, many social, psychological and cultural barriers stand in the way of changing unsafe behaviour.

## 1.3. The African Worldview: Barriers to Behavioural Change

There are significant barriers to changing unprotected sexual contact in South Africa. Besides economic, political, socio-cultural and organisational barriers, a specific worldview of the African people makes it difficult to change sexual behaviour. The African view on condom use and the special position of African women also influence the difficulty in behavioural change.

The traditional African worldview is based on a holistic and anthropocentric ontology, meaning that man is inseparably connected to the cosmos and that everything (including

God, spirits and nature) is seen in connection to mankind. Within this cosmic whole, three levels are recognised that form the traditional African worldview: the macro-cosmos, the meso-cosmos and the micro-cosmos. Insight in these three different levels offers greater understanding in the psychological and social dimensions of AIDS in South Africa (Van Dijk, 2001).

The *macro-cosmos* is the highest level and consists of God, ancestors and the spirits of people who have passed away. In traditional religious systems, God is seen as creator and most powerful being. The spirits of ancestors influence daily life in Africa: ancestors are seen as powerful spirits that either protect the honour, tradition and health of people, or punish them by bringing illness and bad luck.

The *meso-cosmos* is an intervening universe where evil spirits, witches and sorcerers live. Both good and evil exist here to influence human wishes, fears and desires. Almost every form of illness, conflict, suffering, misfortune and death is ascribed to this level. The psychological destiny of individuals is controlled by relationships between people and the invisible but powerful beings in the meso-cosmos.

The *micro-cosmos* represents the daily, social and collective life of people in Africa. Although the existence of Africans is mostly influenced by the macro- and the meso-cosmos, some illnesses have origins in the micro-cosmos. It is generally believed that sexually transmitted diseases are related to bacteria and sexual behaviours (Van Dijk, 2001).

The influence of the African worldview is visible in the perceptions that traditional Africans have of sexuality. The influence of the macro-cosmos, for example, can be seen in the fact that sex is not only important for reproductive purposes, but also as a symbol of immortality. By having many children, traditional Africans achieve personal immortality. Children are also important in the daily micro-cosmic existence because traditional African men can only become wealthy when they have several wives and many children to help them work the land. In the light of this personal immortality and the value of children in the life of Africans, polygamy has a different meaning, which makes it difficult to convince Africans to use condoms, even when they know they are infected with HIV (Van Dijk, 2001).

*Condom Use*
As in many parts of the world, condom use in Africa tends to be low in many populations. There are significant barriers to male condom use in South Africa; such barriers include lack of female control over condom use, costs of condoms, limited availability of condoms, lack of knowledge about the effectiveness of condoms, fear of embarrassment associated with using condoms, lack of knowledge about HIV, perceived lack of HIV risk, decreased condom use in sexual acts following alcohol consumption, and culturally specific stigmas associated with condom use (Shapiro & Kapiga, 2002).

*The Position of Women*
One factor that contributes significantly to the problem of HIV/AIDS in Africa is, as mentioned before, the unequal status of men and women. Today, women are responsible for more than half of the new AIDS cases (Baylies, 2000). Although both men and women are infected with AIDS, most infections occur in women. Women have a special position that makes them more susceptible to this disease than men. First of all, women have a lower status and less power in society. This means that women have limited control over their own lives and are less capable of controlling when and how sexual intercourse takes place. Women are incapable of changing sexual behaviour. A second reason why women are more

vulnerable to HIV infections is because the chance that HIV is transmitted from man to woman is two to four times higher than HIV being transmitted from woman to man. Also women suffer more often from untreated STIs (sexually transmitted infections) which increases the chance of HIV infection (Baylies, 2000).

## 2. Theoretical background

Behaviour is a function of beliefs and subjective evaluation (Conner & Norman, 1996). Several social-cognitive theories and models have proved this function. Ajzen's theory of planned behaviour (1985) is an example of a model that describes certain determining factors in a triad of behaviour, personal factors, interpersonal factors and processes. In previous research (see Chapter 6), attitudes, subjective norms and perceived behavioural control from Ajzen's model were examined to measure their influence on sexual behaviour. The theory of planned behaviour was also used to design the questionnaire in this research.

### 2.1. *Theory of Planned Behaviour of Ajzen*

The theory of planned behaviour (TPB) is a model used for explaining social behaviour. It posits that a person's behaviour is a result of his/her intention to perform a particular action (Ajzen, 1991). The individual's intention to engage in a particular behaviour is supposed to be influenced by three factors: his/her attitude towards the behaviour, the perceived attitudes of important others (subjective norm) and the perceived behavioural control.

*Attitudes* towards a particular behaviour are a result of beliefs about the consequences of engaging in the specific behaviour and subjective evaluations of those consequences. For example, an individual who believes that a condom is likely to prevent HIV transmission and who believes that HIV transmission is undesirable, may be more likely to use a condom (Bogart, Cecel & Pinkerton, 2000).

*Subjective norms* are defined as the individual's perception of social pressure to perform or not perform the specific behaviour. Hence, subjective norms are a result of the likelihood that important others think that an individual should engage in a particular behaviour and the individual's motivation to comply with the desires of important others. For example, if a man believes that his sex partner and his friends would like him to use a condom and he values their opinion, he would be more likely to use a condom (Bogart et al, 2000).

*Perceived behavioural control* reflects the control an individual thinks to have over his/her own behaviour. This factor reflects past experience as well as external factors, such as anticipated impediments, obstacles, resources and opportunities that may influence the performance of the specific behaviour. It consists of two sub-factors: the perceived likelihood of encountering factors that will facilitate or inhibit the successful performance of the behaviour, weighted by their perceived power to facilitate or inhibit performance (Bennet & Bozionelos, 2000).

External variables indirectly influence behaviour through opinions (Fisher & Fisher, 2000). External variables are made up of variables like age, gender, economic status, but also of cultural factors like religion and tradition. These cultural factors, which are important for understanding unsafe sexual behaviour, form the main focus of this research (see Figure 1).

**Attitudes towards behaviour**

**External variables**

**Subjective norms** → **Intention** → **Behaviour**

**Perceived behavioural control**

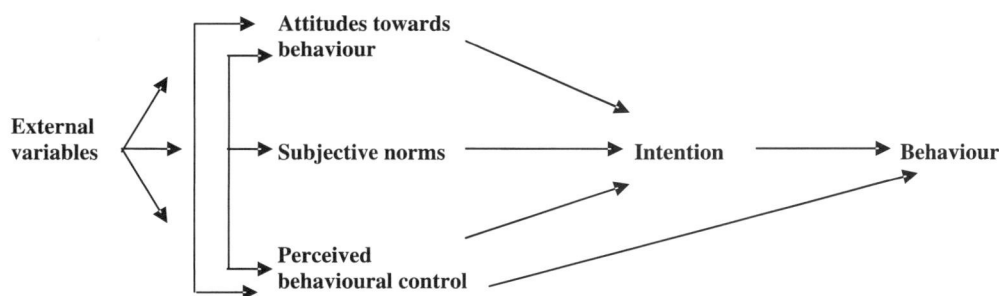

Figure 1: Planned Behaviour Model of Ajzen (1991)

## 2.2. Three-level behaviour model of Eaton et al.

To better understand and explain sexual behaviour in South Africa, it is important to examine the different factors from Ajzen's model on three different levels: within the person, within the proximal context (interpersonal factors and the physical environment) and within the distal context (cultural and structural factors) (see Figure 2).

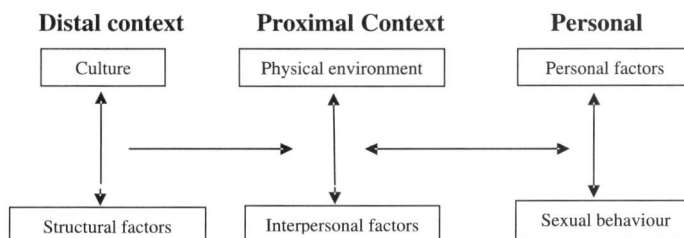

**Distal context**   **Proximal Context**   **Personal**

Culture   Physical environment   Personal factors

Structural factors   Interpersonal factors   Sexual behaviour

Figure 2: Model for the relationship between sexual behaviour, personal factors and the proximal and distal contexts (Eaton et al., 2003)

Personal factors that determine behaviour are knowledge and beliefs, self-efficacy, perceived costs and benefits, intentions and self-esteem. Behaviour is indirectly influenced by interpersonal factors which are part of the proximal context. These interpersonal factors are made up of the following factors: peer pressure, communication with adults, media, talking about risks and access to condoms. Behaviour is influenced in the distal context by cultural and structural factors. In this research, culture is made up out of the following sub-components: religion, myths, tradition, status of man/woman, relationship between men and women, and the goal of sex (Eaton et al., 2003).

*Religion*
77% of all South Africans are a member of one of the many Christian churches. One of the most important Christian values is saving virginity until marriage. African Independent Churches are the second largest religious community in South Africa and can be divided into the Ethiopian and the Zionistic Church. The Holy Ghost, healing and elements from traditional African religion play an important role in these exclusively black churches. The original inhabitants of South Africa had their own native religion before the arrival of white men. Fertility rituals, crop rituals, ancestor worship and a strong belief in the existence of higher powers are common traits of this native religion. A quarter of the black population still practices this religion. Inyangas and sangomas, traditional African healers, still play an

important part in the cultural and religious world of black South Africans, even those in large cities (Dekker, 2000).

### Myths

There are many myths about HIV/AIDS. Wrong conceptions about the transmission of HIV/AIDS, myths about the curability of AIDS and incorrect ideas about the symptoms of HIV and AIDS are examples of beliefs that confuse people and give them a false sense of security.

### Tradition

Belief in ancestors spirits, witchcraft, traditional healers and Initiation School all make up the category of tradition. The African worldview is also an example of tradition.

### Unequal Status of Men/Women

Women have a lower status than men in South Africa. This inferior status makes it more difficult for women to protect themselves by demanding the use of a condom or refusing sex (Eaton et al., 2003). Many women lack economic power, which makes them dependent on men. Men are stimulated to be sexually active and aggressive, without feeling responsible for their actions. Men also feel the need to have more than one partner, and also have the right to satisfy this need, which makes polygamy a common thing.

### Monogamous Relationships Between Men and Women

Violence is a common problem in South Africa. It is a result of cultural male dominance. Men use violence as a way to prove their masculinity and their status in society. Physical violence in a relationship limits a woman's capability to negotiate safe sex.

### Goals of Sex

There are three common goals of sex: pleasure, sex in exchange for material goods, and sex for reproduction. Sex is often seen as medium of exchange; prostitution is not an uncommon way for young girls and women to make money. Besides prostitution, women and especially girls are often convinced to spend time and eventually have sex with older men, called 'sugar daddies', in exchange for money or gifts. Reproduction is very important to Africans, because having many children means a higher status. Girls, adolescents and women often feel pressured into becoming pregnant. Pregnancy is a sign of maturity and fertility (Tillotson & Maharaj, 2001). This contributes to the spread of HIV.

## 2.3. Combined Theoretical Model

The models of Ajzen (1991) and Eaton et al. (2003) were combined to get a clear view on the determinants of sexual behaviour on the three different levels.

This combined model serves as a guideline in answering research questions concerning sexual behaviour. The main question of the research concerns the cultural factors:

*What is the relationship between actual sexual behaviour and the determinants of sexual behaviour and how are they influenced by cultural factors?*

Because the NAAP is aimed at increase of knowledge about HIV/AIDS and a change of sexual behaviour, this question is divided into two sub-questions:

1. *What is the relationship between the respondent's knowledge of HIV/AIDS and cultural factors?*

2.   *What is the relationship between the respondent's sexual behaviour and cultural factors?*

To establish these relationships, the following research questions are posed:

1.   *What is the level of knowledge among the respondents?*
2.   What is the sexual behaviour of the respondents?
3.   What are the values of the determinants of sexual behaviour from the Ajzen model?
4.   What are the values of the cultural determinants from the Eaton model?
5.   What is the relationship between knowledge and cultural factors?
6.   What is the relationship between sexual behaviour and cultural factors?
7.   What is the relationship between intention and the determinants of sexual behaviour?
8.   What is the relationship between intention, perceived behavioural control and sexual behaviour?
9.   What is the relationship between the determinants of sexual behaviour and cultural factors?

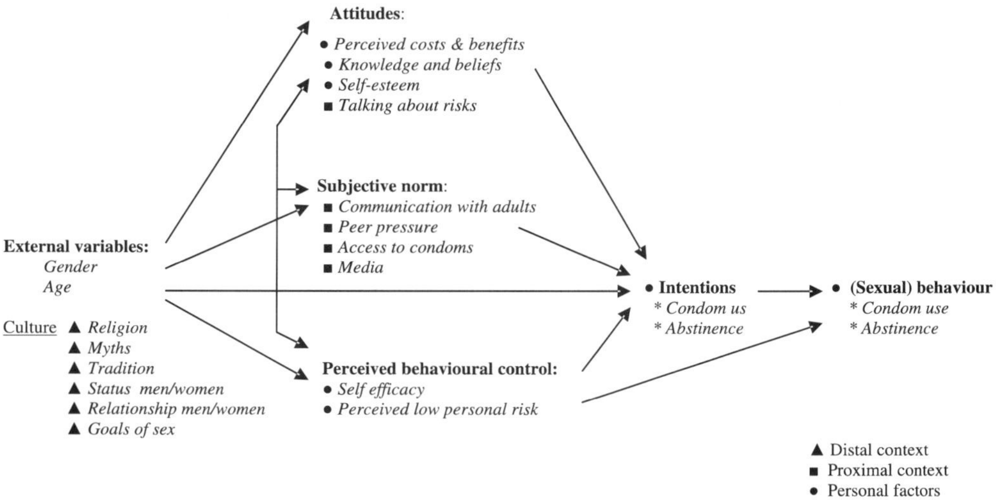

Figure 3: Combined model of Ajzen (1991) and Eaton et al. (2003): Influence of variables on sexual behaviour

## 3. Methods

### 3.1. Subjects

The subjects involved in this research (N=62) are all students between 14 and 18 years old, attending Tagane Primary School in Ntwane, Ramagosetsi Secondary School in Marapong and Sebakanaga and Tlou Kwena Secondary School in Dennilton. The choice of schools, grades and classes depended mostly on the schedule of the NAAP team and on the co-operation of the schools.

In this single a-select sample the students either volunteered or were asked by classroom teachers. The participants were equally divided in six age groups, each consisting of approximately the same amount of girls and boys (see Table 1). To prevent non-response, the surveys were taken in person. In the case of non-response during the questionnaire (for example skipping questions), certain questions were repeated in the interview.

**Table 1: Subject statistics**

| Gender | Age | Frequency | % |
|---|---|---|---|
| Boys | 14 | 7 | 25.0 |
| | 15 | 4 | 14.3 |
| | 16 | 6 | 21.4 |
| | 17 | 5 | 17.9 |
| | 18 | 6 | 21.4 |
| | *Total* | *28* | *100.0* |
| Girls | 14 | 7 | 20.6 |
| | 15 | 6 | 17.6 |
| | 16 | 6 | 17.6 |
| | 17 | 8 | 23.5 |
| | 18 | 7 | 20.6 |
| | *Total* | *34* | *100.0* |

## 3.2. *Instruments*

This research is both qualitative and quantitative. Two forms of measurement were used. A questionnaire, based on the determinants of behaviour from the combined model of Ajzen (1991) and Eaton et al. (2003) (see Figure 3). A self-constructed questionnaire, consisting of 65 two-point-scale statements. The first part of the questionnaire consists of eleven statements measuring the knowledge about the transmission and development of HIV/AIDS. The remaining statements measure views and opinions on HIV/AIDS or self-ascribed behaviours of the respondents (see Table 2). There are three different answering categories, beginning with 'true–false', 'counts for me–doesn't count for me' (derived from the Child Behaviour Check List, 2003) and 'I agree–I disagree'. The reliability analysis that was done in the research preceding this study provided a Cronbach's alpha of .70 on a similar questionnaire. Questions were added to the knowledge part and have a Cronbach´s alpha of .62.

**Table 2: Items of the questionnaire divided into the factors of the Ajzen and Eaton Model**

| Behaviour | | Intention | | Attitudes | |
|---|---|---|---|---|---|
| Condom use | | Condom use | 1 | Perceived costs & benefit | 1 |
| Abstinence | | Abstinence | 1 | Knowledge and beliefs | 11 |
| | | | | Self-esteem | 3 |
| | | | | Talking about risks | 2 |
| *Total* | | *Total* | *2* | *Total* | *17* |
| Subjective norm | | Perceived behavioural control | | Culture | |
| Communication with adults | 4 | Self-efficacy | 3 | Religion | 2 |
| Peer pressure | 2 | Perceived low personal risk | 1 | Myths | 10 |
| Access to condoms | 1 | | | Tradition | 4 |
| Media | 1 | | | Status men/women | 4 |
| | | | | Relationship men/women | 7 |
| | | | | Goals of sex | 7 |
| *Total* | *8* | *Total* | *4* | *Total* | *34* |

The last part of the questionnaire instructs the respondents to put five subjects (health, money, friends, boy/girlfriend and sex) in an order according to the respondent's personal priorities. The goal was to get insight into the value of these subjects among the respondents, especially into the value of sex. Insight in the value of sex leads to better understanding of decisions that are made concerning sexual behaviour.

A qualitative measurement was done with a semi-structured interview that was held with the participants shortly after they finished the questionnaire. The goal of the interviews was to get more detailed and precise information about the answers given in the questionnaires. The subjects of the questionnaire were the guideline for constructing the interview. With the help of the NAAP team, these subjects were reduced to the five (for Elandsdoorn) most relevant topics: tradition, unequal status between men and women, monogamous relationships between men and women, abstinence and communication with adults. The interview provides qualitative, in-depth information.

Before executing the interviews and questionnaires, a pilot was done with ten respondents, to make sure there was sufficient understanding of the questions. After the pilot, several questions from both the questionnaire and the interview were revised.

## 3.3. Design

The main focus is on the subjects' personal thoughts and ideas on HIV/AIDS and sexual behaviour. By doing this two-way research it is possible to get a broader and clearer view of the behavioural and cultural determinants of sexual behaviour. Questionnaires are the best way to measure, describe and explain social issues ('t Hart, Van Dijk, de Goede, Jansen & Teunissen, 1998). The interview is an expansion of the short questionnaire-answers and can be used to establish the validity of the questionnaire. The questionnaire is done one time only. In other words, this study is a one-shot design.

## 3.4. Procedure

The participants were approached personally, after being informed by the school staff. During the interview two researchers were present and, when needed, a translator translated the English questions into both Zulu and Sotho. One of the researchers did the interview, while the other wrote down the answers. Working with a translator gave the child the opportunity to better express him- or herself. Another benefit of doing interviews with the use of a translator is that the answers to the interview questions were validated. This is because the translator has the same cultural background as the respondent and could understand and explain their answers.

The questionnaires were deliberately held with six students at a time to provide sufficient attention and to prevent the respondents from discussing their answers. After the six students had filled in the questionnaire, they were interviewed individually. This was done to create a private atmosphere and make them feel as comfortable as possible. By introducing the researchers and explaining that the interview was not about right or wrong answers, a confidential setting was created.

## 3.5. Statistics

The data obtained from the questionnaire were put into SPSS. The eleven answers to the knowledge questions were recoded into 'right' or 'wrong' answers to gain insight into the level of knowledge on HIV/AIDS. The remaining answers (to the questions on behaviour) were recoded into 'leads to desirable behaviour' or 'leads to non-desirable behaviour'. The means and frequencies of the data of 'condom use' and 'abstinence' were calculated and related to gender and age. 'Being faithful' and 'delay' were not taken into account, because the NAAP paid less attention to these types of desirable sexual behaviour.

The questions of the questionnaire were grouped into sub-components, according to Figure 3. Means were then calculated by adding up the values of the answers. The final value per item was then divided by the number of questions of each sub-component. These scores were added up to form a total score of the determinants of sexual behaviour (intention, attitude, subjective norms, perceived behavioural control). Relationships were calculated between intentions (regarding condom use and abstinence) and the determinants of sexual behaviour to make a comparison with the research done in 2003. Coherence was also measured between sexual behaviour (condom use and abstinence), intentions, perceived behavioural control and the cultural factors, according to the Ajzen model. Knowledge is an elementary component of the factor 'attitude' and was represented by a larger amount of questions than the other sub-components. This is because the NAAP focuses in particular on increasing knowledge about HIV/AIDS. Therefore, during the analysis, knowledge was taken separately from the factor 'attitude'.

Cross tabs were made and the chi-square between the variables was calculated. The data fulfilled the conditions on which chi-square can be calculated. The expected frequencies were all equal to or larger than 1, and a maximum of 20% of the expected cell frequencies was between 1 and 5. The relationship between the separate cultural variables and the variables condom use and abstinence were calculated.

For the analysis of the qualitative part of the research, the answers to the interview questions (according to the five topics) were compared with the results obtained from the quantitative data to check if the answers were similar with or in contradiction to each other.

## 4. Results

### 4.1. Research Question 1: Knowledge
The first eleven questions of the questionnaire measured the respondent's knowledge about HIV and AIDS. The average amount of questions answered incorrectly was 6.3 (see Table 3).

**Table 3: Amount of incorrect answers to the knowledge questions (11)**

|                   | N  | Mean | Median | SD   |
|-------------------|----|------|--------|------|
| Incorrect answers | 62 | 6.34 | 6.00   | 1.35 |

During the interviews, however, the respondents showed that they were well aware of the dangers of HIV/AIDS. Out of the 62 respondents, nine had never been informed about safe sex. Those who did receive information about safe sex had been informed by their mothers. Sex education was told to be based on preventing pregnancy. The main advice given was to abstain from sex. Condom use was also promoted, especially to older and more developed children. In spite of the fact that most respondents had been informed about safe sex by a parent, respondents said they would go to a peer (brother, sister or friend) if they had any questions about sex. In most cases, the respondents admitted the difficulty in talking to parents about sex-related issues. This has several reasons. Talking about sex is considered disrespectful in the African culture. Respondents were also afraid of asking stupid questions, or of getting no answer. Also, adults become suspicious when their children start asking questions about sex. To prevent this suspiciousness and fear, respondents choose to go to peers with questions.

## 4.2. Research Question 2: Sexual Behaviour

Abstinence is practised by 27% of the respondents, 10.7% of the boys and 29.4% of the girls. 17-year-olds abstain the most: 30.8% of them do not have sex. The remaining 73% of the respondents do not practise abstinence. 78% of this group do not always use condoms (see Appendix II, Tables 2-4).

## 4.3. Research Question 3: Determinants of Sexual Behaviour (Ajzen)

Attitude and subjective norms play an important role as determinants of sexual behaviour. Perceived behavioural control has a lower average score; this determinant has a moderate influence on sexual behaviour according to the respondents (see Table 4). The intention of practising safe sexual behaviour is also moderate.

**Table 4: Attitude, Subjective norm and Perceived behaviour control (31)**

| Determinant | Mean | SD | Range |
|---|---|---|---|
| Attitude (17) | 2.00 | 2.68 | 2.68 |
| Subjective norm (8) | 2.73 | 0.62 | 3.00 |
| Perceived behavioural control (4) | 1.02 | 0.53 | 2.00 |
| Intention to use condoms (1) | .53 | 0.50 | 1.00 |
| Intention to abstain (1) | .61 | 0.49 | 1.00 |

## 4.4. Research Question 4: Cultural Determinants of Sexual Behaviour (Eaton et al., 2003)

### Religion

Religion appears to have little influence on the decision to practise abstinence (interpreted as not having sex before marriage), for both boys and girls (see Appendix, Table 5 & 6).

The finding that religion does not particularly stimulate abstinence was confirmed by answers given during the interviews.

### Myths

The respondents show no strong beliefs in myths about HIV and AIDS (see Appendix, Table 5). In contrast to these results, belief in certain myths was unmistakably present in the answers given during the interviews. The question about the cause of AIDS was answered several times with 'AIDS is a curse from God'. When asked to explain this, the respondents said that people were being punished for their behaviour and that AIDS would teach them a lesson. Myths about the dangers of abstinence were also believed: a person who does not have sex will dry out, be in pain, menstruate and/or have an unhealthy mind.

### Tradition

A moderate belief in traditions was found among the respondents (see Appendix, Table 5), except for the 18-year-olds: 92% of them do not believe in traditions like the power of ancestor spirits, witchcraft, traditional healers and Initiation School (see Table 5).

### Table 5: Belief in traditions, by age

| Age | | Frequency | % | SD |
|---|---|---|---|---|
| 14 | .00 | 4 | 28.6 | .47 |
| | 1.00 | 10 | 71.4 | |
| | total | 14 | 100.0 | |
| 15 | .00 | 4 | 40.0 | .52 |
| | 1.00 | 6 | 60.0 | |
| | total | 10 | 100.0 | |
| 16 | .00 | 6 | 50.0 | .52 |
| | 1.00 | 6 | 50.0 | |
| | total | 12 | 100.0 | |
| 17 | .00 | 5 | 38.5 | .51 |
| | 1.00 | 8 | 61.5 | |
| | total | 13 | 100.0 | |
| 18 | .00 | 12 | 92.3 | .28 |
| | 1.00 | 1 | 7.7 | |
| | total | 13 | 100.0 | |

Score 0 = weak beliefs in tradition
Score 1= moderate to strong beliefs in traditions

Answers derived from the interviews, however, showed a moderate belief in ancestor spirits by some respondents. The respondents who believe in ancestor spirits communicate with them in dreams, or through close relatives. This is proof of the fact that traditions *do* play a role in the lives of some adolescents. When asked if ancestors could protect them from getting infected with HIV, all of the respondents answered 'no'.

Two third of the respondents went to Initiation School (I.S.). All respondents were asked to explain why most adolescents who finish Initiation School become sexually active. Most of them said that those who finish I.S. have reached adulthood, which equals being sexually active. Respondents who finished I.S. as well as those who did not go to I.S confirmed this fact. Another reason given for becoming sexually active after I.S. is peer pressure. Boys seem to be especially sensitive to pressure from friends.

### Unequal Status of Men and Women

A total of 29% of the respondents do not believe in the unequal status of men and women. 60.7 % of the boys however, and 73.5% of the girls show strong beliefs in the unequal status of men and women. 14- and 15-year-olds (92.9% and 90%) have the strongest beliefs in the unequal status (see Appendix, Table 5, 7 & 8).

During the interviews, many respondents said to believe that women are inferior to men and that men have the right to have certain expectancies of women. For example, a man can decide when and where sex takes place. Women know they must obey and respect their husbands demands because 'Labola' (dowry) has been paid for them. If the wife does not obey, her husband will become suspicious, violent or decide to leave her.

### Monogamous Relationships between Men and Women

The majority of the respondents (93.5%) disapproves of having multiple sex partners when in a relationship (see Appendix, Table 5 & 9). These thoughts were confirmed in the interviews. When talking about cheating in relationships, however, it was repeatedly mentioned that there was a difference between boys cheating and girls cheating. Boys are allowed to cheat because they like sex more and therefore need more than one girlfriend. They have more powerful feelings and needs, which 'forces' them to have sex. Sex is also more important to boys because they have to become fathers. Boys feel they have the right to cheat on their girlfriends because one girl alone cannot satisfy their needs. If a girl cheats in a relationship, it has to do with wanting money. Although most of the respondents disapprove of polygamy, they admit to seeing it happen quite often in their neighbourhoods, especially by men. Women have no choice but to accept this.

*Goal of sex*
- *Pleasure:* 59.7% of the respondents does not have sex for pleasure. 57.1% of them are boys, and 61.8% girls. All of the 18-year-olds claimed that sex was not for pleasure (see Appendix, Tables 5, 10, 12 & 13).
- *Sex in exchange for material goods:* Sex is not seen as something that can be given in exchange for material goods. None of the respondents admitted to have sex in exchange for clothing, food or better grades (see Appendix, Table 5). During the interview, 'sugar daddies' were discussed. Many of the respondents showed they had a problem with this phenomenon. Sugar daddies are a common problem in and around Dennilton. The main reason given for girls having sex with older men was the need of money.
- *Reproduction:* 45.2% of the respondents (32.1% of the boys and 55.9% of the girls) see reproduction as the goal of sex. Especially the 14-year-olds (86%) and the 17-year-olds (69%) showed high rates of this belief (see Appendix, Tables 5 & 11-13).

The most important information obtained from the interviews was that sex is not important or necessary for children and adolescents. Sex is a part of adulthood, especially because people are supposed to have babies in this stage of life. The age at which the respondents think that adulthood is reached differs from 17 to 21. Information obtained from the last part of the questionnaire (in which the respondents were instructed to put five different values in the correct order, according to the respondent's own interest) also showed that sex had *no* priority among the respondents. Health and money are more important (see Appendix, Table 14). This confirms the results that reproduction is one of the main goals of sex.

## 4.5. Research Question 5: The Relationship between Knowledge and Cultural Factors

As seen in Table 6, a significant relationship is found between knowledge and the goal of sex (pleasure).

### Table 6: Chi-square test for knowledge and cultural factors

|  |  | Knowledge Chi² | p |
|---|---|---|---|
| Religion |  | 9.67 | .09 |
| Myths |  | 9.09 | .11 |
| Tradition |  | 3.81 | .58 |
| Unequal status of men and women |  | 9.89 | .08 |
| Monogamous relationships between men and women |  | 4.49 | .48 |
| Goal of sex | Pleasure | 11.04 | .05 * |
|  | Sex in exchange for material goods | 2.90 | .72 |
|  | Reproductioj | 7.23 | .20 |

0 cells (0%) have an expected frequency of less than 5. * Cramer's V = .42 (power of the relationship)

## 4.6. Research Question 6: The Relationship between Sexual Behaviour and Cultural Factors

No significant relationships were found between sexual behaviour and cultural factors, except for religion and abstinence. Many of those who believe in the importance of religion also practise abstinence (see Table 7).

### Table 7: Chi-square test for sexual behaviour and cultural factors

|  |  | Condom use Chi² | p | Abstinence Chi² | p |
|---|---|---|---|---|---|
| Religion |  | 3.99 | .14 | 10.73 | .00 * |
| Myths |  | 1.67 | .43 | 3.20 | .07 |
| Tradition |  | 1.15 | .56 | .10 | .76 |
| Unequal status of men and women |  | .29 | .87 | .90 | .34 |
| Monogamous relationships between men and women |  | 1.10 | .58 | 2.18 | .14 |
| Goal of sex | Pleasure | 3.63 | .16 | .23 | .63 |
|  | Sex in exchange for material goods | 1.42 | .49 | 2.25 | .13 |
|  | Reproduction | 2.54 | .28 | .50 | .48 |

0 cells (0%) have an expected frequency of less than 5. * Cramer's V = .42 (power of the relationship)

## 4.7. Research Question 7: The Relationship between Determinants of Sexual Behaviour

No significant relationships were found between both forms of intention and the determinants of sexual behaviour (see Table 8).

### Table 8: Chi-square test for the determinants of sexual behaviour and intentions

| Intention | Attitude Chi² | p | Subjective norms Chi² | p | Perceived behavioural control Chi² | p |
|---|---|---|---|---|---|---|
| Condom use | 16.98 | .71 | 13.82 | .31 | 7.79 | .25 |
| Abstinence | 27.89 | .14 | 9.50 | .66 | 11.44 | .08 |

0 cells (0%) have an expected frequency of less than 5.

## 4.8. Research Question 8: The Relationship between Intention, Perceived Behavioural Control and Sexual Behaviour

Several significant relationships were found between intention, perceived behavioural control and behaviour. First, a significant relationship was found between the intention of using condoms and actually using them. Also a significant relationship between the intention of abstaining and practising abstinence was established. A third relationship was found between perceived behavioural control and abstinence (see Table 9).

### Table 9: Chi-square test for the intentions and sexual behaviour

| Behaviour | Intention to use a condom | | Intention to abstain | | Perceived behavioural control | |
|---|---|---|---|---|---|---|
| | Chi² | p | Chi² | P | Chi² | p |
| Condom use | 6.68 | .04 * | 1.67 | .43 | 6.28 | .39 |
| Abstinence | 1.69 | .19 | 10.12 | .00 ** | 13.69 | .03 *** |

0 cells (0%) have an expected frequency of less than 5.  * Cramer´s V = .33 (power of the relationship)
** Cramer´s V = .40 (power of the relationship) .    *** Cramer´s V = .47 (power of the relationship)

## 4.9. Research Question 9: The Relationship between Determinants of Sexual Behaviour and Cultural Factors

No relationships were found between intentions and cultural factors (see Table 10).

### Table 10: Chi-square test for intentions and cultural factors

| The intention to ... | use a condom | | abstain | |
|---|---|---|---|---|
| | Chi² | p | Chi² | p |
| Religion | 3.33 | .07 | .38 | .54 |
| Myths | .02 | .88 | 1.86 | .17 |
| Tradition | 1.62 | .20 | .27 | .60 |
| Unequal status of men and women | .63 | .43 | .12 | .72 |
| Monogamous relationships between men and women | .81 | .37 | .23 | .63 |
| Goal of sex     Pleasure | .77 | .38 | .31 | .08 |
| Sex in exchange for material goods | .16 | .69 | .09 | .76 |
| Reproduction | .32 | .58 | .01 | .93 |

0 cells (0%) have an expected frequency of less than 5.

No significant relationships were found between the determinants of sexual behaviour and cultural factors (see Table 11).

### Table 11: Chi-square test for the determinants of sexual behaviour and cultural factors

| | Attitude | | Subjective Norm | | Perceived behavioural control | |
|---|---|---|---|---|---|---|
| | Chi-square | p | Chi² | p | Chi² | p |
| Cultural factors | 891.43 | .22 | 260.70 | .44 | 542.55 | .20 |

0 cells (0%) have an expected frequency of less than 5.

# 5. Discussion

## 5.1. *Knowledge of* HIV/AIDS *and Cultural Factors*
The first question to be answered in this research is based on the NAAP's attempts to increase knowledge about HIV and AIDS among students in and around Elandsdoorn: *What is the relationship between the respondent's knowledge of* HIV/AIDS *and cultural factors?*

The knowledge measured in this study was quite moderate. On average, 6 out of 11 questions on HIV/AIDS were answered incorrectly. This research focused on the existing level of knowledge of HIV/AIDS among students. Previous research was based on the increase of knowledge after attending the NAAP. Therefore, a comparison is difficult to make. However, it can be stated that knowledge of HIV/AIDS improved significantly after following the AIDS awareness programme more than twice (see Chapter 6). The respondents of the present study were not selected on the number of times they had seen the NAAP, which means that this number was unequally divided among the 62 subjects. If all the respondents were to attend the NAAP more than twice, the average level of knowledge might be higher.

Another explanation for the moderate level of knowledge was discovered during the interviews. Most of the respondents answered they had been informed about safe sex. Surprisingly, only few mentioned the NAAP as a form of sexual education, while they had noted down the number of times they had witnessed a NAAP performance on the questionnaire. A possible explanation for this could be that the NAAP performances are not regarded as sexual education, but as a form of entertainment. The information about safe sex that the respondents mentioned mainly concerned birth control and was given mostly by their mothers. Almost none of the information contained facts about the prevention of HIV/AIDS. This could explain why the level of knowledge was not as high as expected.

A relationship was found between knowledge and the goal of sex (pleasure). This result was quite surprising, but can be explained as follows. A higher level of knowledge leads to the belief that sex is for pleasure. In their performances, the NAAP team spreads the message that it is wrong to have sex in exchange for clothing, good grades and money. In other words, sex should not be exchanged for material goods. The answers to the questionnaires showed that none of the respondents would have sex in exchange for material goods. Answers also showed that only a small amount of respondents practised abstinence, which means that many of them are sexually active. Almost all of the respondents considered themselves to be too young to have children. This leaves pleasure as most important goal of sex for those who are sexually active.

## 5.2. *Sexual Behaviour and Cultural Factors*
The second question concerned sexual behaviour and the determinants of sexual behaviour: *What is the relationship between the respondent's sexual behaviour and cultural factors?*

The number of respondents that practises abstinence is quite low, only 27% of the 14- to 18-year-olds do not have sex. This means that 73% of the 62 respondents is sexually active. When we look at the number of respondents that practises safe sex, the amount is quite low: 22% use condoms. Unfortunately, it is not possible to compare these results with the previous research due to a difference in measurement and analysis. It is, however, possible to compare results found on the relationship between intention and sexual behaviour. Results from this research show that those that have the intention to use condoms also say they actually use them during sex. The same relationship was found between the intention to abstain and practising abstinence. There was also a significant relationship between perceived behavioural control and behaviour. Consistent with these results, previous research also shows a significant relationship between intention and behaviour. Results showed that attitude, subjective norms and perceived behavioural control significantly influence intentions, and that perceived behavioural control directly influenced behaviour.

The importance of cultural factors appeared to be quite low after analysing the answers to the questionnaires. The answers to the interviews, however, showed a strong belief in the importance of cultural factors among the respondents. Certain myths are well believed in by the respondents, as is the existence of ancestor spirits. Initiation School was told to be of great influence on becoming sexually active. Also, polygamous relationships were disapproved of, but they did exist in and around Dennilton. Sex was widely seen as a way of reproduction among the respondents. It had to do with becoming an adult and having children. These seem to be important issues to the respondents.

There was a great contradiction in the answers given to the questionnaire and during the interview. A possible explanation is that the respondents did not understand the questions of the questionnaire very well and gave incorrect answers. Another possibility of the conflicting answers is a positive effect of the NAAP. When answering the questionnaire, respondents were forced to admit their own thoughts, beliefs and behaviour. However, when talking to the researchers during the interview, they had the opportunity to speak about things in a different perspective; they spoke about things they saw in their surroundings, about people they knew, etc. The respondents were able to describe certain cultural factors from a wider perspective, but they did not see these issues as their own. A reason for this could be the knowledge acquired from the NAAP.

No significant relationship was found between the determinants of sexual behaviour and cultural factors. The relationship was also measured between cultural factors and sexual behaviour (regarding condom use and abstinence). The results from the chi-square test showed no significant relationships between the six cultural factors and condom use. The only significant relationship found with abstinence was the cultural factor of religion.

Finally, it should be mentioned that the results showed no significant difference in cultural beliefs among the different age groups. One would expect that knowledge would increase with age, and that beliefs in myths and traditions might decrease accordingly. This was not found to be the case. The reason for this might be the large variation of ages within the different school grades. 14-, 15-, 16-, 17- and 18-year-olds are sometimes all put together in the same grade. This could explain more similarity in the level of knowledge per grade, instead of per age.

## 5.3. Implications for the NAAP

The level of knowledge about HIV/AIDS should have been higher among these subjects. It is important to provide clear and understandable information on HIV and AIDS. More attention should be given to the way sexual education takes place, both in and outside the home. Freshly obtained knowledge should be tested after attending awareness and prevention programmes to see what is remembered and what not.

Abstinence seems to be an important way of protection among the respondents, especially among the younger group. More attention should be given to this safe behaviour, besides condom use.

Condom use is still very important, but given the results of this research, it can be concluded that many of the respondents consider themselves too young to have sex. They choose to abstain and wait until they are mature enough to have sex. Promotion of condom use should be focussed on older adolescents of 18 years plus.

Theory and practice should be intertwined to reach the best effects of HIV and AIDS prevention. Knowledge should be implemented effortlessly in daily life.

# References

Achenbach, T.M. & Edelbrock, C. (1983). *Child Behaviour Checklist.* Burlington: V.T. Queen City Printers.

Ajzen, I. (1985). From intentions to actions: A theory of planned behaviour. In: J. Kuhl & J. Beckman (eds.), *Action-control: From cognition to behaviour (pp. 11-39).* Berlin: Springer.

Ajzen, I. (1991). The Theory of Planned Behaviour. *Organizational Behaviour and Human Decision Processes, 50,* 179-211.

Baylies, C. (2000). Perspectives on Gender and AIDS in Africa. In: C.Baylies & J.Bujra (eds.), *AIDS, Sex and Gender in Africa (pp. 1-24).* London: Roufledge.

Bennett, P. & Bozionelos, G. (2000). The theory of planned behaviour as predictor of condom use: A narrative review. *Psychology Health & Medicine, 5,* 307-326.

Bogart, L.M., Cecel, H. & Pinkerton, S.D. (2000). Hispanic Adult's Beliefs, Attitudes, and Intentions Regarding the Female Condom. *Journal of Behavioural Medicine, 23* (2), 181-206.

Conner, M. & Norman, P. (1996). *Predicting Health Behaviour.* Buckingham, UK: Open University Press.

Dekker, M (2000). *Zuid-Afrika.* Brecht: Gottmer Uitgevers Groep b.v

Dijk, van A.C. (2001). Traditional African beliefs and customs: implications for AIDS education and prevention in Africa. *South African Journal of Psychology 31* (2), 60-66.

Eaton, L., Flisher, A.J. & Aorø, L.E. (2003). Unsafe sexual behaviour in South African youth *Social Science and Medicine, 56,* 149-165.

Elder, J.P. (2001). *Behavioural Change and Public Health in the Developing World.* London: Sage Public inc.

Hart 't, H., Dijk van, J., Goede de, M. Jansen, W. & Teunissen, J. (1998). *Onderzoeksmethoden.* Amsterdam: Boom.

Tempelman, H.A., Lubbe, C.M.M.V.van der, Schinnij M. & Vermeer, A. (subm.). *Evaluation of an Aids Awareness Programme in rural South Africa.*

Shapiro, R.L.& Kapiga, S.H. (2002). Male condom and Circumcision. In: M. Essex, S. Mboub, P.J. Kanki, R.G. Marlink & S.D. Tlou (eds.), *Aids in Africa (498-506).* New York: Academic.

Stadler, J. & Hlongwa, L. (2002). *Monitoring and evaluation of Love Life's AIDS prevention and advocacy activities in South Africa 1999-2001.* Reproductive Health Research Unit, Chris Hani Baragwanath Hospital.

Stillwaggon, E. ( 2001). Aids & Poverty in Africa. *Nation 272,* 22-26.

Tillotsen, J. & Maharaj, M. (2001). Barriers to HIV/AIDS protective Behaviour among African adolescent males in township secondary schools in Durban, South Africa. *Society in Transition, 32 (1).*

# Websites

CDC's HIV and Transmission. (n.d.). Retrieved July 7, 2004, from Centres for Disease Control and Prevention, Division of HIV/AIDS Prevention: Global AIDS Program, From http://www.cdc.gov/hiv/pubs/facts/transmission.htm

Socio-cultural aspects of HIV/AIDS in South Africa. (2003). From www.health24.co.za

*Address for correspondence:*
H.A. Tempelman, MD
Ndlovu Medical Centre
P.O. BOX 1447
Groblersdal 0470
South Africa

# Appendix

## *Knowledge*

### Table 1: Incorrect answers to the knowledge questions (11)

| Amount of questions answered incorrectly | Frequency | % |
|---|---|---|
| 4 | 8 | 12.9 |
| 5 | 7 | 11.3 |
| 6 | 19 | 30.6 |
| 7 | 14 | 22.6 |
| 8 | 12 | 19.4 |
| 9 | 2 | 3.2 |
| total | 62 | 100.0 |

## *Behaviour*

### Table 2: Sexual behaviour

| | | Mean | SD | Range |
|---|---|---|---|---|
| Behaviour | Condom use | .53 | .39 | 1.00 |
| | Abstinence | .79 | .41 | 1.00 |

### Table 3: Respondents who use a condom and/or abstain (behaviour)

| | Condom use | No condom use | Total |
|---|---|---|---|
| Abstinence | 3 = 18% | 14 = 82% | 17 = 27 % |
| No abstinence | 10 = 22% | 35 = 78% | 45 = 73 % |
| Total | 13 | 39 | 62 = 100% |

### Table 4: Condom use and abstinence by gender and age

| Condom use | | | | | Abstinence | | | | |
|---|---|---|---|---|---|---|---|---|---|
| Gender | | Frequency | Percentage | SD | Gender | | Frequency | % | SD |
| Boys | .00 | 8 | 28.6 | .46 | Boys | .00 | 3 | 10.7 | .32 |
| | 1.00 | 20 | 71.4 | | | 1.00 | 25 | 89.3 | |
| | Total | 28 | 100.0 | | | Total | 28 | 100.0 | |
| Girls | .00 | 9 | 26.5 | .45 | Girls | .00 | 10 | 29.4 | .46 |
| | 1.00 | 25 | 73.5 | | | 1.00 | 24 | 70.6 | |
| | Total | 34 | 100.0 | | | Total | 34 | 100.0 | |

"

| Age | | Frequency | Percentage | SD | Age | | Frequency | % | SD |
|-----|------|-----------|------------|-----|-----|------|-----------|------|-----|
| 14  | .00  | 8         | 57.1       | .51 | 14  | .00  | 2         | 14.3 | .36 |
|     | 1.00 | 6         | 42.9       |     |     | 1.00 | 12        | 85.4 |     |
|     | Total| 14        | 100.0      |     |     | Total| 14        | 100.0|     |
| 15  | .00  | 1         | 10.0       | .32 | 15  | .00  | 2         | 20.0 | .42 |
|     | 1.00 | 9         | 90.0       |     |     | 1.00 | 8         | 80.0 |     |
|     | Total| 10        | 100.0      |     |     | Total| 10        | 100.0|     |
| 16  | .00  | 1         | 8.3        | .29 | 16  | .00  | 3         | 25.0 | .45 |
|     | 1.00 | 11        | 91.7       |     |     | 1.00 | 9         | 75.0 |     |
|     | Total| 12        | 100.0      |     |     | Total| 12        | 100.0|     |
| 17  | .00  | 4         | 30.8       | .48 | 17  | .00  | 4         | 30.8 | .48 |
|     | 1.00 | 9         | 69.2       |     |     | 1.00 | 9         | 69.2 |     |
|     | Total| 13        | 100.0      |     |     | Total| 13        | 100.0|     |
| 18  | .00  | 3         | 23.1       | .44 | 18  | .00  | 2         | 15.4 | .38 |
|     | 1.00 | 10        | 76.9       |     |     | 1.00 | 11        | 84.6 |     |
|     | Total| 13        | 100.0      |     |     | Total| 13        | 100.0|     |

Score 1 = these respondents use a condom
Score 1 = these respondents abstain

## Cultural factors

### Table 5: Importance of the cultural factors

| Factor | | N | Mean | SD | Range |
|--------|---|---|------|-----|-------|
| Religion (2) | | 62 | .21 | .41 | 1.00 |
| Myths (10) | | 55 | .36 | .49 | 1.00 |
| Tradition (4) | | 62 | .50 | .50 | 1.00 |
| Unequal status of men and women (4) | | 60 | .70 | .46 | 1.00 |
| Monogamous relationship between men and women (7) | | 62 | .94 | .25 | 1.00 |
| Goal of sex | Pleasure (2) | 62 | .40 | .49 | 1.00 |
| | Sex in exchange for material goods (4) | 61 | .23 | .42 | 1.00 |
| | Reproduction (1) | 62 | .55 | .50 | 1.00 |

The closer the mean is to 1:
the more the respondents abstain according to their religion.
the more the respondents believe in myths.
the more the respondents believe in traditions.
the more the respondents believe in the different status between men/women.
the more the respondents believe in monogamous relationships between men/women.
the more the respondents believe the goal of sex to be pleasure
the more the respondents believe that sex is a way to gain material goods.
the more the respondents believe the goal of sex to be reproduction.

### Table 6: Importance of religion, by gender

| Gender | | Frequency | % | SD |
|--------|-------|-----------|------|-----|
| Boys | .00 | 5 | 17.9 | .39 |
| | 1.00 | 23 | 82.1 | |
| | Total | 28 | 100.0 | |
| Girls | .00 | 8 | 23.5 | .43 |
| | 1.00 | 26 | 78.5 | |
| | Total | 34 | 100.0 | |

Score 1 = the respondents abstain (interpreted as no sex before marriage) according to their religion

### Table 7: Importance of the unequal status of men and women

| | Frequency | % | SD |
|---------|-----------|------|-----|
| .00 | 18 | 29.0 | .46 |
| 1.00 | 42 | 67.7 | |
| Total | 60 | 96.8 | |
| Missing | 2 | 3.2 | |
| Total | 62 | 100.0 | |

Score 1 = the respondents believe the different status of men/women is highly important.

### Table 8: Importance of the unequal status of men and women, by gender and age

| Gender | | Frequency | % | SD |
|--------|---------|-----------|------|-----|
| Boys | .00 | 11 | 39.3 | .50 |
| | 1.00 | 17 | 60.7 | |
| | Total | 28 | 100.0 | |
| Girls | .00 | 7 | 20.6 | .42 |
| | 1.00 | 25 | 73.5 | |
| | Total | 32 | 94.1 | |
| | Missing | 2 | 5.9 | |
| | Total | 34 | 100.0 | |

| Age | | Frequency | % | SD |
|---|---|---|---|---|
| 14 | .00 | 1 | 7.1 | .27 |
| | 1.00 | 13 | 92.9 | |
| | Total | 14 | 100.0 | |
| 15 | .00 | 1 | 10.0 | .32 |
| | 1.00 | 9 | 90.0 | |
| | Total | 10 | 100.0 | |
| 16 | .00 | 7 | 58.3 | .51 |
| | 1.00 | 5 | 41.7 | |
| | Total | 12 | 100.0 | |
| 17 | .00 | 4 | 30.8 | .48 |
| | 1.00 | 9 | 69.2 | |
| | Total | 13 | 100.0 | |
| 18 | .00 | 5 | 38.5 | .52 |
| | 1.00 | 6 | 46.2 | |
| | Total | 11 | 84.6 | |
| | Missing | 2 | 15.4 | |
| | Total | 13 | 100.0 | |

Score 1 = the respondents believe the different status of men/women is highly important

## Table 9: Importance of monogamous relationships between men and women

| | Frequency | % | SD |
|---|---|---|---|
| .00 | 58 | 93.5 | .24 |
| 1.00 | 4 | 6.5 | |
| Total | 62 | 100.0 | |

Score 1 = the respondents believe monogamous relationships between men/women are highly important.

## Table 10: Goal of sex: pleasure

| | Frequency | % | SD |
|---|---|---|---|
| .00 | 37 | 59.7 | .49 |
| 1.00 | 25 | 40.3 | |
| Total | 62 | 100.0 | |

Score 1 = the respondents believe the goal of sex is pleasure

## Table 11: Goal of sex: reproduction

| | Frequency | % | SD |
|---|---|---|---|
| .00 | 28 | 45.2 | .50 |
| 1.00 | 34 | 54.8 | |
| Total | 62 | 100.0 | |

Score 1 = the respondents believe the goal of sex to be reproduction.

### Table 12: Goals of sex, by gender

| Pleasure | | | | Reproduction | | | | |
|---|---|---|---|---|---|---|---|---|
| Gender | Frequency | % | SD | Gender | | Frequency | % | SD |
| Boys  .00 | 16 | 57.1 | .35 | Boys | .00 | 9 | 32.1 | .48 |
|      1.00 | 12 | 42.9 | | | 1.00 | 19 | 67.9 | |
|      Total | 28 | 100.0 | | | Total | 28 | 100.0 | |
| Girls  .00 | 21 | 61.8 | .37 | Girls | .00 | 19 | 55.9 | .50 |
|      1.00 | 13 | 38.2 | | | 1.00 | 15 | 44.1 | |
|      Total | 34 | 100.0 | | | Total | 34 | 100.0 | |

Score 1 = the respondents believe the goal of sex is pleasure

Score 1 = the respondents believe the goal of sex is reproduction.

### Table 13: Goals of sex, by gender

| Age | Pleasure | | Reproduction | |
|---|---|---|---|---|
| | N | Mean | N | Mean |
| 14 | 14 | .36 | 14 | .86 |
| 15 | 10 | .25 | 10 | .30 |
| 16 | 12 | .46 | 12 | .42 |
| 17 | 13 | .27 | 13 | .69 |
| 18 | 13 | .00 | 13 | .38 |
| | | min .00 / max .00 | | |
| Total | 62 | | 62 | |

The closer the score is to 1, the more the respondents believe the goal of sex to be pleasure

The closer the score is to 1, the more the respondents believe the goal of sex to be reproduction.

## *Priorities*

### Table 14: Respondent's priorities

| Gender | | Mean | SD |
|---|---|---|---|
| Boys N = 28 | Money | 2.6 | 1.17 |
| | Health | 1.3 | .66 |
| | Friends | 2.6 | .91 |
| | Relationships | 3.8 | .61 |
| | Sex | 4.6 | .68 |
| Girls  N= 34 | Money | 2.5 | 1.26 |
| | Health | 2.2 | 1.37 |
| | Friends | 2.6 | 1.16 |
| | Relationships | 3.3 | .98 |
| | Sex | 4.4 | 1.10 |

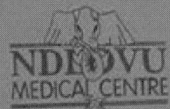

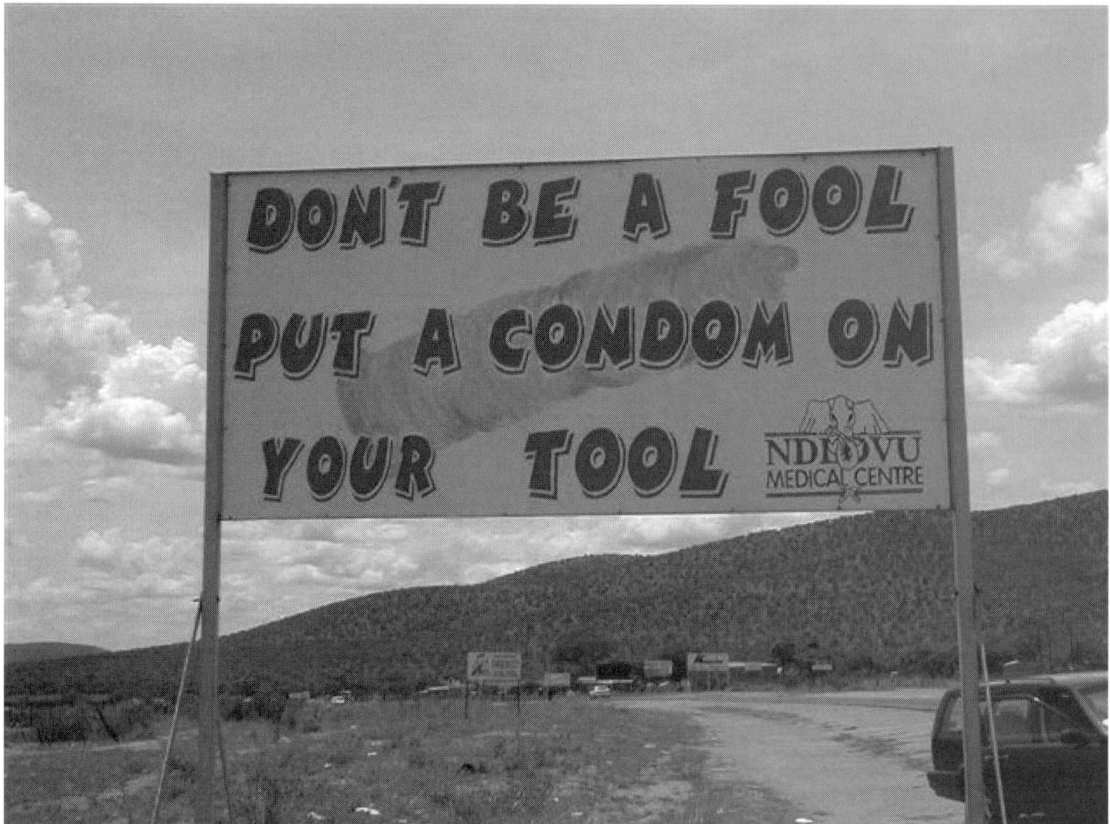

# Chapter 8

# Ndlovu Autonomous Treatment Centre: an Innovative and Integrated Approach towards Rural TB and HIV/AIDS Care

*Hugo Tempelman[1]*

[1] Ndlovu Medical Centre, Elandsdoorn, South Africa

## Abstract

The availability of Highly Active Anti-Retroviral Treatment (HAART) makes it possible to start mass programmes to fight HIV/AIDS. The general HAART concept as a free service roll-out programme was modified and adapted to be effective in the private sector. To this end, the model of an 'autonomous treatment centre' for integrated primary health care, TB and HIV/AIDS care at a local level was developed. The results of the HAART and the PMTCT (Prevention of Mother-to-Child Transmission) programmes are described. Co-operation with the public sector has resulted in an outreach programme and mobile HIV/AIDS care.

## 1. Introduction

The unfortunate timing of the political changes and the upcoming HIV epidemic have caused South Africa to become the epicentre of the HIV/AIDS epidemic (Nattrass, 2004). The political denial by the South African government has led to further damage and confusion amongst the South African population. Whereas in 1990 the prevalence was still 0.8% (antenatal survey)[1], now, in 2005, national HIV prevalence is estimated at 10.8%, with a higher prevalence in women (13.3%) than in men (8.2%). In the age group of 15-49 years the overall prevalence is 16.2%. Mpumalanga has the highest prevalence in this age group, 23.0%, followed by KwaZulu-Natal with 21.9%[2].

An estimated 5-7 million South Africans are infected, but it could be stated that de facto 50 million South Africans are affected. It is impossible to live in this country and not be confronted with the impact of the epidemic. It goes through all layers and colours of this society. We have to realise that ten years of failing to treat HIV/AIDS has made a million victims and that each day we have a thousand HIV/AIDS-related deaths and two thousand people newly infected. Often people appear unimpressed when they hear these figures. To put it differently: If in Europe a Boeing 747 crashes, it is hot news, CNN and BCC World and all newspapers make it their headlines. In South Africa alone, three Boeings crash every day and six new ones are taking off with nobody knowing when they run out of fuel.

When HAART (Highly Active Anti-Retroviral Treatment) became available in the late 1990s, it became feasible to start thinking of treating patients in mass programmes all over the world (Sande & Volberding, 1999). Daring projects like the MSF-Khayalitsha project (near Capetown) were a wake-up call for the government and the NGO fraternity[3].

In 2001, we started thinking about a prevention of mother-to-child transmission (PMTC) programme in our Columbine Maternity Clinic (CMC) and forwarded a proposal to the Dutch fund Stichting Liberty. Three weeks later, a reply arrived in which we were asked: *'Why do you try to save the children and make them AIDS-orphans by not treating the mothers?'* A valid remark, which meant that we had to start thinking in a completely different direction: 'HAART for All'.

As a small non-governmental organisation (NGO), but a pioneer in the fight against HIV/AIDS, the number of patients on treatment at the NMC could never significantly contribute towards the massive task faced by this country. That was the reason why we chose a different track and set our goals to become:
− a care provider to the community;
− a model for ARV roll-out in resource-poor settings;
− a capacity builder for the public sector, NGOs, and other CBOs (community based organisations);
− a capacity builder for in-service training of our own staff and for other NGOs or the public sector.

We dared to make a statement that was quite unconventional: *'Would you agree that HIV/AIDS, with its 7 million victims, is going to be a huge employer in this country?'*

If we accept this statement, we could turn part of this awful epidemic into a tremendous opportunity and you might to understand the concept of our approach.

PharmAccess International (PAI, The Netherlands) is a non-profit organisation that originates from the Academic Medical Centre of the University of Amsterdam. PAI is committed to the treatment of HIV-infected patients in a clinically justified manner and at an affordable cost. It has taken on the task to guide projects in the implementation of ARV roll-out programmes and serves as a consultant for the participating projects. In the 1990's, PAI developed a concept of what they called an 'autonomous treatment centre'[4].

We modified and adapted this concept and formulated it differently as it was not originally developed for a 'free service' roll-out but as a model that works mainly in the private sector, especially in the occupational HIV care to be given by employers within their companies. The modifications made were mainly to serve our purpose to provide a free service for the people who are unable to bear the cost of their own health care. We also extended the services with primary health care and TB care, as we are of the opinion that in a stigmatised environment like South Africa, the only approach is an integrated service, rather than special clinics for HIV management only.

If we accept that HIV/AIDS is going to be a massive employer, we have the great opportunity to address some of the biggest problems of this country at the same time:
− massive unemployment in rural areas is often up to 60-70 %;
− the highest prevalence of HIV/AIDS is also found in rural areas.

If we can connect these problems by bringing HIV/AIDS back to a community level, we could kill two birds with one stone.

Build up the local capacity to fight the epidemic, let job opportunities flow back to the local communities and you will have something very valuable: local people looking after local ill people, often their brother, neighbour, relative or schoolmate. This means that the people involved in providing the care are related to the ones in need of it: committed care in the fight against HIV/AIDS is the most important factor in implementing adherence management. A secondary spin-off is the economic impact of this employment plan for rural capacity building

## 2. Integrated Primary Health Care, TB and HIV/AIDS Care: the Ndlovu Autonomous Treatment Centre

Due to the stigma of HIV/AIDS, especially in rural areas, a combined comprehensive service of primary health care (PHC), TB and HIV/AIDS care appears to be the best approach towards the problem. The service envisaged should be able to provide care for a population of approximately 100,000 - 140,000 people (Moutse and parts of KwaNdebele). Patients of the surrounding townships will be able to reach this service by public or their own transport.

The autonomous treatment centre (ATC) is a concept of creating a 'one-stop centre' for primary health care, TB care and HIV/AIDS care. It brings all services back to a local level and, as said, addresses three major problems of South Africa at the same time. It provides employment in areas with an unemployment rate of approximately 60-70%. It creates local capacity through education, enabling local people to become involved in an important community care project. It brings the care back to the environment where the HIV/AIDS epidemic is at its worst: the rural areas. Our HIV/AIDS prevention and treatment model aims to serve as a model to make ARV treatment accessible for rural South Africa. The aimed capacity of the ATC is approximately 2,500–3,500 HIV positive patients on treatment. The aimed capacity of the laboratory is approximately 4,000-6,000 HIV positive patients on treatment. Growth towards this capacity will take place over several years, but to realise this the hardware has to be in place from the onset of the project. One ATC could serve up to four peripheral 12-hour clinics, each with a capacity of 300-400 patients on ARVs. This would amount to a total of max. 4,000-4,500 HIV patients on ARVs in a well-controlled environment. If we accept that only HIV-positive patients with a CD4 count below 200 are starting on ARVs, the estimation is that 2 out of 10 HIV-positive people need treatment. This means that one ATC with its four satellites can control 20,000 –22,500 HIV-positive people. If we assume the adult HIV prevalence in rural South Africa to be around 20%, it this would mean that the population that could be controlled by one ATC is approximately 100,000 –115,000.

Figure 2 shows the model of the ATC with its possible peripheral clinics. These clinics may belong to other NGOs, the public sector or could even provide the care in places with no medical infrastructure, using a mobile unit . If implemented properly, 99% of the HIV-positive patients can be treated and monitored at a local level, involving local people as caregivers. Those patients who cannot be looked after at local level, need referral to a tertiary centre for their care.

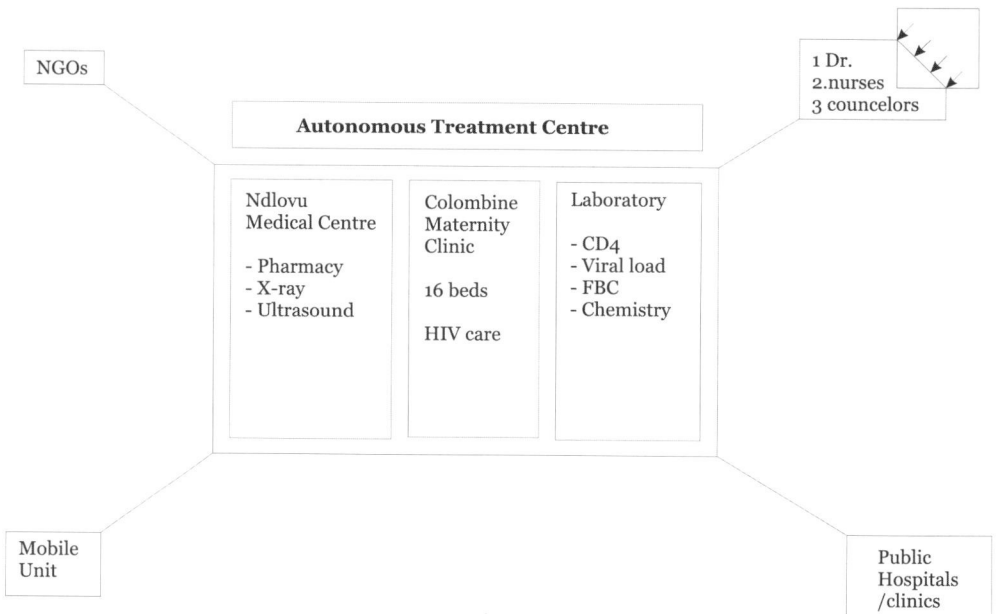

Figure 2: Organisational structure for HIV/AIDS care of Ndvlovu Autonomous Treatment Centre

The ATC consists of four components:

## 1. Twelve-hour Clinic with Pharmacy and X-ray

A well-stocked pharmacy is imperative to provide good PHC, TB and HIV/AIDS care, and the logistics in this regard have to be investigated and implemented in a proper way. The X-ray is necessary in order to diagnose and treat tuberculosis. TB is a co-infection of HIV: in our clinic 64% of the TB patients are HIV-positive managed on an out-patient basis. They temporarily need clinical support because of a reconstitution syndrome, adverse events or opportunistic infection management, etc.

## 2. Maternity Clinic

The obstetrical unit is imperative to provide a good PMTCT programme (prevention of mother-to-child transmission). Nowadays it is possible to reach an almost 0% transmission, also in the most rural areas. This unit will also provide this area with a maternity service, a service non-existing in most rural areas.

## 3. Laboratory

A laboratory specialised in HIV monitoring is a necessity for good HIV/AIDS care at a local level. The advantages of having a laboratory on site are tremendous. First of all, the return time is very short: results are available varying from immediately to a day or two at the maximum. Secondly, the logistics of lab specimen transport in South Africa's hot climate are neglectable. Thirdly, the laboratory on site, together with an integrated IT system, offers the opportunity of a well developed patient follow-up system as well as programme evaluation on compliance, defaulting, viral suppression etc. on site.

Kimera Health Solutions has developed a unique HIV monitoring laboratory, the TOGA-tainer, which is a semi-mobile laboratory built in a sea freight container. They are also the providers of the IT monitoring system

*4. Conference Room/Training Facility*
Because of the fact that the ATC will become a centre of excellence in the area where it is established, we have to assist other stakeholders in the area in their capacity building. Therefore a training centre, in the form of a conference room, is an important part of the ATC.

The clinical services provided through the ATC are:
– a community AIDS awareness programme;
– normal PHC service;
– VCT voluntary counselling and testing;
– HAART clinical and laboratory monitoring;
– PEP, post-exposure prophylaxis;
– prevention of mother-to-child transmission;
– obstetrical and clinical admission facility;
– occupational health service in the lodges and on the farms through a mobile service.

# 3. Results of the Ndlovu HAART Project

The antiretroviral drugs we use are divided in two lines of regimen. In the first line regimen we also adapt the treatment for specific target groups. In the first line we start treatment for naïve patients (patients who have never been exposed to ARVs before). The second line is used when patients 'break through' the first line and develop resistance to the first line of drugs.

*First-line regimen ARVs:*
– 1st choice d4T, 3TC, NVP, female, reproductive age group;
– 1st choice d4T, 3TC, EFV, female, co-infected with TB;
– 1st choice d4T, 3TC, EFV, male.

*Second-line regimen ARVs:*
– resistance testing done in case of treatment failure although the patient is therapy-compliant;
– in case treatment failure occurs and patient is not therapy-compliant;
– AZT, DDI, Kaletra;
– laboratory monitoring done as a routine: VL, CD4, liver functions, renal functions, full blood count, amylase at regular intervals.

In the period 12.02.2004 to 01.11.2005, a total of 3,474 patients were offered a VCT, of whom 1,558 (44.8%) were tested positive for HIV. This figure is not representative as a prevalence figure for our area. The overall prevalence in Mpumalanga for the age group of 15-49 years is 23.0%[5]. It has to be realised that the majority of patients came with clinical suspicion of HIV or clinical complaints therefore testing at our clinic results in a much higher percentage HIV-positive patients.

To be eligible for HAART, patients have to meet a number of social, adherence and biological criteria:

*Social criteria:*
– selected area;
– fixed address;
– patient ready for lifelong treatment;
– patient ready to commit to safe sex;
– patient must identify a treatment assistant in his home;
– counsellors must be allowed to enter the patient's home;
– no medical aid that covers payment of treatment;
– patient will disclose to at least ONE person;
– patient willing to attend support groups.

*Adherence criteria:*
– patient must have been consulting at NMC for at least 6 weeks;
– patient must have been on time for last 4 visits;
– patient has proven adherence to TB treatment or OI treatment.

*Biological criteria:*
– WHO stage 4;
– CD4 cells < 200 cells/µl;
– Karnofsky Performance Score > 40%;
– asymptomatic patients with CD4 cells < 50 cells/µl.

The results shown in Tabel 1 are from our patient population admitted into the HAART project in the period from 18.02.2005 to 01.03.2005, i.e. patients who started ARV treatment during this period and have been on treatment for at least six months. At this stage, patients are admitted into the programme with an average number of 30-40 per month. At the end of November 2005, a total of 515 patients were started on ARVs, of whom 42 are children.

**Table 1: Results from the Ndlovu HAA RT project**

| CD4 | Treated with HAART | | | Not treated | | No show[2] |
| | N Patients | Died (%) | Lost to follow-up[1] | Died (%) | Lost to follow-up[1] | |
|---|---|---|---|---|---|---|
| 0-50 | 114 | 28 (24.6%) | 4 | 13 (11.4%) | 2 | - |
| 51-100 | 46 | 11 (23.9%) | 3 | 1 (2.2%) | 1 | - |
| 101-200 | 74 | 11 (14.9% | 6 | 2 (2.7%) | 3 | 5 |
| >201 | 18 | 1 (5.5%) | 2 | 0 | 0 | 0 |
| 201-350 | 13 | 0 | 0 | 1 (0.9%) | 6 | - |
| >350 | 69 | 0 | 0 | 6 (8.7%) | 9 | 1 |
| Total | 252 | 51 (20,2%) | 15 (5,9%) | 23 (9.1%) | 21 | 6 |

[1] Lost to follow-up: on several accounts not available, no response on home visits or telephonic follow up.
[2] Missed controls but does not yet meet criteria for 'lost for follow-up'.

These results show that too many people come in at a late stage (CD4 counts below 100 and even below 50), both categories have a high death rate after starting HAART due to the fact that these patients often suffers from advanced AIDS. We still have to realise, though, that over 75% of the patients from these categories who started on ARV survived and are now compliant and undetectable and have a good quality of life. This means that a low CD4 count is no reason not to start HAART. A total of 5.9 % of defaulting patients is the result of good compliance management and shows the dedication of our team in creating awareness among the patients about the importance of treatment compliance.

## 4. Results of the PMTCT Project

We have chosen for a prevention of mother-to-child transmission protocol that aims at a very low transmission rate.

HAART is started at a gestational age of 20 weeks, irrespective of maternal CD4s, for all pregnant women. What we would like to achieve is that the pregnant woman's viral load is undetectable at birth. The following routine is used:
– We use our first line regime: D4T/3TC/NVP.
– We strive for a normal vaginal delivery; caesarean section only on obstetrica indication.
– Post partum mother and child remain in the CMC for three days, neonates PEP for one month with syrups of ARVs ( AZT, 3TC).
– The mother is given Dostinex in order to suppress the production of breastmilk.
– Breastmilk is replaced with formula feed that will be provided for one year.
– Six weeks post partum we perform an HIV-DNA-PCR test for the neonate, which will be confirmed at the age of one year.
– The follow-up period for the neonate is one year.
– Pregnant women with an initial CD4> 200 will be weened off of the ARVs and have six-monthly check-ups until they are illegible for lifelong ARVs.
– Pregnant women with an initial CD4 count < 200 will continue lifelong treatment.

During the period September 2003-March 2005 we performed voluntary counselling and testing (VCTs) on all 542 antenatal clinic attendances. 84% out of 542 women agreed to be tested (N=456) and 114 women were tested HIV-positive (25.6%). Until October 2005, out of the 76 women who started their PMTCT programme, 46 are still pregnant.

All women delivered at the obstetrical clinic, one delivered at another institution where she and her infant get the one-month dual therapy with AZT/3TC, although formula feed was given directly after birth. The patient was not lost for follow-up and the child has been confirmed HIV-negative. One neonate died six weeks post partum, due to cot death.

At six weeks a PCR-HIV-DNA test was done on all the infants in order to establish their HIV status. They are all negative for HIV, which is a very promising result. At the age of one year, the PCR-HIV-DNA test will be repeated in order to confirm the child's HIV status.

The 0% transmission rate in our PMTCT programme proves that the slogan 'PMTCT keeps South Africa HIV-free' is not an Utopia. It means the start of a new South Africa that can be raised without being infected with the virus.

## 5. Outreach Programme for Public Sector and NGOS

In view of the enormous backlog of HIV patients in need of ARVs, a speedy roll-out must be facilitated all over the country. Often NGOs are willing to start but do not know how, because they used to be involved in home-based care for the terminally ill. We can offer them assistance.

Government clinics are facing a different problem. They are overburdened, understaffed and not able to handle the extra workload that an ARV programme would entail. We would like to offer assistance to the NGOs and the public sector, so as they can start their programmes as soon as possible.

The government clinics can be assisted by sending them a well-trained team, educated at our ATC, consisting of one medical doctor, two professional nurses, counsellors and an administrator. They will run the ARV service and provide continuous education for the clinic staff. Eventually, the local personnel will be sufficiently empowered to take on this care on their own.

Another important aspect of co-operation with the public sector is that we must never forget that community health care problems, like TB and HIV/AIDS remain primarily the responsibility of the government. NGOs are allowed to assist and contribute but must never claim to take over the care. Therefore we consider it our main task to keep the lines of communication with the government open. When they are willing to accept our assistance, we must be in the position to provide them with the knowledge gathered or offer them the capacity they need in speeding up the national roll-out

For NGOs that are on the verge of starting treatment programmes but do not know how, we offer our assistance in the same way. We assist them in writing their project proposal, try to find funding, assist them in the start-up phase and educate their staff at our ATC.

At this stage, we have assisted two NGOs, and the Department of Health of Mpumalanga, the province we are in, has started dialogue to make use of our services. The ATC has only functioned for three years now and already the success of the formula starts to flourish. At this stage, we are also involved in copying the ATC concept and starting a second project in the Sabie Sand/Bushbuckridge area, in order to serve the community there. This second ATC will be called Ingwe. Ndlovu and Ingwe mean respectively 'elephant' and 'leopard' in Zulu.

## 6. Mobile HIV/AIDS Care

As shown in Figure 2, the ATC organogramme, at least four satellite clinics can be set up in order to create a network of ARV-providing clinics in the area. The other unique component is the mobile HIV care unit that can bring the care to those groups of patients that have no easy access to this kind of care.

We are involved in two mobile care programmes for people who do have a job, but because of the job location cannot reach ARV care as it is simply not available in their environment: agricultural labourers and people working in game lodges in the Kruger National Park area. These are successful programmes in which we first send our NAAP team to the farm or lodge to create awareness and educate people and invite them to do a VCT. Subsequently, a confirmation test and a CD4-count allow us to set out a programme for the farm/lodge concerned.

For the farming community (with a measured prevalence of approximately 30-35%), ARV services are not yet available in the government clinics in the areas where the farms are. The mobile clinic is the solution for this situation. We bring the care to the workplace. The same goes for the Sabie Sand area, where mobile HIV/AIDS care is brought to the different lodges in order to provide care to the lodge personnel. In this way the occupational health threat of HIV/AIDS for all personnel of the lodges can be addressed properly.

Tabel 2: Results from the Ndlovu Farm Project (November 2004 till September 2005)

|  | Farm I (n=500) | Farm II (n=500) |
| --- | --- | --- |
| Permanent workers | 500 | 500 |
| Total VCTs done | 258 (51.6%) | 236 (47.2%) |
| - HIV + | 85 (33%) | 83 (35%) |
| - HIV - | 173 (67%) | 153 (65%) |
| Waiting for treatment | 60 (71.6%) | 53 (64.9%) |
| On treatment | 25 (29.4%) | 30 (35.3%) |
| Defaulting | 7 (28%) | 4 (13.3%) |
| - Died | 2 (8%) | 1 (3.3%) |
| - Lost for follow up | 5 (20%) | 3 (10.0%) |
| Number of HIV+ pt back at work | 81 (95.3%) | 76 (92%) |

Although we have started on only two farms and the amount of patients treated is not very high yet, the results shown are most promising. Within one year after initiating the programme on both farms, we see that respectively 51.6% and 47.2% of the employees agreed to be tested for HIV, of whom respectively 33% and 35 % were tested positive. The slow roll-out, 29.4 % and 35.3% of the HIV-positive employees started on ARVs right away, is due to a long process of de-stigmatisation that has to take place before treatment can be started. Therefore, it is essential to have a good awareness programme preceding the treatment programme. Of the patients that were started on ARVs, respectively 8% and 3.3% died, but the amount of defaulters is relatively high, possibly due to stigma in the community.

The result that respectively 95.3% and 92.0% of the patients treated in our programme are back to work full-time within six months of starting therapy, proves the importance of starting up an occupational HIV/AIDS care programme on the work floor, which is feasible not only for the big co-operates but also for middle-sized companies..

The ATC concept is a concept that is starting to prove its value towards building up capacity with and for other organisations. It also proves to be reproducible and cost-effective. No compromise has been made on quality of care and by involving the local community in providing care to HIV/AIDS patients within their community, there is the plus that compassionate care proves to be very effective from a treatment-compliance point of view.

Ndlovu ATC has become a centre of excellence in the middle of a rural township. It shows that quality care can be given at grass root level with the involvement of local people. The next step for this centre of excellence is to become a centre that will start focussing on education and research.

The focus has to be on education, because we feel that the knowledge gained at Ndlovu Medical Centre is not something we are not allowed to keep to ourselves. Ndlovu Medical Centre can become an educational centre for doctors, professional nurses, councillors, data-capturers, ARV programme managers, etc. It is now a place where people can be trained academically and on the job in our clinical setting and conference facilities. In this way we can provide excellent practical expertise for other ARV roll-out projects and assist them in the starting phase of their programme.

Research is an obligation if one would like to start programmes as described in this chapter. Our experiences deserve it that the outcomes are described and published in order to provide evidence-based material on the basis of which other programmes can start their initiatives. Research will also prove the viability and sustainability of the autonomous treatment centre as a model to deliver TB and HIV/AIDS care in rural resource-poor settings. In order to do so, we will need to scale up our academic staff, managerial expertise and seek out universities that are interested to assist us in this major task.

## 7. Conclusion

Regarding HIV/AIDS as an empowerment tool in the fight against unemployment and for the education of local people creates numerous opportunities, opportunities that we do not always think of when we speak about HIV/AIDS. The existing Ndlovu ATC has proven the concept, Ingwe ATC must prove its reproducibility. This might lead to the Big Five ATC as a model of integrated rural health care, a partnership between public and private sector, for South and Southern Africa.

## References

Nattrass, N. (2004). *The moral economy of AIDS in South Africa*. Cambridge: Cambridge University Press.
Sande, M.A. & Volberding, P.A. (1999). *The medical management of AIDS*. Philadelphia: W.B. Saunders Company.

*Address for correspondence:*
H.A. Tempelman, MD
Ndlovu Medical Centre
P.O. Box 1447
Groblersdal 1070
South Africa
e-mail: tempelman@ndlovumc.org

## Notes

1. www.avert.org\aidssouthafrica.htm
2. www.hsrc.ac.za\media\2005\11\20051130-1factsheet2.pdf
3. Providing Antiretroviral Therapy at Primary Health Care Clinics in resource-pour settings. Preliminary Report: May 2001 – May 2002, Médecins Sans Frontières (MSF), School of Public Health and Primary Health Care, University of Cape Town.
4. A concept developed by PharmAccess International, The Netherlands (002a PAI ATC short.doc.).
5. See footnote 2.

# Part II

# Sizanani Village (Bronkhorstspruit)

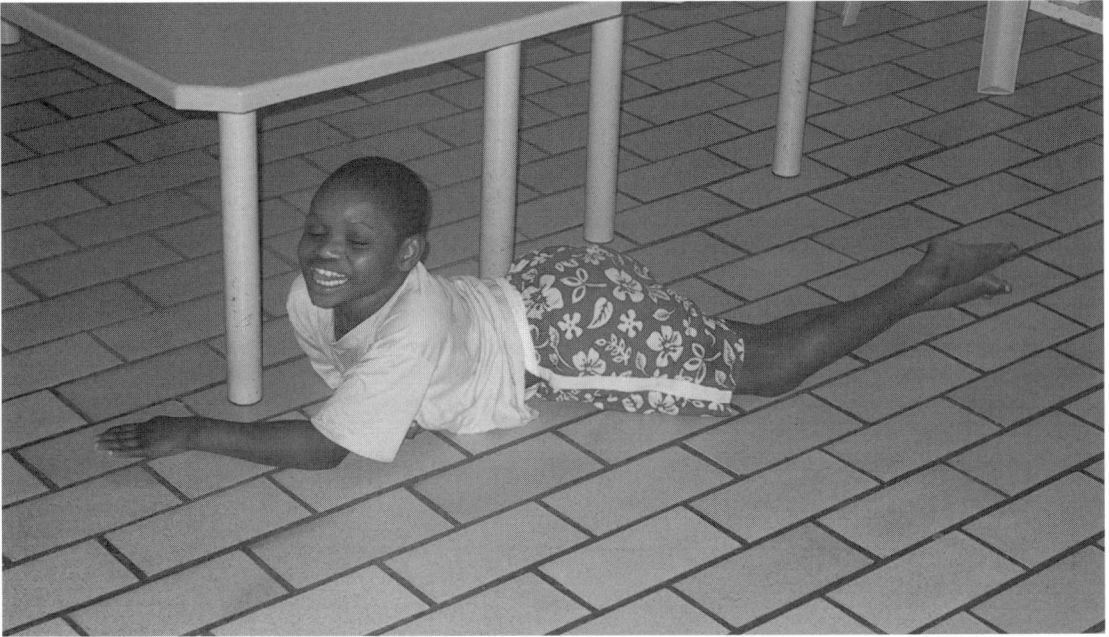

# Chapter 9

# Disability in South Africa: Transformation Efforts at a Home for Children with Developmental Disabilities

*Zsoka Magyarszeky [1], Nthoana Mbethe [1]*

[1] St. Mary's Home, Sizanani Village, Bronkhorstspruit, South Africa

## Abstract

This chapter aims to provide an overview of the evolution of disability theory in developing countries and place it within the context of the transformation process at St. Mary's Home. The Home is a residential facility in rural South Africa for children and youth with neurological disorders, and is in the process of shifting its approach from nursing care towards developing the children's potential to assist them in leading a more independent life.

A developmental programme, Conductive Education, is being established and integrated into the childcare services of the Home by training caregivers in the basic principles of the method. However, the organisation faces various challenges as a result of the historical past of South Africa, the lack of financial and human capital and a cultural mindset that often has a negative impact on the lives of people with disabilities.

The Home is now in the initial phase of transformation focusing on developing its centre-based services. Long-term objectives include the establishment of an outreach programme with the main focus on community-based support. Capacity building, both within the organisation and in the surrounding communities will be crucial for achieving these objectives.

## 1. Introduction

By the end of the 20th century, disability has been increasingly seen as a human rights and development issue. Society as a whole must take the responsibility of integrating its members with disabilities into mainstream activities by rehabilitation, adapting the environment, providing financial support when necessary and by changing the negative attitudes of non-disabled people towards their peers with disabilities. Many of these tools, however, require ample financial resources from both public and private sectors, and this hinders developments in African countries. Unique strategies need to be developed in these communities in order to uphold the rights of people with disabilities and ensure that their quality of life is similar to those without disability.

Any discussion that concerns itself with political, social or economic issues within the African continent cannot be looked at in isolation but must take into account the aspects of cultural diversity and Western influence over traditional values and belief systems. Disability is no exception. The authors of this chapter will therefore first look at how disability theory has evolved on an international level, its influence on how disability is viewed and dealt with in South Africa and then place the transformation efforts of St. Mary's Home at Sizanani Village within this context.

## 2. The Evolution of Disability Theory

Both state policies and the work of non-governmental organisations related to people with disabilities reflect the inherent attitude of a particular country towards disabilities. Although policies vary greatly both historically and geographically, three major approaches can be identified: the isolation, the medical and the now emerging social model (Turmusani, 2003).

### 2.1. *The Isolation Model*
The isolation model is often supported by religious beliefs or superstitious explanations. It is based on the view that disability is a sign of sin and punishment from God or the ancestors. People with disabilities are therefore hidden away from sight in order to prevent the ostracism of the family. This view may also imply the irrelevance of intervention, or the improvement of the condition in any way (Turmusani, 2003).

There are two manifestations of the isolation model that are, although seemingly different, theoretically almost identical. One approach is the traditional way of life in developing countries, where people with disabilities are cared for within the family, but are kept out of sight, and only provided with the minimum necessities for survival. The other approach is the segregation of people with disabilities through residential institutions. In the developing world, many of these have been established by religious organisations that regard people with disabilities as needing care within the context of charity. Although the first approach provides care for disabled people within the community, they have no better chances of participating in mainstream society than they have in residential institutions. Both approaches are based on the assumption that people with disabilities are unproductive members of the community and therefore considered a drain on resources with no possible return on investment.

### 2.2. *The Medical Model*
This model defines disability as a medical 'problem' and therefore implies the need for medical treatment in order to attempt to eliminate or improve the condition of persons with disabilities. This view recognises that people with mild to moderate disabilities have the potential to actively participate in society, and therefore need assistance and training to acquire the necessary skills (Turmusani, 2003). It also acknowledges the need for exercise and stimulation with regard to people with severe or profound disabilities, but often lacks a functional approach that is aimed towards greater independence in everyday activities. The medical model is, furthermore, based on the view that disability is something that is deviant from the norm, as it concentrates on the 'abnormal' or the pathology rather than on the development of the potential of the clients: '…professionals see disability as pathology. They are stuck in the medical model of disability. Using this perspective, professionals do not accept the disabled person for who what he or she is. They become preoccupied in trying to remake the disabled person into a non-disabled one. This does not work … professionals should spend more time identifying and developing the abilities of the disabled person …' (Armstrong & Barton, 1999; p.15). This is quoted from a statement made by a resident in one of the institutions for people with disabilities in Zimbabwe.

## 2.3. The Social Model

This model asserts that it is society that poses restrictions on people with impairments through disabling barriers in the environment. It is society's duty to create an accessible physical and social environment in order for people with impairments to be able to participate in mainstream activities on an equal ground. Some writers identify this view as a socio-political model, emphasising the responsibility of the state to establish policies and legislation that facilitate this enabling process (Turmusani, 2003). While the isolation and medical model can flourish in communities that have lower levels of government intervention, the adoption of the social model requires high state involvement that, in turn, implies higher public expenditure in the initial phase. The model then points out that the inclusion of people with disabilities in the mainstream, including the labour market, will provide in the long-term a high return on investment. The training of people with mild or moderate disabilities will enable them to retain employment, thereby eliminating their need for social grants. People with severe or profound disabilities can also be trained to gain increased independence in their everyday life, and this can result in a reduced need for caregiver or technical assistance. The social model also asserts that people with severe or profound disabilities are also respected and – to a certain extent – active members of a society.

# 3. Disability in South Africa

'The concept of a caring society is strengthened and deepened when we recognise that disabled people enjoy the same rights as we do and that we have a responsibility towards the promotion of their quality of life. We must stop seeing disabled people as objects of pity but as capable individuals who are contributing immensely to the development of society. The emphasis is on a fundamental shift in how we view disabled people away from the individual medical perspective, to the human rights and development of disabled people. As a government we endorse these principles.'

The above is an extract from the Foreword of the *Integrated National Disability Strategy* (*INDS*), published in 1997 by the Office of the Deputy President of South Africa (p. 1). It is apparent that the passage is based on one of the theoretical models of disability, and that the government of South Africa has adopted the social model and intends to put policies in place that will facilitate the implementation of its principles.

The INDS also acknowledges that past government policies and the attitudes of society as a whole have resulted in the severe isolation of people with disabilities.

In the wake of democracy, the Ministry without Portfolio in the Office of the President has developed a policy document, called the Reconstruction and Development Programme, that focuses on the upliftment of the previously disadvantaged population of the country, including black people, women and persons with disabilities. With regard to labour legislation, under Affirmative Action and the Employment Equity Act, 2% of jobs in the public sector have to be occupied by persons with disabilities by 2005. The National Skills Development Strategy prescribes that 4% of learnerships (apprenticeships) have to be awarded to people with disabilities (Rowland, 2001). A commendable achievement of the government, demonstrating its commitment to the social model, is the fact that the National Assembly of South Africa has twelve members with various disabilities. Many agree that these policies and legislation together with the 1996 Constitution of South Africa are highly advanced even according to the standards of the developed world. The foundation has been laid; the government, the public, the private sector and non-governmental organisations (NGOs) must now put in a concerted effort to implement these principles.

The first step is a comprehensive assessment of the needs of people with disabilities across the country in order to develop appropriate services and infrastructure, through which people with disabilities can play a full, participatory role in society.

## 3.1. Prevalence of Disability in South Africa

There is very little statistical information available on the prevalence of disability in South Africa, including the demographic and socio-economic characteristics of people with disabilities, as well as the services available and accessible for them. This poses a significant difficulty for both governmental and non-governmental bodies to develop an appropriate network of services. Statistics South Africa has published a document in 2005, titled *Prevalence of Disability in South Africa,* that draws on the data obtained during the National Census carried out in 2001. These findings, however, cannot be deemed entirely reliable as information was obtained from people directly affected by disabilities and their individual perceptions might vary greatly. Regrettably, besides estimates from NGOs, no objective information is available from health care or social service providers.

According to the above mentioned document, during Census 2001, 5% of the population reported that they had some kind of disability 'that prevented them from full participation in life activities'. This number has corresponded to the estimate of the United Nations Development Programme.

The following statistical analysis was conducted for the purpose of discussion on St. Mary's Home Trust for Children with Disabilities. The analysis aimed to establish the size of the black population in Gauteng Province with intellectual and physical disabilities.

St. Mary's Home caters to children and youth with neurological disorders, however, no information is available on the prevalence of this type of disability. Taking into account that the prevalence of disability among the elderly tends to be higher, this implies that out of the 114,207 persons with disabilities, there are a significant number of people who have acquired physical or intellectual disabilities due to age-related disorders. For the purpose of establishing the size of the population St. Mary's Home caters to, only people with intellectual and physical disabilities under the age of 30 were considered, as shown in Table 1. It can also be assumed that a large portion of these people are disabled due to neurological disorders.

**Table 1: Statistics on the prevalence of intellectual and physical disabilities among the black population in Gauteng Province, under the age of 30 (Source: Statistics SA, 2005)**

| Population group | N | % |
|---|---|---|
| National prevalence | 2,255,982 | 5 |
| Black population | 1,854,376 | 82 |
| Gauteng prevalence | 331,611 | 3.8 |
| Black population | 271,921 | 82 |
| Physical or intellectual disabilities | 114,207 | 42 |
| Under 30 years | 39,972 | 35 |

Note: Calculations were made under the assumptions that the percentage of blacks on a national level is the same as in Gauteng, and that the percentage of physical and intellectual disabilities in the total population is the same as under the age of 30.

According to the calculations in Table 1, there are approximately 40,000 children and youth in Gauteng that could potentially benefit from the services provided by St. Mary's Home. At present, there is limited information available on the service provision and the needs of people with disabilities in Gauteng. A scoping study is therefore planned to be conducted by St. Mary's Home during 2006, the objectives of which will be discussed in more detail later on.

## 3.2. Challenges and Shortcomings on a National Level

The government of South Africa acknowledges the following major challenges to be over-come as described in the *Integrated National Disability Strategy*:

1.  Lack of integration of disability issues among various government departments, such as Health, Education, Labour, Housing and Transport.
2.  Widespread poverty, particularly in rural areas, which contributes to malnutrition, poor housing conditions and low levels of education.
3.  Low numbers of appropriately trained professionals.
4.  Poor access to appropriate health care facilities, assistive devices and early childhood development opportunities.
5.  High levels of bureaucracy, corruption and inaccessibility with regard to social grants.
6.  Cultural beliefs of African people, ostracising families with disabled members.
7.  High unemployment rate even among the non-disabled population.
8.  Physical barriers in the environment, including transport and buildings.
9.  Considerable inequalities between white/urban and black/rural areas.

St. Mary's Home faces each of the above challenges every day. Plans and strategies for the future can only be developed with the full understanding of the external environment in which the organisation operates. Moving away from the isolation and medical models to the social model will therefore be a long and strenuous process, but St. Mary's Home is committed to the transformation these principles entail.

The following is a discussion on the background of and the strategies put in place by the organisation.

## 4. St. Mary's Home for Children and Youth with Disabilities at Sizanani Village

### 4.1. History

St. Mary's Home is situated within Sizanani Village in Bronkhorstspruit, 60 km east of Pretoria. Sizanani, meaning 'help each other', was started by an Austrian catholic priest, Fr. Charles Kuppelwieser, as a mission in 1989. Wanting to help the communities around former KwaNdebele (one of the so-called bantustans during the apartheid government), he employed the research results that were offered by students from the Medical University of South Africa, and opened a residential care facility for children with neurological disorders. After the research was conducted, the quota showed a high number of children with neurological disorders who were kept at home with mothers who did not know what to do with them.

Sizanani Home was then opened in March 1993 and has been operating under the St. Vincent de Paul Society. Sizanani Village Trust (SVT) was established in May 2000 to take over the programmes established by St. Vincent de Paul. These programmes included the home, crafts workshops, a conference centre, HIV/AIDS programmes, farming projects, and a school for learners with special educational needs. The crafts shops and the conference centre were built to generate funds for the running costs of the Home. The founder also became the major donor of the institution as the funds raised by him from overseas constituted more than 50% of the Home's total income.

Because of the complexity of running the various projects as they expanded, SVT decided to unbundle them into independent, separate legal units to enhance their effective and efficient management. Sizanani Village Trust remained the owner of the fixed property and the Home was incorporated into St. Mary's Home Trust, registered in April, 2004.

St. Mary's Home now has a capacity of 250 and is licensed to render residential care for children and young adults with severe and profound neurological disorders, who are distributed through eight units used as their dormitories or houses. The majority of the children and youth have families in the surrounding communities but have limited contact with them.

The South African government encourages NGOs to provide health care and welfare services due to the lack of state funds. As St. Mary's Home continuously meets the standards set by the Government, under the Department of Health – Mental Health Directorate, it is provided with a licence which is renewable annually and is subsidised per child admitted. At present, the government subsidy covers approximately 50% of the running costs of the Home.

Since its establishment in 1993, the core function of the Home has been nursing care. Nursing sisters were employed in supervisory posts, who oversaw the work of the caregivers, the majority of whom had no relevant qualifications. They were responsible for taking care of the children 24 hours a day, including feeding, bathing, dressing, nappy changing, and any other activities related to the physical well-being of the children. The Home also employed 1-2 therapists who had the responsibility of providing treatment for all 170-210 children, with the help of 3-4 occupational therapy assistants. They have tried to reach as many of the children as possible but found it difficult to involve caregivers in the application of therapeutic gains within the children's daily routine.

All of the above indicate the strong presence of the isolation model and traces of the medical model. From around 2003, however, various external factors have influenced the management of the Home to reconsider the strategic direction of the institution and implement major structural and operational changes.

## 4.2. The Shift from the Isolation and Medical Model towards the Social Model

In 2002, Sizanani was visited by the wife of the former Prime Minister of The Netherlands. Seeing the programmes run in Sizanani, she promised to contribute to the welfare of the children in whatever way. Through her efforts, support came from the Utrecht University in the Netherlands, offering a needs analysis concerning the development of the children and the working conditions of the caregivers (see Chapter 10). The study concluded that, although the children are very well taken care of, the introduction of a developmental programme would be very beneficial for the entire organisation. The children needed training in order to function more independently which could increase the possibility of reintegrating them into their communities. It was also realised that the childcare workers needed to be more involved in the development of the children and see it as the main purpose of their work. The organisation itself needed to restructure in order to facilitate this change.

Shortly after the introduction of the developmental programme Conductive Education (CE), the founder-donor of the Home announced his retirement. This put a considerable strain on the financial situation of the organisation and forced its management to attempt to expand its donor base and fundraise more intensely. This has resulted in the establishment of contacts with various local and international aid organisations as well as corporate sponsors. Their condition of financial support is generally the same: the development of children with disabilities to facilitate their increased participation within the mainstream society. Most of these organisations have adopted the social model and are reluctant to offer funds for only the operational costs of residential facilities. They want to provide support to organisations that train, educate or provide assistance for people with disabilities to help them lead a more active and self-sufficient life.

The Gauteng Department of Mental Health that subsidises the children in the Home has also started to shift its approach towards the social model. The new set of criteria that is used to evaluate NGOs now includes items concerning the development of the children and youth in residential facilities. A comprehensive inspection is carried out annually to ensure that only organisations that meet these criteria will be subsidised the following year.

Responding to the above mentioned changes in the external environment, the Home has started a transformation process that involves all areas of the organisation. Two Conductive Education practitioners have been contracted to train the caregivers in the basic principles of the method; a fundraiser has been recruited to assist with the expansion of the donor base, and the organisational structure has been changed to provide an internal environment that is conducive to the realisation of the new vision, mission and objectives of the Home.

*Vision*

The vision of St. Mary's Home Trust is to be a centre of excellence for the diffusion of child-care, development and training, for people with mental and physical disability, within the context of a catholic Mission, in service of humanity.

*Mission*

The mission of St. Mary's Home Trust is:
1. To have an established regulatory framework and a professional management team which plans, organises and controls the operations and ensures that the organisation is adequately resourced with human and financial capital.
2. To have a sustainable and integrated service range that grows according to the demands of the external environment.
3. To move the organisation from a centre-based to a home-based approach, establishing relevant links with the surrounding communities and providing assistance to families or small, community-based organisations (CBOs) in need.

*Objectives*

The objectives set by St. Mary's Home Trust are:
1. To have a full complement of trustees to serve on the Trust, representing a range of relevant skills and expertise.
2. To have a fully functioning management team that is in possession of the necessary managerial and functional skills in order to operate the Home effectively and efficiently.

3.  To establish an organisational structure conducive to the developmental needs of the children and youth in the Home.

4.  To implement Conductive Education throughout the Home by training caregivers in the basic principles of the method and assisting them to establish a daily routine for the children that facilitates their physical, social, cognitive and emotional development.

5.  To establish an accredited training programme in CE in order to transfer skills to the local community.

6.  To establish an outreach programme in our region that will entail the re-integration of young adults into their communities, assisting local CBOS and establishing 'mother and child' group sessions in the communities.

*Conductive Education*

Conductive Education is a training programme for children and adults with neurological disorders. It was developed by Prof. Andras Peto, a neurologist, in Hungary, after world war II (Coles & Zsargo, 1998). The programme is in line with the social model approach of disabilities for the following reasons:

1.  It promotes functional independence, teaching skills that are necessary in everyday activities, such as mobility, dressing, bathing or feeding.

2.  It treats clients in a holistic manner, including all areas of development: motor, cognitive, social, communication and emotional.

3.  It actively involves parents or caregivers, training and educating them on how to best assist the development of persons with neurological disorders and encouraging the application of learned skills in the client's home and community environment.

The implementation of Conductive Education at St. Mary's Home is unique in the sense that it focuses on the training of childcare workers. The responsibility of the two specialists currently contracted is not, in principle, to train the children, but to train childcare workers how to best utilise their time with the children to create educational opportunities and to educate them on the importance of helping children reach their full potential. Fourteen childcare workers have been trained by the end of 2005 within a small group setting of ten children. The objective of the programme for the forthcoming two years is to implement the basic principles of the method throughout the entire home, adapting it in accordance with the varying needs of children. Once CE is consolidated within the organisation, it is planned to provide the basis of an outreach programme in the future.

The Conductive Education programme is evaluated by means of a longitudinal research, conducted by Master Degree students from the Utrecht University (see Chapter 11). This provides the management of the Home with insight into the progress made by both children and childcare workers, facilitating the planning and implementation of short- and long-term strategies.

## 4.3. Present-situation, in the Initial Phase of Transformation

The Home currently caters to 166 children and youth with mild to profound physical and intellectual disabilities, with ages ranging from 3 to 24 years. Figures I and II provide a general picture of their age in relation to their level of functioning.

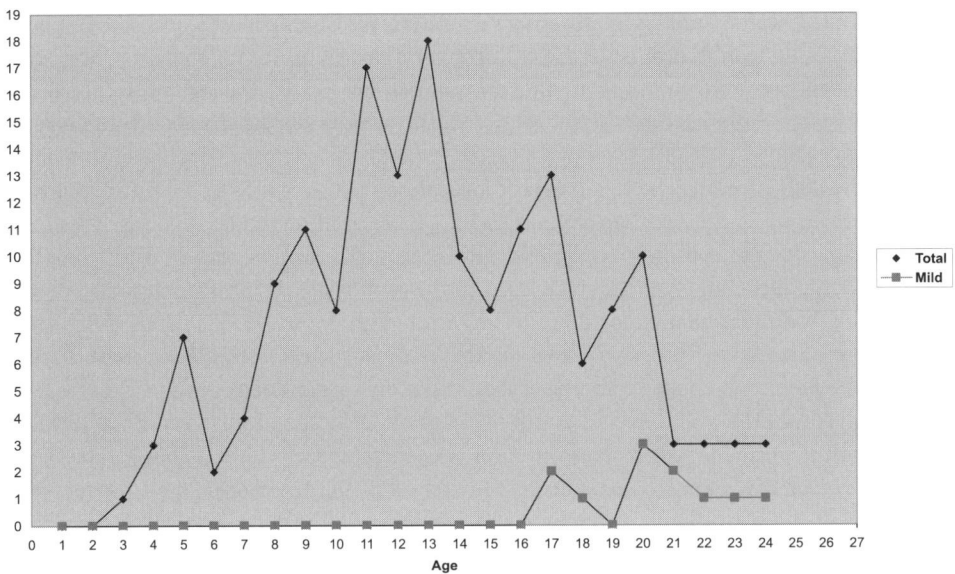

Figure I: The number and age of children with mild disabilities in proportion to the total population of St. Mary's Home.

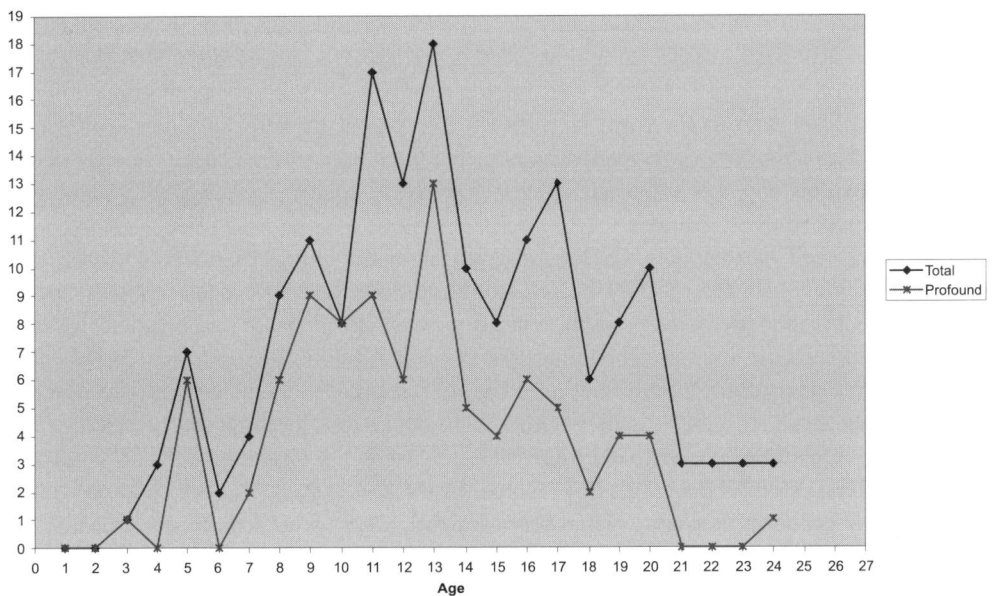

Figure II: The number and age of children with profound disabilities in proportion to the total population of St. Mary's Home.

There are three major conclusions that can be drawn from the two figures. The first is that the majority of the children are above the age of 12, in fact constituting 64% of the total population. Further analysis shows that 21% are young adults, as they are above the age of 18. Secondly, it is also noticeable that the majority of the children have profound, while only a few children have mild disabilities; 53% and 7% respectively. The remaining children – not shown on the graphs – are either severely or moderately disabled, 29% and 11% respectively. Thirdly, it can be seen that most of the children with profound disabilities are younger, while all of the children and youth with mild disabilities are above the age of 16. This can be explained by the organisation's admission criteria, which will be discussed in more detail later on.

All of the above findings have important indications with regards to the future plans of the Home. A relatively large number of young adults have mild or moderate disabilities, making it more likely for them to be reintegrated into their communities and to find some type of employment. On the other hand, since most of the children have profound or severe disabilities, there is a limited chance for them to be re-integrated into society successfully. It seems most likely that taking into consideration the poor socio-economic backgrounds of their families, the Home will have to accommodate them on a permanent basis.

Around 25% of the children and youth are orphaned or abandoned and have virtually no contact with the outside world. The situation is exacerbated by the fact that Sizanani Village is located on a farm, 5 km from the nearest town and 25 km from the largest township in the area, making it very difficult to include the residents of the Home in regular community activities. As there are no group homes in the surrounding area and no service infrastructure available for people with disabilities living on their own, the Home will most likely have to provide a permanent placement for these residents as well. An appropriate plan needs to be put in place that addresses their needs to lead an active life within the premises of Sizanani.

The advancing age of the children also causes difficulties with regard to rehabilitation. Early intervention is crucial to acquire necessary skills and prevent secondary impairments. However, internal statistics show that most of the children on admission to the Home are already over the age of 8, without ever having received any therapeutic or educational interventions. They often come from families with very poor housing conditions, are malnourished and already have developed various deformities. Their home environment offers them no stimulation and this often has irreversible effects on the cognitive, social and physical development of these children.

Besides the Conductive Education programme of the Home that aims to equip children with life skills, only 28% of the children attend school. The only special school in the area is located within the premises of Sizanani but run by the government and is mainly for children with intellectual disabilities. The school has its own admission criteria that exclude children with severe or profound disabilities as it has no resources to cater to them. Despite government policies which aim to include children in education, the high teacher-learner ratio in special schools makes it virtually impossible to provide quality education to children with varying levels of disability. This has resulted in the fact that 72% of the children residing at the Home cannot access educational services at all. Even those who do attend school have a very low level of literacy and numeric skills.

*Admission criteria*
Since the Home receives around 50% of its total funds from the government, it is necessary to follow admission criteria established by the Department of Health. All children who submit an application for admission must be assessed according to these guidelines. The government classification system is based on four levels – mild, moderate, severe and profound disability – and all assessments must be conducted by using a measurement developed by government officials. The measurement is non-standardised and does not consider differences in age-appropriate functioning. It includes items on mobility, self-care, communica-

tion, intellectual abilities and emotional stability. Staying in line with the social model, encouraging community-based care, only children with severe and profound disabilities are subsidised in residential institutions. The young adults of the Home with moderate or mild disabilities were admitted before the government started to support the Home.

The experiences gained during assessments indicate significant inconsistencies between government policies and the reality. The Home is often forced to turn down applications of children with moderate disabilities, despite of the desperation of the parents. Due to the lack of health and educational services in rural areas, the majority of these children stay at home, placing a considerable burden on families, usually preventing the mother from retaining employment. Furthermore, families do not receive appropriate support or information on how to best handle a child with disability at home, how to involve family members, or how to deal with the negative attitude of their communities.

Although the Home recognises the benefits of government policies, and itself is planning to move towards community-based care, it is unrealistic to expect that a large number of children could be discharged from the Home in the near future. The profoundly and some of the severely disabled children and orphans will have a very slight chance of leaving Sizanani, and therefore the combination of a centre-based and community-based approach will be needed.

## Human Resources

The Home currently employs 126 staff members to provide comprehensive, 24-hour care for 166 children and youth. The educational levels of employees are shown below, in Table 2.

**Table 2: Educational levels of employees**

| Level | Auxiliary | Childcare workers | Professionals | Managers | Total |
|---|---|---|---|---|---|
| Gr. 8 | 36 | 5 | 0 | 0 | 41 |
| Gr. 10 | 4 | 12 | 0 | 6 | 22 |
| Matric[1] | 3 | 30 | 6 | 12 | 51 |
| Level 5[2] | 0 | 0 | 5 | 2 | 7 |
| Level 6[3] | 0 | 0 | 0 | 3 | 3 |
| Level 7[4] | 0 | 0 | 1 | 1 | 2 |
| Level 8[5] | 0 | 0 | 0 | 0 | 0 |
| Total | 43 | 47 | 12 | 24 | 126 |

Note[1]  High School Diploma
Note[2]  2-year tertiary qualification
Note[3]  Bachelors Degree
Note[4]  Honours Degree
Note[5]  Masters Degree or higher

It is clear from Table 2 that the Home struggles with recruiting the necessary intellectual capacity needed to successfully complete the transformation process. As a NGO, the organisation finds it difficult to compete with the public or corporate sector with regards to salary packages, particularly now that the founder-donor has retired and the Home is just starting to get back on its feet financially.

As the Home began the transformation process outlined earlier, it was realised that the structure of the organisation must change as well, to reflect the shift from nursing to childcare and development. Childcare workers have been promoted to supervisory and middle management positions to take responsibility for their own department. Therapy, CE and childcare have been integrated into one department to ensure the holistic development of the children. A separate Health Services department has also been established with a professional nurse in charge, and is now regarded as a support function. With the nurses' station established, nurses can now take full responsibility and accountability for quality nursing care, while childcare practitioners focus on the training and development of children. They are proud to work with nurses as team members instead of being their subordinates. It is also clear that the children residing at the Home do not necessarily need nursing or medical intervention to solve their disability problems but need to be trained and their potential to be developed in order for them to be able to execute activities of daily living more independently, and thus improve their quality of life.

Capacity building is now the main objective of the Childcare Department, both among line workers and within the supervisory level. Since the establishment of the organisation, caregivers have been recruited from the surrounding communities, with no previous experience or qualifications. Furthermore, the high unemployment rate in the area (around 40%) has resulted in a workforce that is not passionate about their field of work, but only take the job in order to feed their families. The situation is further exacerbated by the lack of precise job descriptions and policies that would provide guidelines and set clear expectations for employees. The establishment of these guidelines is currently the highest priority for the top management. Performance appraisals, based on precise job descriptions, will also assist management to identify areas where training is most needed.

The transformation process has clearly resulted in staff members being insecure about their job and uncertain of the expectations of the management. The organisation currently struggles with labour relations difficulties and considerable time is spent on negotiations with trade unions. Various tools have been put in place to assist the communication between staff and management in order to regain the trust of employees and involve them as active participants in the process of transformation.

*Future plans: Outreach Programme*

'... *Some claim that communities will and do take care of children with disabilities. But first and foremost, communities are not all the same. Secondly, very often the community contributes to the exclusion of the children with disabilities. Third, many of the material needs of children with disabilities are not available to the community where the child lives. This does not mean that there is no role for community-based rehabilitation but rather acknowledges the limitations of the community, and the need to find indigenous solutions from within communities, rather than a viewpoint being forced on communities by well-meaning outsiders.' (McClain, 2000, online).*

Indeed, there are various factors that contribute to the difficulties St. Mary's Home will face on initiation of its outreach programme. The following challenges will need to be addressed when considering the reintegration of young adults with disabilities or establishing day-programmes for children and their parents.

Most rural communities still have superstitious or religious beliefs, including the causes of disability. It is still seen as a stigma, a curse, the manifestation of sin or disgrace in the family and this affects the attitude of the society towards disability and limits their participation in the development and rehabilitation of children with disabilities (Onasanya, 2002). People with disabilities are usually isolated by being hidden away from society or placed in institutions. Integration becomes ineffective unless the mindset of the society changes. Introduction of any developmental programme, such as Conductive Education, should be within the African model for it to be effective. When introducing such programmes to mothers and at day care centres, there are cultural considerations to be made as well. Issues such as individualism vs. grouping, collective responsibility vs. independence, medical treatment vs. traditional healing, are important to consider. Priority is also given to ancestral direction or prescription over any Western way of intervention.

Many live in poverty, with often only one breadwinner for an extended family and several dependents to take care of. '… Family caretakers become poor themselves, many need care and the problem of the disabled person is no longer amongst the priorities for investment or action. … In poor societies we need to support the strongest before we can speak about the rights of the weakest.' (Vanneste, 2003). Other factors, such as the HIV/AIDS epidemic, play a role in the fact that often grandmothers are left alone to care for children with disabilities.

The unemployment rate in the country is very high, especially in rural areas where most of the young adults of the Home come from. Unemployment is already a major concern for non-disabled people with a low standard of education and a lack of skills needed in the job market. People with disabilities, therefore, find it extremely difficult to find employment, also due to the inaccessibility of buildings and the lack of reliable public transportation. The Home plans to investigate the possibility of establishing sheltered workshops in the community and provide relevant vocational training for young adults.

When considering the reintegration of young adults, the Home must also consider their safety when living within the community. The sexual, physical and emotional abuse and the exploitation of vulnerable people in communities are common, and monitoring becomes difficult with no adequate social services available. Frequent home visits and the ongoing provision of comprehensive assistance will be essential to ensure that the quality of lives of reintegrated young adults will not decline after leaving the Home.

A scoping study will be conducted by the Home in the surrounding communities in the first half of 2006, before the initiation of outreach projects. This is essential in order to provide relevant and effective services that will have a long-term positive impact on the lives of people with disabilities.

Taking into consideration that the majority of the children and young adults currently residing in the Home will need to stay permanently, the establishment of an outreach programme will entail the expansion of services, rather than simply the different allocation of current resources. The organisation will have to ensure that it is in possession of the necessary financial and human capital in order to achieve its objectives.

The new South African government is facing the challenge of distributing resources equally throughout its entire people in order to improve the quality of life of those who were adversely affected by apartheid. St. Mary's Home is also aware of these challenges and therefore determined to play a role in contributing to the improvement of the quality of life of people with disabilities.

## References

Armstrong, F. & Barton, L. (1999). *Disability, Human Rights and Education: Cross-cultural perspectives.* Palo Alto, CA: University Press.

Coles, C. & Zsargo, L. (1998). Conductive Education: towards an 'educational model'. *British Journal of Special Education, 25,* 70-74.

McClain, C. (2000). Presentation to the Cape Town workshop, May 2000: *Human Rights: Social Assistance for Children with Disabilities.* Retrieved 17 November 2005 from http://www.sahrc. org.za/human_rights_focus.htm

Office on the Status of Disabled Persons (1997). *Integrated National Disability Strategy.* Pretoria: Office of the Deputy President.

Onasanya, A. (2002). *Pearls of Africa: Disability in Africa.* Retrieved 17 November 2005 from http://www.pearlsofafrica.org/htmlDIA.html

Rowland, W. (2001). *Nothing about us without us: Inside the Disability Rights Movement of South Africa.* Pretoria: UNISA Press

Statistics SA (2005). *Prevalence of disability in South Africa.* Pretoria: Statistics South Africa.

Turmusani, M. (2003). *Disabled people and economic needs in the developing world: a political perspective from Jordan.* Aldershot: Ashgate Publishing.

Vanneste, G. (2003). *The impact of HIV/AIDS and disability in Africa.* Retrieved 18 November 2005 from http://www.rehab-international.org/publications/ Vanneste.htm

*Address for correspondence:*
Mrs. N. Mbethe, Home Director
Sizanani Village
P.O. Box 1372
Bronkhorstspruit 1020 GP
South Africa
www.sizanani.org, info@sizanani.org, director@sizanani.org

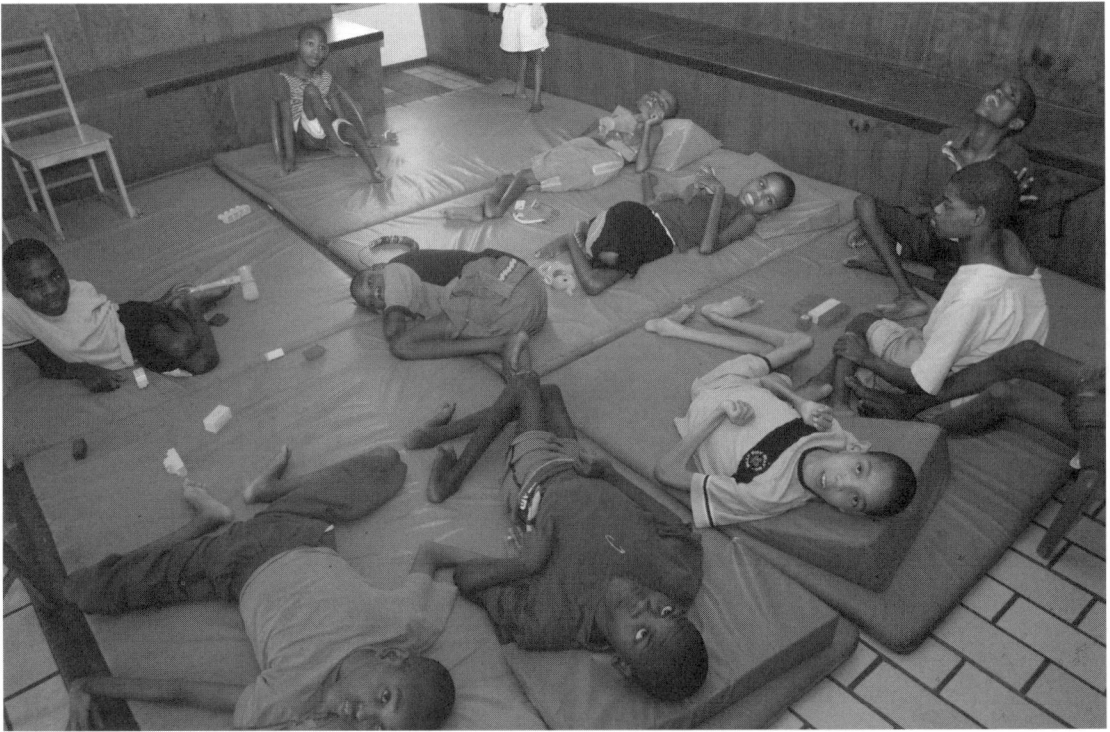

# Chapter 10

# The Need for a Developmental Programme in a Home for Children with Developmental Disabilities

*Thirza Tamboer[1], Gunilla Groenhuijzen[1], Nthoana Mbethe[2], Adri Vermeer[1]*

[1] Department of Educational Sciences, Utrecht University, Utrecht, The Netherlands
[2] St. Mary's Home, Sizanani Village, Bronkhorstspruit, South Africa

## Abstract

This study was conducted in a centre for children with developmental disabilities, where developmental stimulation is lacking for of all kinds of reasons. The goal of this study was to consider if implementation of a developmental programme would be possible and which programme this should be.

A report of the current situation in the Home was made, describing the disabilities of the children, observing the level of guidance the children receive from their caregivers and asking the caregivers what needs, problems and wishes they have regarding their work.

Restrictions in the activities of the children did not always seem to be in line with their physical capabilities, which could be indicative of a lack of stimulation and learning opportunities. During the activities of feeding, bathing and dressing it was found that there was hardly any interaction between child and caregiver. The level of guidance a child received from a caregiver proved to be unrelated to the severity of the disability of that child. The caregivers do say that they want more time to interact with the children although no daily activities mentioned as an opportunity for this could be observed.

Conductive Education, a developmental educational and training programme, focusing at what children with neurological disorders need to learn to cope with the daily demands at home, at school and in their leisure time, seems to be a suitable programme to introduce in this Home, although implementation will only succeed with sufficient commitment of the caregivers.

## 1. Introduction

In 1993, a centre for children with physical disabilities, in particular children with neurological disorders, and HIV patients, was founded as a mission in Bronkhorstspruit (South Africa) by an Austrian priest, Fr. Charles Kuppelwieser. The centre is closely located to a number of townships where more than 100,000 people live. The centre attracts children and their caregivers mainly from these townships. The centre consists of a church, craft workshops, 'rondavels' for guests, a restaurant, a conference centre, a recreation park, a hospice for HIV patients, and a home for children with physical disabilities. After the start, the centre has grown to be a home for almost 200 children with physical and intellectual disabilities, caused by neurological disorders, between the age of 2 and 24 years. They are taken care of by approximately 110 employees for the whole centre, among them two fully qualified nurses, one occupational therapist with three assistants, one social worker en one physiotherapist, who works as a volunteer. There is one childcare worker for every seven children .

Taking a look around in the Home, one would observe that the children are very well taken care of. Despite this, the amount of treatment and education they receive is not sufficient, due to a shortage of paramedical and educational staff and a high childcare worker-child ratio. As a result of this, the disabilities of the children cannot be sufficiently treated and numerous developmental problems exist. Disability is defined as the restriction in the execution of daily activities (WHO, 1980).

At this moment it is very important for the Home to get a perspective on the future. As it is now, once children have come to the home, they stay there. At the time this research took place, they did not show levels of independence, which could be reached. If children only come and never leave, the Home will become overcrowded. What is needed is a way to stimulate the children in their development so that not only the Home itself, but also every individual child gets a perspective on the future. This is why this study aims to consider if the implementation of a developmental programme would be possible and which programme this should be. To this end, the following research objectives were set:

1. to describe the disabilities of the children;
2. to describe the daily care situation in the centre;
3. to identify the needs, problems and wishes of the childcare workers;
4. to use all this information to give an advice about the implementation of a developmental programme.

Emphasis was placed on the needs, problems and wishes of the childcare workers, as previous projects, for example to better the feeding of the children, remained without any improvement, because it involved only benefit for the child, not for the caregivers. According to the fact that any newly introduced developmental programme will need to have the full support of the childcare workers to survive implementation, a new programme needs to directly meet the problems the workers have to deal with. Only then, there will be sufficient motivation to not only implement but also sustain a new programme, which aims at more independence of the children than could be realised now.

## 2. Methods

### 2.1. Participants
The children live in seven blocks of which two blocks were left out of the study because the children living there have a high level of independence already. Therefore, they do not need much attention from the caregivers with respect to their daily functioning. Each block provides a home for twenty to thirty children who are placed there according to their mental age. One block is a 'baby block': this is where the youngest children live. Another block is specifically for children with behavioural problems. Two blocks are for children with moderate disabilities and one is for the really severely disabled and dependent children. The total number of children participating in this study is 133, of which 59% is male and 41% female. The average age of the children is 12, ranging from 2-24 years.

The number of caregivers working on a block depends on the level of independence of the children living there, ranging from three to six. For the childcare workers, the only inclusion criterion for the study was that they had to have worked in the Home, on one of the seven blocks, for at least three months, so they had enough experience to participate in the study. The average age of the childcare workers is 34.8 years, with a range from 24-54 years. The average working experience is 6 years, with a range from 1-10 years. A total of 36 childcare workers participated in the study.

## 2.2. Instruments

### Classification of Disability

To get a good picture of the children living in the Home, first an inventory was made of the block files and data that were present. Emphasis was placed on dates of birth, diagnoses and information about the way the child had been treated until then. Because it was expected that the files would not be complete and updated, a standardised instrument, the Activities of Daily Living Questionnaire (ADLQ; Thorburn, Desai & Davidson, 1992; Thorburn & Marfo, 1994) was also used to assess the actual functioning of the children. The ADLQ was developed to screen children in developing countries for problems in development, viz. functional disabilities. The instrument consists of 21 yes/no items, which means that the minimum score of 0 indicates that a child has no functional difficulties at all. A score of 21 means that the child has functional difficulties in all the activities of daily life mentioned in the ADLQ. The ADLQ proved to be sensitive to identify the presence, absence and severity of a functional disability in children in developing countries (Thorburn, 1994). Of course, the determination of the child being disabled was unnecessary in this case, but the instrument is very useful to get more specific information about the functional (dis)abilities of the children. A childcare worker who knew the child best answered the questions of the ADLQ, and for the more specific questions, those concerning motor activity, the knowledge of one of the therapists was used. The ADLQ was only completed if the child was in the room so that, while the ADLQ was being filled in by the caregiver, the researchers could observe the child and use their knowledge as an extra check-up.

### Level of Guidance

Using the results of the ADLQ, for every block the three children who scored highest on the ADLQ (i.e. who are most dependent) were selected for observations of feeding, bathing and dressing. As mentioned, the blocks differ widely with regard to the functional level of the children, so by selecting the three most dependent children of the different blocks a large variety in dependency level was assured. The method used for the observation was a standardised, qualitative observation, concerning the guidance of the childcare worker in respect to the child. To this end an observation method constructed by Vermeer (Vermeer, Vos, Lindeman, Van Alphen & Snel, 1989; Vermeer, Westra, Benig, Beks, Diemel & Van den Brink, 1990) was used (see Figure 1).

The instrument offers a framework for categorising the teaching strategies that professionals use to bring a child to an independent performance of a task during therapeutic and other activities. Next to these interventions, also educational actions of the professional can be observed. The intervention categories that are used cover a continuum from 'field-guidance' to 'self-guidance'. In the case of 'field-guidance', guidance is external, coming from the environment or the professional to the child. In the case of 'self-guidance', the independent contribution of the child in the execution of a task is increased. The following classification of intervention levels is made:

1.  guidance of body parts: the intervention is directed to a part of the body;
2.  guidance through physical object: physical objects are used to evoke and guide the movement;
3.  guidance by means of rhythm, music, singing or tone: rhythm is used to evoke and guide the movement;
4.  guidance by means of structuring the immediate environment: the arrangement of the immediate environment evokes and guides performance;
5.  guidance through demonstration: a (visual) representation of (a part of) the movement is given;
6.  verbal guidance: verbal actions are used to evoke or guide the performance of the movement (questioning, explaining, encouraging, etc.);
7.  free exploration after a given task: an instruction to perform a movement is given, the performance is left to the individual.

The following classification is used for the educational actions of the professional:

1.  evaluation: questions and remarks referring to present and/or previous sessions as well as to experiences in everyday life;
2.  personal contact: 'nice weather talk', hugging, 'rough and tumble play'.

The reliability and validity of the instrument were proven in two studies (Vermeer et al., 1989; Vermeer et al., 1990), the first of which was conducted in a setting with children with cerebral palsy and the latter in a setting with persons with mental retardation. Intra- and inter-observer reliability (kappa >.80) and concurrent validity ($r_s$ >.74) proved to be good.

The instrument is a direct observation method using time sampling. For this research though, event sampling was used. This way the scoring was done continuously throughout the activity. The main reason to do this was the fact that most activities only lasted a few minutes and as much information as possible needed to be gained from those minutes.

Before starting the observations, a try-out with the observation instrument was conducted to see if the researchers got the same scores on the instrument while observing the same activity. There was a maximum level of agreement.

The observations of the feeding were done two times for every child. After this, a stability test was conducted. It was found that, even though the second observations of the feeding of the children were done at a different time of the day and with a different caregiver assisting them, 12 of the 15 children scored exactly the same on the level of intervention scale, with Spearman's rho being .65 (p < 0.01). It was therefore decided that the observations of the bathing and dressing would be conducted only once. This decision was prompted by the fact that the observations led to a tense relationship between researchers and caregivers. To not jeopardise the relationship any further, the amount of observations was reduced to a minimum of two for the feeding and one for bathing and dressing.

After the observations of the feeding were completed, the researchers themselves fed every observed child. This was done firstly to gain a better understanding of the way the caregivers work, secondly to personally experience which difficulties the feeding involved and, thirdly, to build a more trusting relationship between the researchers, children and caregivers.

| time sample | 1 | 2 | 3 | 4 | 5 | 6 | 7 | etc |
|---|---|---|---|---|---|---|---|---|
| *field-guidance/self-guidance* | | | | | | | | |
| 1 of body parts | | | | | | | | |
| 2 through physical objects | | | | | | | | |
| 3 through rhythm, music, etc | | | | | | | | |
| 4 structuring environment | | | | | | | | |
| 5 demonstration | | | | | | | | |
| 6 verbal guidance | | | | | | | | |
| 7 free exploration | | | | | | | | |
| 0 no judgement | | | | | | | | |
| *educational actions* | | | | | | | | |
| a evaluation | | | | | | | | |
| b personal contact | | | | | | | | |
| c no judgement | | | | | | | | |

Figure 1: Observation instrument (Vermeer et al., 1989, 1990)

*Needs, Problems and Wishes of the Childcare Workers*

A questionnaire was used to determine the needs, problems and wishes of the childcare workers. The questionnaire was specially developed for this situation and consisted of questions about the work of the caregivers, the problems encountered during feeding, bathing and dressing of the child, but also questions about what has to be changed in the Home, to make it a better home for the children, as well as a better place to work for the caregivers. As the questionnaire was in English, it had to be found out if this would lead to any problems in understanding the questions. Therefore, a test-session was held. From this, it was learned that language was not going to be a problem for most of them, but the collecting of the questionnaires after a few days did not have the desired result. Of the seven questionnaires, not one was handed in at the appointed time. Therefore, the procedure was changed. The questionnaires had to be filled in in presence of one of the researchers, who could then immediately collect them afterwards. This also yielded the advantage that, if a childcare worker met a difficulty in understanding a question, this could be clarified. That the researcher was present also made it possible to prevent the caregivers from discussing the questions among themselves, which could lead to 'unanimous' answers, instead of the individual, personal answers that were aimed for.

## 2.3. Procedure and Statistics

The management of the Home gave permission for this study and allowed the children to be part of it. The staff was instructed by the management to give their full support to this research and help the researchers when needed. Although contact with the children was easily established, it took the researchers almost two months to build a trusting relationship with the caregivers. Still the majority of the caregivers was reluctant to co-operate and really needed to be persuaded to give their co-operation. This can be explained partly by the history of South Africa, black people still have problems with giving trust to white people, trust needs to be earned. On the other hand the reluctance to co-operate was fed by the idea that it would not matter whether or not they co-operated, nothing could be done to change the way things are going in Sizanani. To overcome this reluctance, the researchers took the time to get acquainted with the staff and slowly introduced the research in the Home, taking time for discussion and 'small talk' before starting the research activities.

This research must be considered as a description of the actual situation of the Home and therefore uses mainly descriptive statistics.

## 3. Results

### 3.1. Description of the Disabilities of the Children
The screening of the existing block files of the children gave information about date of birth and date of arrival in St. Mary's Home. Diagnoses as 'mental retardation' and 'cerebral palsy' were mentioned in most files, but without any record of a physical and/or mental examination of the child. It was found that no standard file existed, every file looked different and consisted of different kinds of records, most of them dated. The procedure of the assignment to the Home is done by the district medical doctor.

The ADLQ was conducted for the children of the five mentioned blocks, to get a better overview of the abilities of the children. Table 1 gives an overview of the data of the complete group and of the separate blocks, to get insight in the level of functioning of the children from the different blocks.

Block A and B are homes for children with minor disabilities, as can be seen from Table 1. But these blocks also show the widest range on scores for ADLQ, which means that the differences in the children's level of functioning is big within the group. In the children's blocks C, D and E, the children are dependent in several activities of daily life and the difference between them is not so big.

**Table 1: Data on the ADLQ of the children of 5 blocks (A-E)**

| Block | N | Average score ADLQ | SD | Range (min-max) |
|---|---|---|---|---|
| A (Thembaletu) | 22 | 10.27 | 3.44 | 14 (2-16) |
| B (Tsakane) | 25 | 10.56 | 4.69 | 16 (2-18) |
| C (Leseding) | 23 | 14.26 | 1.89 | 8 (11-19) |
| D (Botshabelo) | 33 | 15.82 | 2.08 | 9 (10-19) |
| E (Thokozani) | 30 | 16.33 | 1.63 | 8 (12-20) |
| Total | 133 | 13.76 | 3.83 | 18 (2-20) |

Figure 2 gives the results of the ADLQ per item for the whole group (N=133). On the item 'takes part in family activities', all children scored a 'no', because the children are not living with their families. A striking result is the fact that over 80% of the children are able to move their arms, but that this, obviously, does not give them any independence in functional tasks like brushing their teeth or eating. Over 50% of the children understand what is said to them, but again, this does not seem to help them in fulfilling activities of daily living. Although only less than 40% of the children are able to express emotions and feelings, the caregivers' impression is that over 75% of them have pains and aches, especially in their joints due to spasms.

### 3.2. Level of Guidance
For every block, three children were selected who (1) had the highest score for the ADLQ and (2) scored a 'no', i.e. are dependent, for the items bathing, dressing and feeding. If more than three children fulfilled these conditions, the oldest ones were chosen. Table 2 gives an overview of the children that participated in the observations. The letters A to E refer to the blocks as mentioned in Table 1.

**Results ADLQ**

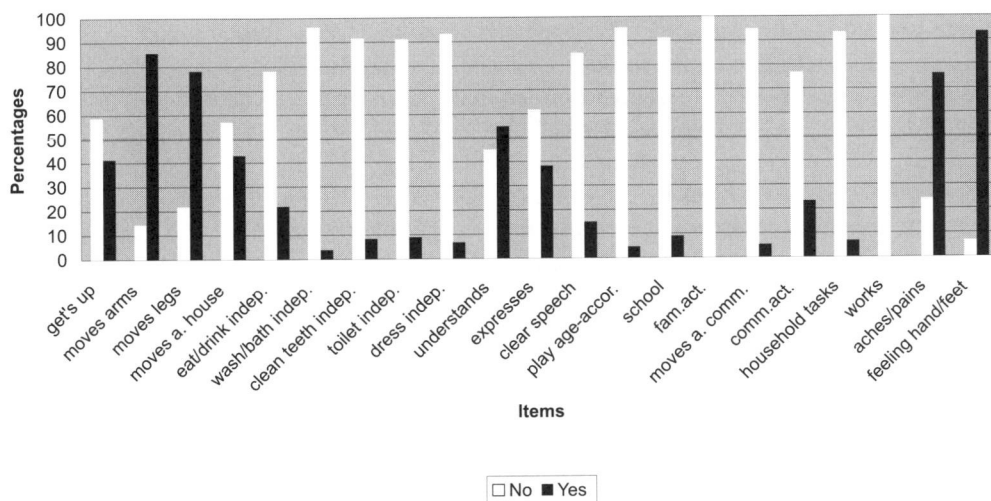

Figure 2: Scores of the total group (N=133) on the items of the ADLQ

Table 2: Children (N=15) participating in the observations

| Child | Score on ADLQ, mean of 1-3 | Age (years) | Gender |
|---|---|---|---|
| A1 | 16 | 9.42 | Male |
| A2 | 14 | 7.58 | Male |
| A3 | 13 (14.3) | 19 | Male |
| B1 | 18 | 14.67 | Female |
| B2 | 17 | 17.5 | Female |
| B3 | 15 (16.7) | 7.58 | Female |
| C1 | 19 | 12.67 | Male |
| C2 | 16 | 12.08 | Female |
| C3 | 16 (17) | 8.58 | Male |
| D1 | 19 | 13.17 | Male |
| D2 | 19 | 17.58 | Male |
| D3 | 19 (19) | 16.42 | Male |
| E1 | 20 | 7.42 | Male |
| E2 | 19 | 12.5 | Male |
| E3 | 19 (19.3) | 11.5 | Female |

*Feeding*

The 15 children were all observed twice and fed once by one of the researchers. The difference in level of functioning of these children and also the difference between the blocks becomes clear when looking at the time it takes to feed the children. For block A this ranges from 2 to 8 minutes, for block B from 5 to 22 minutes, for block C from 5 to 8, for block D from 5 to 15 and for block E the time to feed a child ranges from 12 to 16 minutes.

Five children were fed sitting in their wheelchair, which was tilted backwards. One child was sitting in her wheelchair, which was in an upright position. Six children were sitting on regular 'highchairs' while being fed. One child was fed lying on her back on a puff, one child was sitting independently on the floor and one child was fed lying on the floor with a wedge-shaped pillow under her head.

As can be seen in Table 3, 24 times a score 2 was given, viz. the interaction between caregiver and child took place through a physical object, in this case a spoon. This means that the child was expected to know what to do just by seeing or smelling the food, seeing the spoon or feel it touch his mouth. Only two times educational actions were observed in the form of 'nice weather talk', which means that 28 times no educational actions of the caregiver were observed.

The main problem with feeding the children is the fact that most of them have difficulty opening their mouth, chewing and/or swallowing. Because of this, feeding the children can be exhausting and as a consequence time-absorbing. In such cases there is often too little time for careful feeding. The caregivers consider this their biggest problem, because there are so many children that need to be fed.

*Bathing*

Fifteen observations of bathing were done. The bathing lasted a minimum of 2 and a maximum of 5 minutes. The bathing was always done by one caregiver, only the lifting in and out of the bath of the bigger children was done with assistance of a colleague. Most children were lying on their back in the tub, unable to sit up unassisted. The washing was done in the tub all the times except for one time, when this particular caregiver used the dressing table to wash the child and only rinsed the child in the tub. She did this with every child she washed because she felt it was safer. Most children looked comfortable in the tub, two really expressed this by singing and laughing, only one cried during the bathing.

During the observations, the children were always safe and secure. The caregivers always made sure there was not too much water in the tub and the children were placed with their feet in the deep end of the tub. Temperature was always checked first. Two times, a child that was observed had an open wound. In this case the caregiver made sure the bathing was as little painful as possible. As for the caregivers, most of the time they looked comfortable although they usually work in a high, hurrying tempo. Lifting the children from their chair or from the ground onto the dressing table is straining. Then lifting the child from the dressing table into the bath as well. When the child is in the bath, the caregiver has to bend forward to be able to wash the child, which is really hard on the lower back. During the observations, no equipment was used to support the child or caregiver.

Using the observation instrument of Vermeer et al. (1990), nine times a score 1 was given. This indicates that no information about the bathing was given to the child, the child was just put passively into the right position. Of these nine scores, with 6 of them a score 2 was given on 'educational actions'. Although the caregiver was not communicating with the child about the activity they were doing, she was talking to the child about more general subjects, the so-called 'nice weather' conversations. Two times a score 3 was given: the caregiver used singing to stimulate the child in sitting actively in the tub. Four times a score 6 was given. This was done when the caregiver really told the child what she expected of him during the bathing and gave him instructions. These four caregivers did not talk to the child about other issues, however, so they scored a 0 on educational actions.

Spasms and stiffness of the children cause the biggest problem during the bathing. Also the lifting of the children puts a major strain on the caregivers.

*Dressing*
Fifteen dressing observations were carried out for the children mentioned in Table 2. The time it takes to dress the children ranges from 2 to 5 minutes. The dressing was done by one caregiver, sometimes assisted by a colleague for the lifting. The children are always dressed on the dressing table. This is a high sort of table; it is a good height for the caregivers to work on. The only difficulty is the lifting on and off the table. In all cases the child and caregiver looked comfortable. The child was always safe although the only protection from falling of the table is the caregiver. When she turns away to get something or when she has to give attention to another child, a dangerous situation *could* be created, but this has not been observed. There was no equipment used to support child or caregiver.

Ten times a 1 was scored with the observation instrument, which means that the caregiver interacts with the child through body parts. She touches and turns him to dress him. Because the child knows the routine, he knows what is going to happen and 'goes with the flow'. Of these ten times, only one time the caregiver talked to the child. Not about the activity but 'nice weather talk'. Five times a 6 was scored. In these cases the caregiver gave the child verbal information about what she was going to do or what she wanted him to do. All these five times the caregiver also talked to the child about other things, or played with him while dressing him, which leads to a score 2 on the second scale. In four occasions the caregiver stimulated the senses of the child by calling his name, responding to sounds he made etc. The biggest problems caregivers encounter in dressing the children are their struggles with the children's spasms and stiffness.

**Table 3: Field-guidance/self-guidance during feeding, bathing and dressing**

|  | Feeding obs. 1 | Feeding obs. 2 | Bathing | Dressing |
|---|---|---|---|---|
| 1 Of body parts |  |  | 9 | 10 |
| 2 Through physical objects | 13 | 11 |  |  |
| 3 Rhythm, music | 1 |  | 2 |  |
| 4 Structuring Environment |  | 2 |  |  |
| 5 Demonstration |  |  |  |  |
| 6 Verbal guidance | 1 | 2 | 4 | 5 |
| 7 Free exploration |  |  |  |  |
| 0 No judgement |  |  |  |  |
| Total | 15 | 15 | 15 | 15 |
| *educational actions* |  |  |  |  |
|  | Feeding obs. 1 | Feeding obs. 2 | Bathing | Dressing |
| 1 Evaluation |  |  |  |  |
| 2 Personal contact | 1 | 1 | 6 | 6 |
| 0 No judgement | 14 | 14 | 9 | 9 |
| Total | 15 | 15 | 15 | 15 |

### 3.3. Relationship between Extent of Disability and Level of Guidance

To establish if there was any relationship between the extent of the disability of a child (expressed by an ADLQ score) and the way the caregivers interacted with this child (expressed by the score on the observation instrument), this relationship was calculated for the feeding, bathing and dressing. The correlation (Pearsons r) between ADLQ score and the scores on the observation instrument of the first observation of the feeding (Table 3) is .18 (p> .05). For the ADLQ score and the second feeding observation it is .15 (p> .05). The correlation ADLQ-bathing is .10 (p> .05), the correlation ADLQ-dressing is .09 (p > .05). All results are far from significant (p> .05), which means that there is no relationship between the level of functioning of a child, or in other words, the level of independence, and the way the caregivers interact with this child during feeding, bathing and dressing.

### 3.4. Needs, Problems and Wishes of the Childcare Workers

#### The Caregivers and their Work

The results of the questionnaires first gave information about the age, working experience and the block in which the childcare workers are working at the moment. For the questionnaire, the childcare workers were asked how they experience the work on the two blocks that were not included in the study (Ekukhanyeni and Leratong). Besides this general information, the questionnaire provided information about how the caregivers experience their work, what kind of problems they encounter during their daily tasks and what has to be changed for the Home to improve.

During the daily work, the childcare workers have to deal with several tasks. After the morning ritual of bathing, dressing, feeding and tooth brushing, there is time for play, exercise and stimulation of the children. After their nap until two o'clock in the afternoon and after the children's snack at three o'clock, there is spare time to play with the children and stimulate them. The childcare workers were asked if they were able to finish their work on time. 50% of the childcare workers say that they are able to finish their work on time, based on the regimes they have developed. The other 50% say that they did not finish on time due to shortage of staff, too many children, too much work and because of not being able to spend time with the children.

#### Experience of Workload per Block

As mentioned before, the children are placed in different blocks according to their mental age and the disabilities they have. This means that every block has a different group of children with different kinds of problems. The researchers wanted to know if there were childcare workers that had working experience on another block than the block where they were working now and how they experienced their work on the different blocks.

This question was asked to get an idea about the connection between the composition of the group in a particular block and the way they experience working on that block. 34 childcare workers (94.4%) have experience working on different blocks. Two childcare workers simply did not have experience on different blocks. To answer this question they could mark the weight of their experience for every block (see Table 4). The percentages are calculated over the total number of childcare workers per block. The childcare workers of the blocks F (Ekukhanyeni) and G (Leratong) who were not involved in the study, received a questionnaire too. Their results are also included in Table 4

Table 4:  Experience of workload per block

|  | Real hard | Hard | Good to do | Easy | Very Easy |  |  |
|---|---|---|---|---|---|---|---|
|  | 1 | 2 | 3 | 4 | 5 | Total % | Total N |
| Block A | 7.2% | 50.0% | 32.1% | 10.7% | - | 100% | 28 |
| Block B | 12.5% | 18.8% | 37.5% | 18.8% | 12.5% | 100% | 32 |
| Block C | 55.2% | 27.5% | 3.5% | 3.5% | 10.3% | 100% | 29 |
| Block D | 57.6% | 30.3% | 12.2% | - | - | 100% | 33 |
| Block E | - | 54.6% | 22.7% | 5.0% | 18.2% | 100% | 20 |
| Block F | 45.8% (1) | 37.5% | 8.3% | 4.2% | 4.2% | 100% | 24 |
| Block G | 9.5% | 14.3% | 33.3% | 28.6% | 14.3% | 100% | 21 |

Block C and D are regarded as 'real hard' blocks. Block C is a big girls' group. The children here are very dependent. Block D is mentioned as the heaviest block to work on. It is a diverse block with a lot of small and not very heavy children, but the children are very difficult to be fed. In block A, the children are not so big and heavy what particularly makes lifting easier. Block B consists of less disabled children. The scores 3-5 are given because a lot of the children are considered to be independent in comparison with the children of other blocks. Block F is a big boys' block and 45.8% scored 'real hard'. The difficulty had to do with the weight of these boys. They are heavy and big and have to be lifted during bathing, bringing to bed etc.

*Options for Improving the Work of the Childcare Workers*
Many aspects will influence someone's feeling if he/she likes his/here job. First, it was asked how the childcare workers (N=36) experience their work. The answering possibilities ranged from 'Don't like it' (1) to 'I love it' (5). 40 % of the childcare workers loves their job, 22.8% really likes it, 20 % likes it, 14.3% says 'it is OK' and only one childcare worker (2.8%) 'doesn't like' her job.  Secondly, the childcare workers were asked to give their opinion about 15 options that could improve their work as a childcare worker if the option was introduced (see Table 5).

Table 5: The options to improve the work mentioned by the childcare workers

|  | Options | % of yes |
|---|---|---|
| 1 | More staff | 100.0% |
| 2 | Better salary | 94.4% |
| 3 | Course about the disabilities of the children | 77.7% |
| 4 | Course about organisation | 75.0% |
| 5 | More responsibility | 72.2% |
| 6 | Course about child communication | 66.6% |
| 7 | Course about staff communication | 66.6% |
| 8 | Feeding course | 63.8% |
| 9 | Course first aid | 61.1% |
| 10 | Course about entertaining children | 61.1% |
| 11 | More swaps in the working schedule | 58.0% |
| 12 | Course about nutrition | 52.7% |
| 13 | Toilet training course | 52.7% |
| 14 | Dressing course | 50.0% |
| 15 | Washing course | 36.1% |

The results are clear. In the first place, the childcare workers would like to have improvements of their working circumstances (personnel, salary). Thereafter, improvements of the contents of their word are mentioned.

After getting an idea about what the childcare workers think would improve their job, it was asked what kind of suggestions the childcare workers had about improving the working in the Home. 'Better communication will improve the Home', is the suggestion given by 66.6% of the childcare workers. Communication is divided in communication between staff members and communication between management and staff. Of the caregivers that mention communication as an issue for improvement, 57.5% thinks that communication between staff and management needs change. They want the management to be more involved in the work of the caregivers so that the management will better understand the problems they encounter. An example given here is the problem of lifting. Better lifting equipment is desired for the washing of big children. The childcare workers also wish to have recognition from the management for their work and for what they know about the children. A way to get that recognition is to be involved in important matters like providing the social worker with information that can help the parents of the child. In this way, the childcare workers' knowledge and voice would count.

There is a wish for programmes about making children more independent. It was also asked if the childcare worker thought that her work would become less difficult if a child needs less help in daily activities. 80 % of the childcare workers thought it would make their work less difficult. Introducing new programmes also requires a great deal of motivation on the part of the childcare workers.

*Practical Problems*

Questions also were asked about the problems experienced with the children during the daily activities like bathing, dressing, feeding and going to the toilet. It is necessary to respond to the problems experienced by the childcare workers, before introducing a new programme.

*The main difficulties when bathing the children:* Lifting the children in and out of the bathtub is more rule then exception and causes a lot of back problems. Besides the weight of the children, there is the safety problem. One childcare worker has to wash seven or more children by herself and is lucky when she is helped by a colleague. Stiffness and spasms of the child also provide problems with opening the hands, moving the legs and arms outwards in order to wash the child properly. Most of the children are lying in the bathtub and when a child moves his head aside because of uncontrolled movement, it could swallow some water and easily choke on it. The other children are waiting for their turn on the floor of the bathroom. It has happened that one child was lying in the bathtub and the child sitting on the floor was getting a fit. Apart form all the problems mentioned above, there is the trouble of dividing the children. Some staff members do not want to wash children at all and others will only wash the easy ones.

*The main difficulties when dressing the children:* Dressing is only a problem with children suffering from stiffness, spasms and restlessness. Sometimes, the legs are so crossed that it takes a long time before relaxation is realised and the trousers can be put on or the nappy changed. Sometimes the dressing would be easier if the clothing had more stretch. When a child is restless, it is difficult to dress because the child keeps on moving and jumping around, so that a colleague is needed for assistance.

*The main difficulties when feeding the children*: There are many problems with feeding the children. Some children do not chew and others can not chew properly, and a lot of the children are slow eaters. There are children who will push the food out of their mouth with their tongue and others are coughing or spitting the food out. Some cannot open their jaws easily and others will keep the jaws locked. It also happens that a child opens his or her mouth but locks it before the spoon is out and it takes some time before the spoon is released. A common consequence of being fed in a lying position is coughing and choking on food.

*The main difficulties when helping the children going to the toilet:* Most of the children need help getting on and off the toilet seat. Picking up the child from the ground, and putting the child on the toilet is a heavy job and cannot be done alone when a child is very heavy, which makes the childcare worker dependent on her colleague. It can take a while before the child is finished, and because the child cannot say for himself that he is finished, it happens that a child is sitting on the toilet for half an hour, not noticed by anyone. The smaller children with spasms will lower through the toilet seat with their pelvis. It gives them stability, but this position requires more strength from the childcare worker to take the child off the toilet. After using the toilet, there is the trouble of dressing the child because the child cannot stand on his or her own feet and the childcare worker has to struggle to get the clothes back on.

## 4. Conclusions and Discussion

Considering the fact that this research was descriptive, a great deal of information was gathered about the Home which allows a number of conclusions to be drawn. In this report, only the conclusions that are relevant to the goal of this study, viz. the introduction and implementation of a developmental programme, are drawn and discussed.

### 4.1. Diagnostic Information and Treatment Records

From the description of the existing block files, it can be concluded that no structure exists in file-keeping. Taking into account that at the time of this research the treatment in the Home relied on therapists who came as volunteers, the lack of diagnostic information and treatment records could be a problem. Volunteers mostly stay for only one year and are then replaced by another volunteer. Without properly keeping record of the care and development of a child, a new therapist will have to start all over again making his own examination of a child. In this way, valuable time is wasted. If all children would be examined using the same instrument, for example the Top Down Motor Milestone Test (Bidabe & Lolar, 1990), the Gross Motor Function Measure (Russell, Rosenbaum, Gowland, Hardy, Lane, Plews, McGavin, Cadman & Jarvis, 1993) or the Pediatric Evaluation of Disabilty Inventory (Haley, Coster, Ludlow, Haltiwanger & Andrellos, 1992), this would offer a good guideline from which to start treatment. This would also provide a solution to the problem that every new therapist comes in with his own ideas about the treatment and care of the children. The therapist is not inclined to continue the treatment of his predecessor, because it does not fit in with his ideas and no proper report of the treatment is available. The Home should have a protocol for the care and the development of the (dis)abilities of the children, which would assure the continuity of the care and, as a result, provide better outcomes. This should be agreed on with new therapists before accepting them as volunteers.

## 4.2. *Extent of Disabilities and Level of Guidance*

A surprising result is that, according to the ADLQ, most children can use their arms, but are unable to eat. For a major part this can be explained by the fact that the ADLQ inquires after any movement of the arms and this is possible for almost every child, even the severely stiff or spastic ones. Of course, eating requires fine motor skills. But this does not entirely explain the fact that almost 80% of the children are not able to eat independently. It was noticed during the observations that there is no time for the child to explore. This was seen during the feeding, but also during bathing and dressing. There is almost no time to take a minute to smell or taste the food, to feel the water and play with it, or to try to put your sock by yourself. No time for the child to explore also means that caregivers have no time for this. No time is taken to observe if the child could possibly do the task, or small parts of the tasks, by itself. In one case, however, it was observed that the caregiver stimulated a child to come into the tub by himself, instead of lifting him into it. Just seeing this child, one would not expect him to be able to do so. Obviously, the caregiver found out that he was able to do this by just trying and teaching him, probably motivated by the fact that this particular child is very big and heavy and that it is not possible to lift him alone. Another explanation is that the caregiver has learned to know what this child is able to do.

The fact that the children are not being stimulated to co-operate was especially clear in the observations of the bathing. In 12 out of the 15 cases, the child was sitting in the bath completely passively. Only with four children active interaction was sought after during the bathing, for example, letting them try to get into the bath by themselves, after lift their arms when they needed to be washed etc. In one case, the child was actively working against the caregiver because he did not want to be bathed.

By exploring and using the full potential of every child, the caregivers would not only make their job more pleasant, but also more challenging and motivating. For a child, no matter how severely disabled, it is important to always have the feeling that he is learning new things and being stimulated to do so.

The most striking result of the observations during the feeding is that 24 out of 30 times, there was no verbal interaction between child and caregiver, only interaction through the spoon. If a caregiver talks, it is usually to colleagues, not to the children. This does not mean that the caregivers are not focused on the child they are feeding. Although eye contact is very rare, most of the caregivers look at the child to see if he is taking the food well and to make sure the mouth is empty before offering the next spoonful. If these observations are compared with the results of the questionnaires, in which caregivers express their wish to have more interaction with the children, it is strange that the feeding should be done in this impersonal way.

## 4.3. *Needs, Problems and Wishes of the Childcare Workers*

### Needs and Wishes

One of the results of this study is that that the caregivers are of the opinion that more staff is needed. The caregiver-child ratio is 1:7, which is too high, especially during washing and feeding and mostly for the blocks with the older, bigger and more severely disabled children.

A striking result is that the options for introducing courses about dressing, feeding, washing and toilet training scored the lowest of all possible options. The childcare workers do not see the benefit of receiving courses about Activities of Daily Life (ADL), and that is remarkable, because practical problems of ADL are mentioned by all childcare workers. They do need information and skills to make their work less difficult and heavy, and to learn how to make the children more independent.

In general, the answers to the question how the work of the childcare workers could be improved are not easy to interpret. The best way is to consider them for what they are: the answers give an impression of a way of thinking. All kind of arguments can be put forward to falsify some answers by confronting them with reality. However, this was not a purpose of this research. One of the - in fact indirect - purposes was to involve the childcare workers in a reflection about their work. Accordingly, they may say what they think. This is the perspective from which the answers of the childcare workers have to be considered.

*Problems*
The main problem is the lifting of the bigger, older and more severely disabled children.

Stimulating the children to be independent should not take place when they have become too heavy or too restricted in their activities. The children in the Home could be trained years earlier, e.g. to get into the bathtub by themselves. Childcare workers have to clearly understand that when they learn new skills, sometimes these are skills for prevention, skills with a long-term goal. They will not see the benefit immediately because the skills are for preventing children becoming too dependent and childcare workers getting lower back problems. The toilet training course had the highest score. A lot of the children wear nappies. Toilet training requires some equipment which, when implemented, will prevent the child to get lower into the toilet and enable him getting on and off the toilet independently.

Another issue worth mentioning is the repeatedly problem of positioning. Many of the children with severe disabilities, for example, are being fed in a lying position and with a lot of difficulties like coughing and choking. After being fed, they are still lying down and therefore experience the world from a lying position, even if they have some motor abilities. These children could use some training in order to systematically acquire motor skills needed for a relatively independent life at home and community environments.

To make the child's life more independent and the caregiver's work worker easier, investment becomes a condition. Investment means more time for the children and consulting one another as colleagues and as management and employee. 50% of the childcare workers, however, cannot finish the daily care of the children within the required time. This means there is no time for extra stimulation of the children. The childcare workers would like to have more personal contact with the children, playing games, going out to explore, etc. It appears that daily care on the one hand and personal contact, play, going out to explore on the other, are regarded as separate matters. However, these apparently different kinds of activities have to be integrated in the daily interaction between caregiver and child. Exploration, playing games and exploration of one's own capabilities in interaction with the environment during the performance of daily activities can be done within the framework of the newly to be introduced developmental programmes.

## 4.5. Suitable Developmental Programmes
The term 'developmental programme' refers to a programme that stimulates a child in every aspect of its development.

On the basis of information that was gathered from previous visits to the Home and interviews with staff members prior to this study, two programmes were selected which, in principle, could be suitable for the Home. These programmes are the Mobility Opportunities via Education (MOVE) Programme (Bidabe & Lolar, 1990), and Conductive Education, also called the Petö-Method (Hari & Akos, 1988; Cottam & Sutton, 1988; Van der Hoek, De Groot & Vermeer, 1992).

MOVE is a top-down, activity-based curriculum, designed to teach students basic, functional motor skills needed for adult life in home and community environments. The programme is suited for children who have not developed the physical skills necessary to sit independently, bear weight on their feet or take reciprocal steps. For MOVE, special equipment has been constructed. It places the children in positions for performing functional activities and at the same time allows the staff to physically manage the child, while teaching appropriate movement patterns. Although the equipment facilitates the outcomes of the programme, the programme can also be conducted without it.

Conductive Education is a method to stimulate the development of children with a non-progressive cerebral palsy, developed by the Hungarian pedagogue and neurologist András Petö. The strength of this method is that it does not divide the child's disability into different problems, but sees it as a whole. The main goal of Conductive Education is to teach the child to be as independent as possible. This is done by a conductor, a professional who combines a number of different disciplines, like physiotherapy, occupational therapy and special education. Children usually work in small groups, depending on age and the severity of the disability, with a maximum of five children per group, guided by a conductor. Conductive Education not only challenges the children but also provides tranquillity and structure for them. They are no longer confronted with all kinds of different therapists and disciplines. Conductive Education is suited for all non-progressive brain damages (cerebral palsy and spina bifida). There is no age limit but the child needs to be able to understand some basic things. A big advantage of this programme is also that parents and caregivers are involved in the execution of the training activities.

It was arranged that two staff members of the Home could visit The Netherlands to see these two programmes in practice at different centres for children with severe disabilities. After this, the current study was conducted to make a definite decision about the suitability of different developmental programmes.

It was concluded that Conductive Education and MOVE would both fit well in the situation of the Home. Preference is given to Conductive Education because this is an integrated training programme, which involves parents and caregivers, fulfils the immediate needs of the Home and requires less expensive equipment.

## References

Bidabe, L. & Lollar, J.M. (1990). *MOVE: Mobility Opportunities Via Education*, Kern County Superintendent of Schools, Bakersfield.

Cottam, P. & Suton, A. (1988). *Conductive Education, a system to overcome motor disorders.* London: Croom Helm Ltd.

Haley, S.M., Coster, W.J., Ludlow, L.H., Haltiwnger, J.T. & Andrellos, P.J. (1992). *Pediatric Evaluation of Disability Inventory.* Boston: New England Medical Center.

Hari, M. & Akos, K. (1971). *Conductive education.* London: Tavistock –Routeledge.

Hoek, A. van der, Groot, L, de, Vermeer, A. (1992). *De Petö-methode: Een geïntegreerde opvang van het hersenbeschadigde kind.* Amsterdam: VU Uitgeverij.

Thorburn, M.J. (1994). Achievements of the Ten Questions and possibilities for its practical use. In M.I.M. Schuurman (ed). *Assessment of childhood disabilities in developing countries (pp 78-86).* Utrecht: Bisschop Beckers Intitute.

Russell, D, Rosenbaum, P.L., Gowland, C., Hardy, S., Lane, M., Plews, N., McGavin, H., Cadman, D. & Jarvis, S. (1993). *Manual for the Gross Motor Function Measure.* Hamilton, Canada: McMaster University.

Thorburn, M.J., Desai, P. & Davidson, L. (1992). Categories, classes and criteria in childhood disabilities. Experiences from a survey in Jamaica. *Disability and Rehabilitation, 14,* 122-133

Thorburn, M.J. & Marfo, K. (1994). *Practical approaches to childhood disability in developing countries.* Tampa (Fl): Global Age Publishing.

Vermeer, A., Vos, H.W.C.M., Lindeman, A.TH., Alphen, J. van, & Snel, J. (1989). Observing the interventions of teachers and therapists in the movement rehabilitation of cerebral palsied children. *Journal of Rehabilitation Sciences, 2,* 25-32.

Vermeer, A., Westra, T., Benig, T., Beks, C., Diemel, T., & Brink, C. van den (1990). Validation of interventions in Adapted Physical Activities for Mentally Retarded Residents (pp. 85-93). In: A. Vermeer (ed.), *Medicine and Sport Science, 30.* Basel: Karger AG.

WHO (1980). *International Classification of Impairments, Disabilities and Handicaps.* Genova: World Health Organisation.

Wolf-Vereecken, M.J. (1993). *Cerebral Palsy in Africa. Early identification and intervention.* Amsterdam: Tool Publications.

*Address for correspondence:*
Mrs. N. Mbethe
St. Mary's Home
Sizanani Village
P.O. Box 1372
Bronkhorstspruit 1020
South Africa

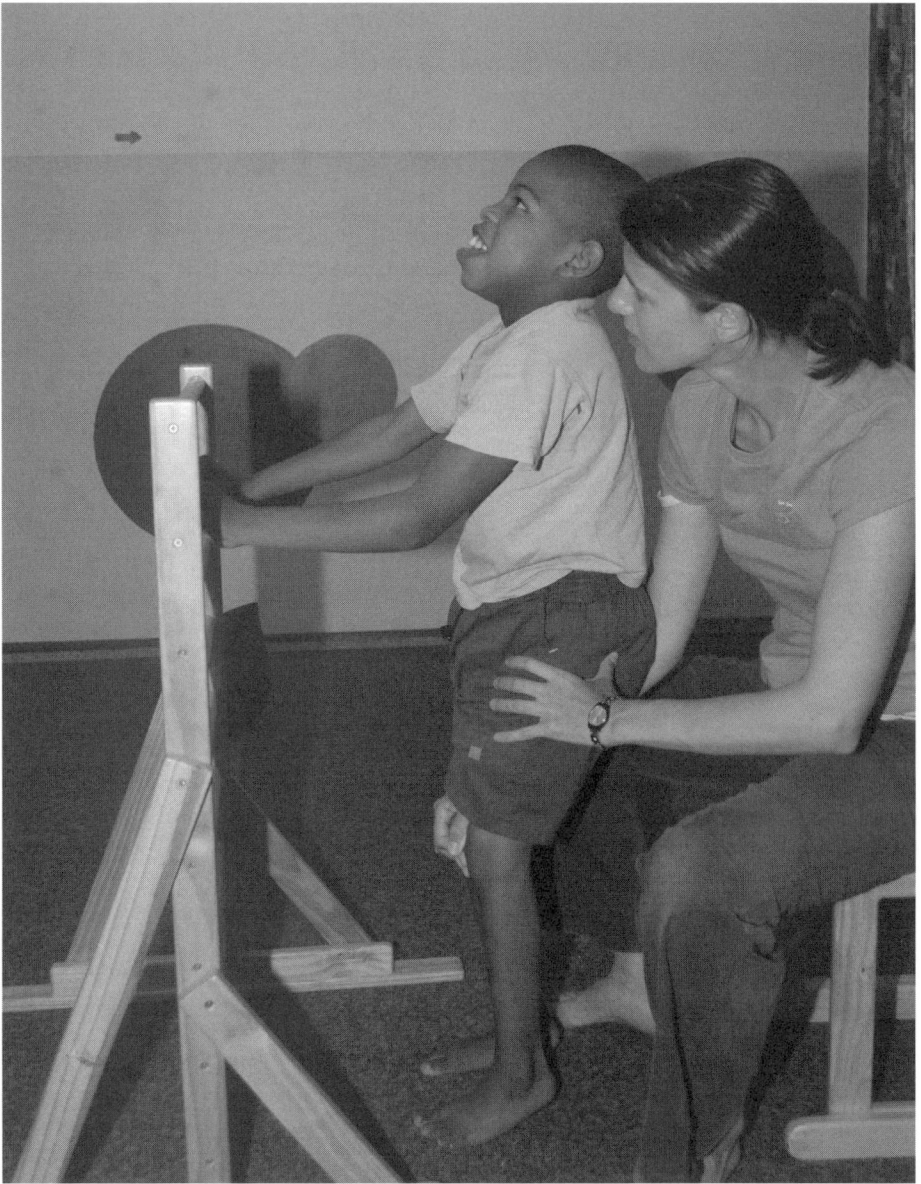

# Chapter 11

# Effects of Conductive Education in a Home for Children with Developmental Disabilities[*]

*Adri Vermeer[1], Lex Wijnroks[1], Zsoka Magyarszeky[2], Nthoana Mbethe[2,**]*

[1] Department of Educational Sciences, Utrecht University, Utrecht, The Netherlands
[2] St. Mary's Home, Sizanani Village, Bronkhorstspruit, South Africa
[*] An earlier version of this article has been published in *Recent Advantages in Conductive Education*, (2006) 4 (2) 9-20.
[**] This research has been conducted over a period of two years by Marischa Fox, Carly van Velzen, Diana van den Broek, Karin Peters, Nyomi Cairo, Emilie Hoogendoorn and Lisa de Bruin

## Abstract

The results of a two-year pilot intervention study into the effects of Conductive Education (CE) on children with developmental disabilities are presented. All participants in the study live at St. Mary's Home, a home for children with physical and intellectual disabilities in South Africa. The design of the study was a pretest-posttest quasi-experimental design with four follow-up measurements. The experimental group of 10 children was individually matched with another group of 10 children, which formed the control group. The experimental group received a daily training in CE and the control group followed the daily routine of the Home. Differences between the two groups were expected for functional abilities (PEDI), quantity (GMFM) and quality of motor skills (GMPM) of the children and for the childcare workers' interaction style (Intervention Observation Instrument) and their attitude towards the new programme (MPOC-SP). No significant results could be established over time. Nevertheless, the experimental group showed more progress than the control group on 22 of the 24 measured variables. Explanations are given for these results. Already at the start of the CE programme, the childcare workers showed a positive attitude towards the new programme and continued to do so during the intervention period. In an Appendix, account is given of the process of implementation of the CE programme in the Home.

## 1. Introduction

In 1993, an Austrian priest founded a centre for children with disabilities in Sizanani Village, Bronkhorstspruit, South Africa. The centre, named St. Mary's Home, is located near a number of townships, in which more than a 100,000 people live. Most of the children and childcare workers come from these townships. Sizanani Village consists of more than only a Home for children and young adults with physical and intellectual disabilities. There is also a church, a meditation centre, a craft work shop, a conference centre, a restaurant, rondavels (round straw-roofed huts) for guests, a recreation park, a special education school and a centre for people infected and affected by HIV/AIDS.

After the start in 1993 the centre has grown to be a home for 170 children with physical and intellectual disabilities, caused by neurological disorders. Their level of dependence ranges from mild to profound and their age ranges from 2 to 31 years, with an average of 15 years. All children and young adults live in one of the seven buildings (blocks) on the premises, grouped according to their age and developmental level. Childcare workers take care of the daily needs of the children, with nurses and occupational therapy assistants supporting them. St. Mary's Home has 67 childcare workers. The number of caretakers working on a block, ranging from two to eight, depends on the level of independence of the children. The average working experience of the childcare workers is 7 years, ranging from 2 to13 years. The children in the Home are well taken care of, but due to a shortage of paramedical and educational staff, the children still do not get enough specialised treatment and education. A previous study in this setting revealed that this would lead to several problems (see Chapter 10). First, the children would not reach a point of relative independence, causing them to stay in the Home. Second, the children would become too heavy to handle as they get older. Difficulties would arise when lifting the children into the bathtub, helping the children with going to and using the toilet and lifting the children onto the dressing table. Third, would be the struggle with the spasms, contractures and restlessness of the children when dressing them.

Depending on the availability of physiotherapists and speech therapists it was possible for at least some period of time to provide the children with additional care. It became clear that this type of care was needed to increase the independence of the children and relieve the childcare workers' workload. To this end Groenhuijzen and Tamboer (see Chapter 10) made an inventory of the disabilities of the children, a description of the daily care situation and a description of the problems and wishes of the childcare workers. They advised the introduction of Conductive Education, a developmental stimulation programme, on a permanent basis. Implementing this programme in St. Mary's Home was expected to enhance the independence of the children and the mastery of daily skills.

## 1.1. Conductive Education

Conductive Education (CE), developed by the Hungarian neurologist and educationalist Dr. András Petö, is a method for children and adults with motor disorders resulting from cerebral palsy[1] and other brain disorders. CE aims to promote a broad spectrum of development, communication, motor, social and daily living skills. All areas are equally important (Bairstow, Cochrane & Hur, 1993). CE places the motor disability in an educational, instead of a medical context and points out that the children often have the potential to achieve various developmental milestones such as sitting and walking. The children often fail to achieve these milestones, because their early efforts are frustrated or the intuitive teaching relationship between parents and children may have been disturbed (Coles & Zsargo, 1998). The main goal of CE is 'orthofunction' which is regarded as an aspect of one's personality (Hari, 1991). An orthofunctional individual is a person who is able to adapt, to cope with and to be creative in any situation in order to find a solution to a problem. CE helps to develop the child's orthofunction by using the whole day as a learning situation, in which the children find solutions to the problems they encounter. Attitude is an important part of orthofunction. Attitude is the ability to solve problems by applying solutions learned from one situation to another. Any good education at any level will submit this (Sutton, 1988), but CE is unique because it applies these learning principles to motor and cognitive development for children with cerebral palsy.

The starting point of CE is that the children have chronic, non-progressive disorders; hence the training is directed at improving their skills in daily functioning, not in treatment of the disorder. Children with cerebral palsy or spina bifida[2] can be included in Conductive Education. The central principle of the method, based on learning theories, is that a motor disorder is a learning difficulty which can be – to some extent – successfully overcome. The learning process focuses on operant conditioning by repeating various tasks in a structured environment. In the end, the learned movement should become an automatism (Van der Hoek, de Groot, & Vermeer, 1992). This way CE teaches children of different age groups to cope with daily demands at home, at school and in their spare time. The CE programmes are always in connection with parents, caregivers or teachers and are executed in a daily schedule. The task series (exercises) are led by the conductor, a professional who combines different disciplines, like physiotherapy, occupational therapy, speech therapy and education. This would be an advantage, because the children are no longer confronted with different therapists and disciplines, therefore CE provides the children continuity and structure. By means of 'rhythmical intention' the execution of the exercises are guided. Rhythmical intention (e.g. counting or singing a song) enables the child to learn normal movement patterns and functional abilities eventually without the help of the conductor. The CE programme also uses specially designed equipment such as beds, benches, chairs and tables to teach children different movements and skills.

## 1.2. Implementation of the CE Programme

The programme started in September 2003. The implementation was in two phases of one year each. In the first phase, that was from September 2003 till September 2004, CE was given to ten children and unit managers were trained in the principles of CE on a daily basis. They learned to apply CE sessions to the ten children, directed by the conductor. The second phase was to start in September 2004 and had to be the training as many childcare workers as possible. This would be done by the trained unit managers supervised by the conductor. Implementation of CE with the children in all the blocks started in September 2005. This study account is concerned with the implementation period from September 2003 till September 2005.

## 1.3. Research

The research to evaluate the effects of CE was conducted as a pretest-posttest quasi-experimental design with four follow-up measurements. The research started with a pretest measurement in September 2003 and ended with the last posttest measurement at the end of August 2005. An experimental group of 10 children received CE four days a week, three hours a day. A control group of 10 children, living in the same setting, followed the normal daily routine of the Home. During each wave the same assessments were executed and the differences between the two groups were compared over time. It was expected that CE would show positive programme effects on the children's level of independence. A selected group of unit managers and childcare workers were trained in the principles of CE. It was expected that after intensive daily training they would show more and more positive involvement with the children.

During every wave the implementation process was evaluated and the improvements and problems were reported and later on used to discuss the implementation on the blocks.

This account is divided into two parts. Part I is concerned with the effects of CE on children and childcare workers. Part II provides a description of qualitative aspects of the implementation process.

The aim of Part I is to assess the effects of the CE programme on both the children and the childcare workers. The effects of CE were expected in several areas. For the children, gains were expected on their functional abilities, quantity and quality of motor movements and their needed level of intervention. For the childcare workers, changes were expected in their attitude towards the new programme. The following research questions had to be answered:

*a. What are the long-term effects of Conductive Education on the children's:*
– development of functional abilities;
– quantity of motor movements;
– quality of motor movements.

*b. What are the effects of Conductive Education on the childcare workers':*
– level of intervention with the children;
– level of involvement in the new programme.

The aim of Part II was to evaluate the process of implementation of the CE programme. Through bi-weekly meetings held with the management and the conductor the evaluation has been kept up to date. Part II is included in the Appendix of this chapter.

## 2. Methods

### 2.1. Subjects
At the start of the study 20 children were selected by the conductor on their potential and suitability to take part in the CE programme. It is important to note that these children were not representative for all children in St. Mary's Home, because the children were not randomly selected from the total population. These 20 children were then divided into two groups of 10 children. The children of both groups were individually matched on five criteria: age, gender, kind of cerebral palsy (CP), diagnosis and school attendance. The children were then randomly assigned to an experimental and a control group. There were no significant differences found between the experimental and the control group on any of the matched variables. The age of the children ranges from 10 to 20 years, with an average of 14 years (Table 1).

**Table 1: Characteristics of the experimental and the control group**

|  |  | experimental | control |
|---|---|---|---|
| age | Mean (SD) | 13,5 (2,7) | 12,0 (2,7) |
|  | Range | 7,9 | 8,0 |
| kind of CP | Di | 2 | 1 |
|  | Quadri | 6 | 8 |
|  | Other than CP | 2 | 1 |
| gender | Boys | 5 | 5 |
|  | Girls | 5 | 5 |

By the end of the study, we had complete data of 9 children in the experimental group and of 9 children in the control group. Two children, one of each group, had to be excluded from the research. One of them had an operation on his leg and the other child stayed at home in the township for a period of three months.

Childcare workers were selected by the conductor and the manager of the Home to receive training in CE. They received the CE training in three groups. In the first two groups there were in total eight unit managers and one childcare worker, in the third group there were five childcare workers. The participants had about the same level of education, but varied in age and years worked in Sizanani. Their ages ranged from 30 to 41, with an average of 35 years. Their work experience ranged from 7 to 12 years, with an average of 9 years.

## 2.2. Design

The research took place over a period of two years. A repeated measurement design was used, with a pretest and a series of posttests and an interval of four months between the waves. The first measurement was a pretest measurement. During the intervention period the experimental group of 10 children received CE training, four days a week, three hours a day. The control group of 10 children, who are living in the same setting, followed the daily routine of the Home.

## 2.3. Instruments

### Paediatric Evaluation of Disability Inventory (PEDI)

To administer the development of functional abilities the Paediatric Evaluation of Disability Inventory (PEDI) was used. It is a standardised assessment instrument for children with a variety of disabling conditions with an age range of 6 months to 7.5 years (Haley, Coster, Ludlow, Haltiwanger & Andrellos, 1992). The PEDI can be used to detect functional deficits or delays, to evaluate individual or group progress and also to assess outcome measure for programme evaluation. A number of studies support the PEDI as a reliable and valid assessment instrument of functional performance for children with disabilities. The PEDI can be administered by professional clinicians and educators familiar with the child or by structured interview with parents or caregivers.

The inventory is designed to identify the child's functional ability on three scales, each scale divided into three domains: self-care, mobility and social function. The first scale, the 'Functional Skills' scale, consists of questions concerning the typical functional skill level of the child. All questions can be answered with 'yes', meaning able, or 'no', meaning unable. The second scale, the 'Caregiver Assistance' scale, consists of questions concerning the physical assistance a child needs to carry out functional activities. The amount of assistance is measured on a six-point scale, ranging from independent to total assistance. The third scale is the 'Modifications' section. This is not a true measurement scale, but a frequency count of the type and extent of modifications the child depends on to support functional performance.

In this research the PEDI was used to measure the effects of Conductive Education on the functional abilities of the children and also the amount of assistance needed from the childcare workers (CCWS), corresponding with the first two scales. Some items were deleted because they were found unsuitable for the Home in its South African setting. The deleted items consist of those on the domains of hair brushing and climbing or descending full flights of stairs. The first because all children have very short afro hair, the second because no full flights of stairs are available in the Home. No new reliability and validity testing were done because the changes were thought to be small. Part three of the PEDI (Modifications scale) is not used in this research, because of the lack of specialised equipment in the Home.

This was thought to be no problem because each PEDI scale is self-contained and can be left out, without affecting the other scales.

The raw scores of the Functional Skills scale and the Caregivers Assistance scale are converted into scaled scores. These scores range from 0 to 100. A higher score represents a higher level of functional performance, respectively a higher level of independence.

### Gross Motor Function Measure (GMFM)

The quantity of motor skills was assessed by the GMFM. This instrument is a clinical measurement designed to evaluate change in gross motor function in children with cerebral palsy (CP) up to 16 years of age (Russel, Rosenbaum, Avery & Lane, 2002). The instrument allows children to demonstrate various motor skills and focuses on how much of the activity the child can perform unaided. The GMFM has shown to be valid and responsive to change in gross motor function for children with CP by multiple studies.

There are two versions of the GMFM, the GMFM-66 and the GMFM-88, each with a corresponding number of questions. For this research the GMFM-88 was chosen, because it gives more detailed information and is preferable for children with severe motor disabilities, as is the case in the Home. With its 88 items the GMFM-88 focuses on five different domains: lying & rolling, sitting, crawling & kneeling, standing & walking, running & jumping. All items have a four-point scoring system (0: No attempt, 1: Makes an attempt, 2: Partial performance, 3: Complete performance). For each of the five domains percent scores are calculated as well as a total score (which is the average of the five domains). A higher score represents a larger quantity of gross motor movements by the child. The instrument is used to measure the magnitude of change in motor skills over time.

All measurements were carried out by the same qualified occupational therapist, experienced in treating children with neuromotor dysfunction. She was familiar with the GMFM from her work.

### Gross Motor Performance Measure (GMPM)

To evaluate change in gross motor performance over time, i.e. the quality of functional motor skills, the GMPM was used. The GMPM is designed to use in conjunction with the GMFM. For every GMFM item with a score higher than 0 the performance of the movement is assessed with the GMPM. The instrument can be used for children with cerebral palsy from 5 months up to 12 years of age (Boyce, Gowland, Rosenbaum, Hardy, Lane, Plews, Goldsmith, Russel, Wright, Potter, & Harding, 1998). Studies show good reliability for the instrument for total scores (intra-rater .96; inter-rater .92; test-retest .96). Scores for single attributes were less reproducible (Gowland, Boyce, Wright, Russell, Goldsmith, & Rosenbaum, 1995).

With 20 items on a five-point scale the GMPM assesses five attributes (or qualitative features) of gross motor performance: alignment, coordination, dissociated movement, stability and weight shift. Average percent scores are calculated for the five attributes and the total score (which is the average of the five attributes). A higher score represents a better quality of gross motor movements by the child. In this study the instrument is used to evaluate change over time in gross motor performance.

All measurements were carried out by the same qualified occupational therapist, experienced in treating children with neuromotor dysfunction. She was familiar with the GMPM from her work.

*Levels of Intervention Observation Instrument*
The levels of interaction between the childcare workers and the children were assessed with the Levels of Intervention Observation Instrument (Vermeer, Westra, Benig, Beks, Diemel & van den Brink, 1990). The instrument can be used in various (rehabilitation) settings for children with disabilities. There is no known age limit. The instrument is a direct observation method using a time sampling method of 30 seconds. The reliability and validity of the instrument were proven to be good in two studies, one with persons with mental retardation (Vermeer et al , 1990) and one with children with cerebral palsy (Vermeer, Vos, Lindeman, van Alphen & Snel, 1989).

The instrument, based upon an action-psychological classification of mother-child interactions, provides a framework for categorising the teaching strategies used by professionals to bring a child to an independent performance of a task. The intervention categories cover a continuum from 'field-guidance' to 'self-guidance'. In case of 'field-guidance', guidance is external, coming from the environment or the professional. In case of 'self-guidance', independent children act according to their own plan. The following classification of levels of intervention emerges:

1. Guidance of body parts: the intervention is directed to a part of the body.
2. Guidance through physical objects: physical objects are used to evoke and guide the movement.
3. Guidance by means of rhythm, music, singing or tone: rhythm is used to evoke and guide the movement.
4. Guidance by means of structuring the immediate environment: the arrangement of the immediate environment evokes and guides performance.
5. Guidance through demonstration: a (visual) representation of (a part of) the movement is given.
6. Verbal guidance: verbal actions are used to evoke or guide the performance of the movement.
7. Free exploration after a given task: an instruction to perform a movement is given, the performance is left to the individual.

The score of a particular event is the sum of the highest score of the samples (maximum score = 7). A higher score indicates a higher level of interaction with the child. Contrary to the manual, for the time samples a duration of two minutes per interval was chosen. In fact, in this study this resulted in a kind of event sampling, because several interactions between childcare workers and child did not last longer than two minutes (e.g. bathing, clothing).

In addition to these interventions the instrument also observes the spoken educational actions of the professional. For the educational actions the following two categories are discerned:

1. Evaluation: questions and remarks referring to present and/or previous sessions as well as to experiences in everyday life.
2. Personal contact: 'nice weather talk', hugging, 'rough and tumble play'.

In this research it was chosen not to score the educational actions of the childcare workers. The main language spoken in the Home between childcare workers and children is Zulu. Because of this language barrier between researchers and childcare workers, it was not possible to interpret the verbal instructions.

*Measure of Processes of Care for Service Providers (MPOC-SP)*
To evaluate the attitude of the childcare workers towards the new programme, which re-
quires higher involvement in the stimulation of the children, the Measure of Processes of
Care for Service Providers (MPOC-SP) was adapted to the situation in the Home. The
MPOC-SP is a self-assessment questionnaire, designed to measure the attitudes, behaviours
and visions of paediatric caregivers (Woodside, Rosenbaum, King, & King, 2001). The
MPOC-SP has been adapted from the widely used Canadian measurement for parents in
paediatric rehabilitation, the Measure of Processes of Care (MPOC). The MPOC has been
shown to be well-validated, reliable and able to discriminate amongst various programmes of
service known to operate differentially (King, King, & Rosenbaum, 2004). The MPOC-SP
has also shown to have good psychometric properties (Woodside et al., 2001). The authors
(Woodside & Rosenbaum, 1996) report good internal consistency (Cronbach's alphas across
scales varied from .79 to .82) and good test-retest reliability (ICC's across scales varied from
.80 to .89).

With 27 items that can be answered on a seven-point scale, the instrument has a structure
of four dimensions that reflect the essential features of family-centred service:
– Showing interpersonal sensitivity (10 items)
– Providing general information (5 items)
– Communicating specific information about the child (3 items)
– Treating people respectfully (9 items).

For each of the four dimensions mean scores can be calculated, which can vary between 1.00
(never) and 7.00 (to a very high extent).

In this study the instrument is used over time to examine changes in attitudes, behaviours
and visions of childcare workers. The questionnaire had to be modified, since most of the
children do not have families and for the ones who do, contact with the families is sparse. In
all questions 'parents' has been changed into 'childcare workers in the block the child lives
in'. Because not all items were suitable for the Home in its South African setting, twelve
items were structurally changed and three items were replaced by new ones. Although the
reliability and validity of the modified MPOC-SP can no longer be based on the original tool,
no new reliability and validity testing has been done. As the changes in the questionnaire
were thought to undermine the structure of the list, it was chosen not to maintain the four
dimensions of the original version. Therefore only the total score of the questionnaire has
been calculated and analysed over time. The total score can vary between 1 and 7. A higher
score resembles better attitude, behaviour and vision of service of the childcare workers.

The questionnaires were handed out to the childcare workers and filled in immediately
thereafter and then returned.

## 2.4. Procedure
After a little exploratory period, the assessments of the instruments were first practised with
a few children and childcare workers to see what problems were encountered. All assessments were done in English. For a period of three weeks, each day started with assessing the
Levels of Intervention. Every day a few children were observed in interaction with the childcare workers. The observations took place in the morning during bathing, tooth brushing,
toileting, dressing and breakfast. In the afternoon the PEDI was administered for the same
children as were observed during the morning. The childcare worker who knew the child
best was interviewed when he or she had some time left between the daily tasks.

After these measurements the research continued with the assessment of the Gross Motor Functional Measure (GMFM) and the Gross Motor Performance Measure (GMPM). The assessment had to take place during the one-week stay of a qualified therapist flown in from The Netherlands.

## 2.5. Statistical Analyses

The assessments were done by two researchers during each wave at the same time. It was not possible to measure the level of agreement between all researchers, since the researchers did not stay at the Home at the same time.

All data were entered and analysed in SPSS 11.0. To test the effects of the CE programme, change scores between two waves were calculated. Change scores were used, because inspection of the pretest scores revealed that the two groups were not equal at the start of the study, despite our effort to match both groups as well as possible. The experimental group outperformed the control group on most of the tests. To correct for this difference, differences in gain scores between the two groups were tested using t-tests for independent samples. A series of subsequent comparisons were conducted , i.e. each wave was compared with the previous wave. Due to the small sample size, the power of the study was low, therefore the overall α was set on p<.10.

To analyse the effects of CE on the functional development of the children the following domain scores of the PEDI were used: self-care, mobility and social function of the Functional Skills section and self-care, mobility and social function of the Caregivers Assistance section.

To analyse the effects of CE on the quantity and quality of movement, the scaled scores of the GMFM and GMPM were calculated. For the GMFM the scores of the domains lying, sitting, crawling, standing, walking and the total score were used. For the GMPM the percent scores of the domains dissociated movement, coordination, performance-alignment, weight shift and the total score were entered.

To analyse the effects of CE on the levels of intervention the interval scores on the Levels of Intervention instrument were calculated. The scores represent mean scores of the interaction style of the childcare workers observed whilst bathing, dressing, eating, tooth brushing and toileting. Finally, the total score was calculated.

## 3. Results

### 3.1. Examination of the Data Characteristics

The analyses on all tests and sub-tests showed no negative or positive outliers on any of the scores of the children. It was therefore decided to include all 9 experimental and 9 control subjects in the analyses.

### 3.2. Longitudinal Group Analyses

Table 2 shows the differences in mean scores of the experimental and control group on the 1st wave compared to the 2nd, the 3rd and the 5th wave. Although all differences between the waves could be calculated, the most interesting are the differences between wave 1 and 5. Also the differences between wave 1 and 2 are important to register, because these measurements give insight into the differences between the two groups of children at the start of the intervention experiment. Because of organisational reasons, these two measurements were executed with an interval of two months. Next, it is interesting to consider the results about half-way through the experiment, i.e. the differences between wave 1 and 3.

A score above zero means the group has made progress on that particular variable. A score below zero means a decrease in the abilities of the group on that variable. The last column of each wave shows whether the differences between the waves were significant at a level of 10 percent.

## Functional Abilities
The PEDI focused on the functional abilities of the children and the amount of caregiver assistance on the domains self-care, mobility and social function.

Comparison between wave 1 and wave 5 shows that the experimental group made some progress, except on the mobility domain. But all these results are not significant.

Comparison between wave 1 and wave 2 shows that the experimental group made significant progress only on social function (CCW). This progress disappeared between wave 3 and 5. However, the control group made significantly more progress on the mobility domain than the experimental group.

## Quantity of Motor Movements
The GMFM focused on the quantity of motor movement of the children. Analyses were made for the total GMFM score and for the domains lying, sitting, crawling, standing and running.

Comparison between wave 1 and 3 demonstrated that the experimental group showed significantly more progress on the total GMFM score than the control group. All other differences between the two groups were not significant.

## Quality of motor movements
The GMPM focused on quality of motor development within the five domains of the GMFM. Analyses were conducted for the total GMPM score and for the domains dissociated movement, coordination, alignment, weight shift and stability. No significant differences between de groups were found.

## Levels of intervention
The Levels of Intervention Observation Instrument was used to determine the level of interaction of the childcare workers in daily activities. There were no significant differences found (Table 2).

## Measure of Processes of Care for Service Providers
On all five waves the mean scores are between 5.20 and of 5.59 (SD = 0.6). No significant changes between the waves were found. This score resembles a good attitude, behaviour and positive vision towards the children amongst the childcare workers involved. In addition, no significant change in satisfaction was measured, meaning that the level of satisfaction is stable, possibly due to a ceiling effect.

Table 2: Mean change scores on Level of Intervention, GMFM, GMPM, and PEDI, of the experimental and the control group across waves 1, 2, 3 and 5.

| | | Difference wave 1 and 2 | | | | | Difference wave 1 and 3 | | | | | Difference wave 1 and 5 | | | | |
|---|---|---|---|---|---|---|---|---|---|---|---|---|---|---|---|---|
| | | exp. group mean | (sd) | control group mean | (sd) | T-test | exp. group mean | (sd) | control group mean | (sd) | T-test | exp. group mean | (sd) | control group mean | (sd) | T-test |
| **Levels of intervention** | bath | 0 | 0,06 | 0,02 | 0,1 | n.s. | 0,08 | 0,29 | -0,09 | 0,07 | n.s. | 0,01 | 0,22 | -0,01 | 0,21 | n.s. |
| | dressing | 0,04 | 0,13 | 0,04 | 0,13 | n.s. | 0,04 | 0,15 | 0,02 | 0,17 | n.s. | 0,07 | 0,17 | -0,03 | 0,34 | n.s. |
| | eating | -0,01 | 0,16 | 0 | 0 | n.s. | -0,01 | 0,09 | -0,02 | 0,08 | n.s. | -0,04 | 0,39 | -0,05 | 0,06 | n.s. |
| | toothbrushing | 0,05 | 0,16 | 0,04 | 0,12 | n.s. | -0,03 | 0,08 | -0,01 | 0,22 | n.s. | -0,08 | 0,05 | -0,001 | 0,19 | n.s. |
| | toileting | 0 | 0 | -0,04 | 0,13 | n.s. | 0,06 | 0,18 | 0,002 | 0,06 | n.s. | 0,1 | 0,16 | 0,06 | 0,32 | n.s. |
| | total | 0,02 | 0,06 | 0,01 | 0,02 | n.s. | 0,03 | 0,12 | -0,02 | 0,07 | ns | 0,01 | 0,13 | -0,01 | 0,11 | n.s. |
| **GMFM** | total | 3,8 | 7,75 | 4,85 | 6,78 | n.s. | 10,41 | 11,68 | 0,86 | 6,36 | P<0.05 | 17,07 | 12,81 | 11,89 | 8,98 | n.s. |
| | lying | 12,34 | 27,06 | 11,76 | 21,42 | n.s. | 21,18 | 22,68 | 10,05 | 15,99 | n.s. | 30,39 | 24,55 | 21,21 | 18,49 | n.s. |
| | sitting | 3 | 11,8 | 7,5 | 20,09 | n.s. | 9,63 | 11,09 | 0,4 | 12,91 | n.s. | 18,67 | 19,97 | 20,33 | 23,07 | n.s. |
| | crawling | 4,05 | 16,5 | 6,19 | 11,51 | n.s. | 13,33 | 20,82 | -0,01 | 9,63 | n.s. | 10,64 | 22,81 | 5,08 | 13,43 | n.s. |
| | standing | 0 | 15,99 | -2,05 | 6,49 | n.s. | 8,53 | 23,25 | 0,56 | 16,88 | n.s. | 4,99 | 8,17 | 1,71 | 4,53 | n.s. |
| | walking | -0,3 | 6,15 | 0,86 | 3,24 | n.s. | -0,01 | 0,04 | -1,39 | 4,17 | n.s. | 21,26 | 21,98 | 11,18 | 16,32 | n.s. |
| **GMPM** | total | 12,65 | 11,86 | 13,54 | 10,26 | n.s. | 12,44 | 11,41 | 9,5 | 13,07 | n.s. | 0,28 | 0,16 | 0,15 | 0,19 | n.s. |
| | dissociated movement | 7,8 | 12,88 | 5,4 | 20,05 | n.s. | 2,96 | 18,41 | 4,57 | 17,54 | n.s. | 0,22 | 0,2 | 0,11 | 0,29 | n.s. |
| | coordination | 9,96 | 14,35 | 14,1 | 16,23 | n.s. | 5,17 | 10 | 8,6 | 19,72 | n.s. | 0,23 | 0,21 | 0,14 | 0,22 | n.s. |
| | performance-alignment | 39,76 | 14,55 | 32,16 | 19,51 | n.s. | 38,29 | 16,9 | 31,95 | 19,75 | n.s. | 0,56 | 0,19 | 0,32 | 0,29 | n.s. |
| | weight shift | 2,78 | 14,89 | 1,74 | 14,5 | n.s. | 13,09 | 23,79 | 1,59 | 18,16 | n.s. | 0,26 | 0,23 | 0,08 | 0,23 | n.s. |
| | stability | 7,38 | 17,33 | 9,87 | 12,1 | n.s. | 2,96 | 15,31 | 1,07 | 13,25 | n.s. | 0,14 | 0,14 | 0,12 | 0,15 | n.s. |
| **PEDI** | functional skills | 2,95 | 6,2 | 0,62 | 6,62 | n.s. | 3,89 | 8,16 | 6,32 | 4,21 | n.s. | 7,76 | 7,1 | 6,91 | 8,61 | n.s. |
| | mobility | 1,17 | 6,4 | 4,67 | 3,15 | n.s. | 10,84 | 7,25 | 15,57 | 7,17 | n.s. | 9,48 | 8,8 | 10,62 | 8,94 | n.s. |
| | social function | 3,61 | 11,93 | 1,96 | 10,18 | n.s. | 9,13 | 11,19 | 7,43 | 10,71 | n.s. | 12,99 | 16,31 | 8,6 | 20,78 | n.s. |
| | functional skills (ccw) | 7,63 | 13,01 | 3,15 | 9,16 | n.s. | 4,62 | 16,41 | 7,24 | 9,49 | n.s. | 17,04 | 16,18 | 9,04 | 17,13 | n.s. |
| | mobility (ccw) | -1,38 | 16,96 | 2,08 | 17,43 | n.s. | 4,29 | 11,24 | 17,67 | 13,75 | P<0.05 | 4,96 | 25,56 | 2,88 | 18,35 | n.s. |
| | social function (ccw) | 13,12 | 17,96 | -3,3 | 20,95 | P<0.05 | 15,1 | 16,1 | 10,61 | 15,89 | n.s. | 22,73 | 21,12 | 7,24 | 30,25 | n.s. |

**Table 3: Total mean score and sd of the MPOC-SP on all waves**

|        | mean | sd  |
|--------|------|-----|
| wave 1 | 5.35 | 0.9 |
| wave 2 | 5.59 | 0.6 |
| wave 3 | 5.21 | 0.9 |
| wave 4 | 5.40 | 0.6 |
| wave 5 | 5.20 | 0.6 |

### 3.3. *Longitudinal Group Descriptives*

Table 4 gives a summary of the differences between the experimental and the control group between wave 1 and 2, wave 1 and 3, and wave 1 and 5 for the PEDI, GMFM, GMPM, and Levels of Intervention. Group comparisons were made on a total of 24 variables. At wave 5, the experimental group demonstrated more progress than the control group on 22 of the 24 variables. For only 2 variables the control group showed more progress.

If we consider the differences between wave 1 and 2, the experimental group performs (already) better on 12 of the 24 variables. In this period, the control group performs better on 11 variables and on one variable they are equal. When comparing the 1st and the 3rd wave, it becomes clearer: on 17 of the 24 variables the gains were larger for the experimental group than for the control group (Table 4).

A sign-test demonstrated that the experimental group scored higher than the control group comparing the scores on wave 1 and 3 ($z=2.04$, $p<.05$) and those of wave 1-5 ($z=3.67$, $p<.01$)

**Table 4: Gains and decreases per wave 1, 2, 3 and 5**

|              | exp < control | exp = control | exp > control | total N variables |
|--------------|---------------|---------------|---------------|-------------------|
| wave 1 and 2 | 11            | 1             | 12            | 24                |
| wave 1 and 3 | 7             | 0             | 17            | 24                |
| wave 1 and 5 | 2             | 0             | 22            | 24                |

As could be seen in Table 2, it will be clear that the majority of the functional changes are not significant ($p<.10$). Given the number of statistical tests conducted, the few significant changes could be the result of chance. Nevertheless, it has to be noticed that all changes - although not significant - are in the expected direction (see Table 4). And, that alone cannot be the result of chance.

## 3. Conclusions and Discussion

The results of about two years of CE for a group of 10 selected children did not show significant results for the functional performance of the children. When considering the descriptive data, there is nevertheless a positive trend: the experimental group showed more progress over time than the control group. The gains are small, but in the expected direction. There are several points to make about the results.

First, it could be discussed whether large changes could be expected in this group of children. The majority of them are over the age of 12 and have severe disabilities. Until the start of the CE programme, they had hardly any training and the majority has developed quite strong contractures.

Secondly, the study suffered from a lack of power. Only 10 (later on 9) children were compared with another 10 (respectively 9) children. The differences between groups would have had to be spectacular to reach significance.

Thirdly, it appeared that the children differed in the kind of disabilities and in the severity of the disability within the groups. This might have affected the results negatively.

Fourth, the researchers who conducted the study, were not blind for the group membership of the children. So, one cannot exclude the possibility that even the very small gains shown by the experimental group were due to (unconscious) manipulations by the researchers.

Fifth, small gains in the scores may not automatically mean that the children's abilities also showed minor changes. Most instruments are not sensitive enough to detect very small changes in abilities, so when scores do change, even when not significantly, it still might be clinically relevant.

Sixth, the instruments are valid to use, but none of them has been validated for use in South Africa.

Seventh, it might be that the PEDI was not used in a reliable way. Between the waves, different childcare workers were interviewed, causing a further decline of reliability. In future research, one should use the same respondent per child.

It is striking that the only significant result was found with the GMFM. This can be explained in two ways. First, the assessments of the GMFM and GMPM were undertaken by the same qualified occupational therapist, probably resulting in more reliable results. Secondly, these measurements were directly measured on the child, not based on information from a third person, in this case the childcare worker.

Finally, analyses of data about the attitude and involvement of the childcare workers towards the children did not show any effect. Already at the start of the intervention experiment, the childcare workers appeared content and involved with the new programme. With the relatively high scores already established during wave 1 and 2, progress could not be expected. Nevertheless, the process evaluation which took place at the same time (see Appendix) showed the other side of the coin. When expanding the programme great emphasis should be placed on a positive mindset amongst childcare workers. Getting them involved will create a willingness to co-operate, a necessity for the programme to be successful.

## Notes

1. Cerebral palsy is a coordinated term for a group of non-progressive, but often changing syndroms with motor limitations secondary to abnormalities or laesies in the brain, the origin of which springs from the early stages of the brain's development (Rosenbaum, 2003).
2. Spina Bifida is a neural tube defect that happens in the first month of pregnancy when the spinal column does not close completely (www.sbaa.org).

## References

Bairstow, P., Cochrane, R. & Hur, J. (1993). *Evaluation of Conductive Education for children with cerebral palsy (final report).* London: HMSO.

Boyce, W., Gowland, C., Rosenbaum, P., Hardy, S., Lane, M., Plews, N.,Goldsmith, C., Russel, D., Wright, V., Potter, S. & Harding, D. (1998). *Gross Motor Performance Measure Manual (GMPM).* Kingston: MacMaster University.

Coles C. & Zsargo, L (1998). Conductive Education: towards an 'educational model'. *British Journal of Special Education, 25,* 70-74.

Gowland, C., Boyce, F., Wright, V., Russell, D., Goldsmith, C. & Rosenbaum, P. (1995). Reliability of the Gross Motor Performance Measure (GMPM). *Physical Therapy, 75,* 597-613.

Haley, S.M., Coster, W.J., Ludlow, L.H., Haltiwanger, J.T. & Andrellos, P.J. (1992). *Pediatric evaluation of disability inventory (PEDI).* Boston: New England Medical Centre

Hari, M. (1991). Intention: the principle hypothesis of Conductive Education. *Lege Artis Medicinea, 1,* 9-10.

Hoek, A.M. van der, Groot, L. de & Vermeer, A. (1992). *De Petö-methode. Een geïntegreerde opvang van het hersenbeschadigde kind.* Amsterdam: VU Uitgeverij.

King, S.M., King, G.A. & Rosenbaum, P.L. (2004). Evaluating Health Service Delivery to Children With Chronic Conditions and Their Families. *Children's Health Care, 33,* 35-57.

Rosenbaum, P.L. (2003). Cerebral Palsy: what parents and doctors want to know. *British Medical Journal, 326,* 73-96

Russel, D.J., Rosenbaum, P.L., Avery, L.M. & Lane, M. (2002). *Gross Motor Function Measure (GMFM-66 & GMFM-88) User's Manual.* Cambridge: Mac Keith Press.

Sutton, A. (1988). Conductive Education. *Archives of disease in childhood, 63,* 214-217.

Vermeer, A., Vos, H.W.C.M., Lindeman, A.Th., Alphen, J. van & Snel, J. (1989). Observing the interventions of teachers and therapists in child rehabilitation. *Journal of Rehabilitation Sciences, 2,* 25-29.

Vermeer, A., Westra, T., Benig, T., Beks, T., Diemel, T., & Brink, C. van den (1990). Validation of Interventions in Adapted Physical Activities for Mentally Retarded Residents. *Medicine and Sport Science, 30,* 85-93.

Woodside J.M. & Rosenbaum, P.L. (1996). *The Measures of Processes of Care for Service Providers (MPOC-SP): A Means for Health Care Professionals to Assess Their Own Family-Centered Behaviours.* Hamilton, Ontario, Canada: Neurodevelopmental Clinical Research Unit, McMaster University.

Woodside, J.M., Rosenbaum, P.L., King, S.M. & King, G.A. (2001). Family-Centered Service: Developing and Validating a Self-Assessment Tool for Paediatric Service Providers. *Children's Health Care, 30,* 237-252.

*Address for correspondence:*
Prof. dr. A. Vermeer
Utrecht University
Department of Educational Sciences
Heidelberglaan 1
3584 CS Utrecht
The Netherlands
e-mail: a.vermeer@fss.uu.nl

# APPENDIX: PROCESS EVALUATION

## 1. Introduction

Part II of this research focuses on the process of implementation of the CE programme. The progression of the Conductive Education training was carefully monitored. The problems and setbacks that might have had a negative influence on the programme results were systematically discussed and recorded.

## 2. Method

To evaluate the implementation process, bi-weekly meetings with the manager of the Home and the conductor were held. The process evaluation focuses on the problems met and solutions found during the execution of the CE programme. The results are a descriptive evaluation report that is based upon the implementation evaluation made by the first researchers and the follow-up evaluation of the following researchers. The progress evaluation focuses on the childcare workers, the children and the conductor, the Conductive Education training itself and the materials used.

## 3. Results

### 3.1. Childcare Workers

By the end of January 2005, the second group of unit managers had almost finished their training. Finishing the training created mixed feelings amongst the childcare workers. On the one hand, they really liked participating in the training and regretted it had to end. On the other hand, they were relieved. They all experienced the training as physically and mentally demanding. It was hard to combine the training with the daily tasks of a unit manager. Mentally they were challenged, because learning the principles of Conductive Education required a whole new way of thinking and acting. The unit managers also expressed their worries. They were afraid of forgetting the information they had learned before CE could be implemented on the blocks. The implementation had been delayed several times and the unit managers were convinced that the implementation would not be starting any time soon. Apparently they were not aware of the fact that the implementation of CE would be starting in September 2005.

By the end of the training the unit managers also expressed their concerns about assisting the conductor during the implementation. They specifically expressed their worries about changing the mindset of the non-involved childcare workers. Most childcare workers do not see a disabled child as a person able to improve or develop, whilst CE is about treating a disabled child as an able person. Because it will be the task of the trained unit managers to convince their non-involved colleagues otherwise, they feel they are facing a difficult task.

Other factors also play a role. It will be difficult to get everybody positively involved in the programme. Even though the majority of the childcare workers claim to be positive about the programme, they still feel threatened by it, afraid of losing their job. In their view CE helps the children to gain more independence, meaning less staff will be needed. Furthermore, the non-involved childcare workers feel neglected and upset for not being able to participate in the training. This causes resistance to co-operate with the CE programme. Also, not all childcare workers accept the leading position of the selected, sometimes less experienced, unit managers. Negative feelings, like jealousy and anger, will make it even more difficult for the unit managers to gain the trust needed to change the mindset and to get everybody positively involved.

## 3.2. Children
At the beginning of the research 20 children were selected. A year-and-a-half later two children, one from the control group and one from the experimental group, had to be excluded. The boy from the experimental group continued his training in the programme, but he was excluded from the research because, due to an operation on his hips, it was not possible to execute the measurements. Almost every day the children in the experimental group took part in the CE programme. Unfortunately, during the Easter and Winter holidays a large number of sessions had to be cancelled. A number of children went home and thus were not able to participate in CE.

## 3.3. Conductor
Between January and August 2005 there was one conductor in the Home. She was not only responsible for the CE training, but she got more responsibilities in the Home as her stay prolonged. Her responsibilities included involvement in the organisation and management of the Home. Due to her busy schedule several training sessions had to be cancelled.

With the upcoming implementation of CE on the blocks and the extra responsibilities of the conductor it was decided to place a vacancy on the internet for a second conductor. The first round of applications ended without a new conductor. The one suitable candidate withdrew her application after reconsidering the dangers of HIV/AIDS. It was decided to place a new vacancy and finally a suitable applicant came forward. The search for this new conductor took a lot of time.

## 3.4. Conductive Education Training
After the second group of unit managers had completed the Conductive Education training, a third group of childcare workers had to be selected. Since all unit managers had finished the training, their assistants had to go through the selection procedure. This took more time than expected. It was very difficult for the conductor and the management to select new people, keeping jealousy to a minimum and getting a motivated group. Negotiations with the Union concerning one of the childcare workers caused a further delay in the selection procedure. Eventually the new group of assistant unit managers and a childcare worker was selected.

Before the new group had been selected, already a period of approximately one month had passed. During this month the CE programme was given in an adapted form. Instead of all children being trained on a daily basis, only half of the children were trained each day. The conductor did not feel able to train all the children without the help of childcare workers assisting her. For a period of one month the children had less CE training.

## 3.5. Furniture
Some of the wooden furniture used in the daily CE training had broken down. They had to be repaired by the carpenter. This took quite a while, but eventually the materials came out fixed and even stronger. Although some materials could not be used for a while, this did not have a negative impact on the programme. The conductor adjusted training when necessary.

One of the unit managers repeatedly requested CE furniture. She wanted to start working with CE on her block, afraid of forgetting what she had learned. Eventually one table and some chairs were made available for this block. This way the children of the experimental group could also practice CE during the rest of the day. Although this is a good initiative, it also caused more jealousy amongst the unit managers at the other blocks. They felt neglected and could not understand why they got nothing.

## 4. Conclusions

Overall it can be concluded that the process implementation of the Conductive Education programme was minimally affected. The elements that did affect the progress are summarised here. Solutions and recommendations are given.

The worries expressed by the involved childcare workers will probably not affect the results at the moment, but might play a role in the future. It is suggested that extra support should be given to the involved unit managers during the implementation of CE. The negative feelings amongst the non-involved childcare workers might already have negatively influenced the results as they are not supporting their involved colleagues. If the non-involved childcare workers feel more important and if they get more involved, their negative feelings might be minimalised. To realise this, it is necessary to provide extra information about CE and to start its implementation in the entire Home as soon as possible.

Excluding two children from the research is seen as a setback. Although the number of children in the experimental and the control group is still equal, it will further lower the power of the statistics. The exclusion is thought not to have negative influence on the programme results.

The busy schedule of the conductor is thought to have a small influence on the programme results. Until the new conductor is admitted, it is advised to keep cancellation of the sessions to a minimum. The delay of the selection of the new group is also thought to have a negative impact on the programme results. For one month, the children got half of the training and the continuity of the programme was affected. The same goes for the Easter and Winter Holiday. The breaking down of the materials did not have a negative impact on the programme, due to adjustments made.

# Part III

# Southern African Catholic Bishops' Conference AIDS Office (Pretoria)

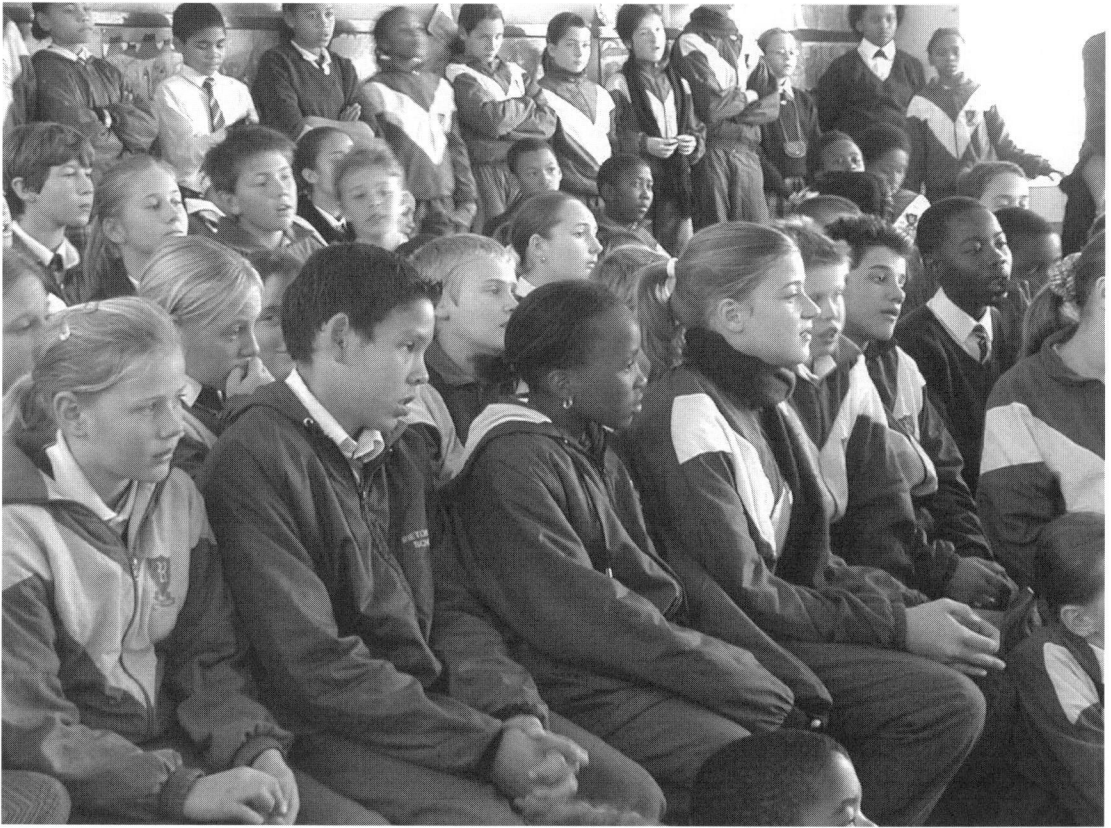

# Chapter 12

# The ARV Therapy Distribution Project

*Ricus Dullaert* [1]

[1] Southern African Catholic Bishops' Conference AIDS Office, Pretoria, South Africa

## Abstract

This chapter describes the reasons and vision of the Southern African Catholic Bishops' AIDS Office behind the initiation of their ARV therapy distribution project. It also draws the political context in which this roll-out is taking place. Next, an outline is given of the admission criteria for the patients at two points of service, St. Joseph's Care and Support Centre at Sizanani, Bronkhorstspruit, and Nazareth House, Johannesburg, both in the Gauteng province. Based on the accounts of the projects, it can be stated that the assumption of the SACBC AIDS Office that ARVs can be introduced successfully in resource-poor settings has been proved.

## 1. Political Context

As is common knowledge among persons who regularly read the South African and Dutch press, the roll-out of antiretroviral (ARV) therapy by the government of South Africa via public health institutions is very slow.

End 2003, the South African Cabinet announced the large scale roll-out of antiretrovirals (also called HAART: highly active antiretroviral therapy) in the public health sector. Ambitious plans were published. The government promised that before the national elections of April 2004, at least 54,000 HIV-positive South Africans would benefit from antiretroviral therapy in the public health sector. This treatment would be handed out for free. Many people did not have much confidence in these announcements, due to the often denialist attitude of President Thabo Mbeki and his Health Minister Dr. Manto Tshabalala-Msimang in the years prior to this announcement. In October 2003 for instance, President Thabo Mbeki told *The Washington Post*: 'I don't know anyone with HIV....... Personally I don't know anyone who died of AIDS'.[1,2] On the International AIDS Conference in Bangkok, July 2004, President Mbeki was not present, although he is the political leader of the country with the highest number of HIV-positive people in the world: 5.3 million people infected with HIV were living in South Africa in 2004.[3] When the Mail & Guardian evaluated Mbeki's Cabinet in January 2005, Health Minister Dr. Manto Tshabalala Msimang got an F-mark (meaning 'you are fired') for her performance in the fight against HIV/AIDS.[4] Many saw the promise to provide ARVs to 54,000 people living with AIDS before 1 April 2004 as a move to gain votes and also feared that after the elections the 'dog would be laid asleep' again. Because South Africa has no strong opposition parties and because 60-70% of the electorate vote for the ANC, the opposition against the government often has to come from civil society, trade unions, churches, action groups and NGO coalitions.

Also 54,000 people on ARVs might sound impressive, but in a country like South Africa with an estimated number of 5.3 million HIV-positive citizens on a total of 44 million inhabitants, 600,000 of whom need ARVs urgently and 300,000-400,000 of whom die yearly from AIDS-related illnesses, 54,000 is still a rather bleak figure.

In hindsight the worst fears regarding the government roll-out came true. After the April 2004 elections, the target to reach 54,000 patients on ARVs by April 2004 was shifted to April 2005 and to date (October 2005) the target of 54,000 people on treatment in public health facilities in SouthAfrica has not been reached yet.

Dr. Manto Tshabalala-Msimang, the Health Minister, goes on preaching that garlic, beetroot, olive oil, African potatoes and spinach are helpful against AIDS.[5] Also she promotes dangerous persons like Dr. Matthias Rath from Switzerland, who states that ARVs are dangerous and toxic and promotes vitamins to prevent dying from HIV/AIDS, which have never officially proven to be effective.[6] President Mbeki hardly speaks about HIV/AIDS and declared that he personally knows no one with HIV/AIDS. This is in strong contrast with the braveness of former President Nelson Mandela who declared in January 2005 that his only surviving son Makgatho had died of AIDS.[7, 8]

## 2. Accreditation Process

In order to reach the above mentioned targets, the South African government started from November 2003 an accreditation process to sort out which hospitals were equipped to start the ARV roll-out. The initial aim was to have in each province at least a few hospitals accredited. It turned out that only hospitals with their own laboratory facilities, their own pharmacies and sufficient trained medical staff had a chance to be accredited and that the pace of accreditation was very slow. End 2004, 54 hospitals nation-wide should have been accredited to start ARV roll-out. In March 2004, only thirteen sites had been accredited, all of them in the Western Cape province. This left AIDS patients in eight out of nine provinces of South Africa with no option than to pay for ARVs from their own pocket, or to die.[9]

## 3. ARVs in Recourse Poor Settings

This is where the SACBC AIDS Office came in. The SACBC AIDS Office wanted to prove that also in *resource-poor settings*, i.e. settings without a pharmacy, a laboratory and a full-time doctor, an ARV project could be successfully implemented. The backbone of these ARV projects would be a well-trained home-based caregivers team. Members of a home-based caregivers team under the SACBC AIDS Office in general have a 69-day government-approved training. Each home-based caregiver has a workload of around twenty HIV patients who are visited once or twice a week. The home-based caregivers are supervised by a professional nurse and work twenty hours a week on a voluntary basis. They receive a stipendium for their work. These home-based caregivers identify the patients who need ARVs, help to educate them about ARVs (drugs literacy training), encourage them to disclose their status to one or more members of their household, and do an adherence follow-up once the patients are on treatment.

The SACBC AIDS Office would undertake to provide a centrally co-ordinated laboratory service, a centrally co-ordinated pharmacy service and a centrally co-ordinated training. And most important, centrally co-ordinated funding. With this trial, the SACBC AIDS Office was following the example of a project of Medicines Sans Frontières in Kayelitsha in Capetown, where a similar trial turned out to be a success.[10]

## 4. Aims of the SACBC AIDS Office

The SACBC AIDS Office is an office put in place by the Roman Catholic Bishops of Southern Africa (including South Africa, Namibia, Botswana, Lesotho and Swaziland). The office, seated in Pretoria, aims to make the Roman Catholic Church in all its structures - parishes, women's leagues, schools, communities of religious life and so on - more active in the battle against HIV/AIDS and its devastating effects on the population. The SACBC AIDS Office disseminates publications[11] about HIV/AIDS and funds grass-root level projects, like orphan care projects, home-based care projects, hospice projects and ARV projects.

The SACBC AIDS Office wanted to prove that a successful ARV roll-out would be possible in resource-poor settings. The SACBC AIDS Office was driven by the desire to save lives in areas where the government hardly had any medical infrastructure and where people would surely die of AIDS given the slow pace of roll-out of the South African government. The Catholic Church wanted to use its infra-structure in rural and remote areas where missions could reach the people that could never be reached by government hospitals. The Roman Catholic Church in Southern Africa could use its human resources in these areas, mainly home-based carers, who were already trained in the 69-day training approved by the government. During this course, the trainees, mainly women without a job, receive training in basic nursing skills, bed-bathing, wound dressing, palliative care and spiritual care for patients, mainly AIDS patients. The South African government sees training of home-based caregivers as the only way to cope with the growing burden of terminally ill AIDS patients. Hospitals cannot take the terminally ill anymore, they are already overburdened. Therefore patients have to be cared for at home as long as possible.

It cannot be denied that the SACBC AIDS Office had a desire to challenge the South African government to keep its promises and not to fall back to denialist attitudes after the April 2004 elections. The SACBC AIDS Office always kept good contacts with critical movements like the South African Clinicians Society[12], the Treatment Action Campaign[13] and the Trade Unions (COSATU)[14] and wanted to encourage the government with its ARV roll-out programme not to fall asleep. On the other hand, the SACBC AIDS Office aimed not to remove responsibility from the government. It negotiated with the government for permission for the roll-out in each of the nine provinces of South Africa and promised in these negotiations to follow the same protocol and medicine regiments as the South African government would use for the hand-out in public health facilities.

## 4. Admission Criteria

The admission criteria for people living with AIDS who want to qualify for ARVs at points of service of the SACBC AIDS Office are:
- Patients must have a CD4 count < 200[15] or be in clinical stage 4 of HIV according to WHO guidelines.
- Patients must be prepared to follow drugs literacy training.
- Patients must be prepared to take the ARVs lifelong and have to sign a consent form in which they agree to do so.
- Patients have to disclose their status to at least one member of their household.

- Patients must agree to be followed up by home-based caregivers or peer counsellors after they have started their treatment.
- Patients must live in the areas served by the home-based care teams or peer counsellors.[16]
- Patients must practise a lifestyle that goes with taking ARVs (no excessive smoking or drinking and safe sex).
- Patients must collect their treatment in person once a month and pay for their own transport.
- Patients must come for a blood check every six months.
- The whole project is on a 'first come, first serve' basis.

## 5. Granters of the ARV Project

End 2003, the SACBC AIDS Office and Memisa/Cordaid[17] agreed that the first five sites[18] would be funded by Memisa/Cordaid in The Netherlands. This very basic funding provided for:

- The laboratory costs for CD4 count and viral load tests as a baseline test and henceforth the same tests every six months (including courier costs for sending the blood samples to a central laboratory in Johannesburg).
- Training costs and salaries for a nurse, a part-time doctor and a part-time co-ordinator for each site.
- Additional budget for transport, training and office equipment.
- A small budget for medicines for opportunistic infections (like TB, pneumonia, candida, shingles, meningitis, etc.).

With the help of Memisa/Cordaid the first five projects could start in February 2004.

Later in the same year, a memorandum of understanding was signed with PEPFAR (Presidential Emergency Plan For AIDS Relief)[19] from the USA via CRS (Catholic Relief Services)[20] which made it possible to scale up to 22 projects in South Africa. The Memisa/Cordaid funding was shifted to points of service in Swaziland and Botswana, also under the auspices of the SACBC AIDS Office.[21]

## 6. Two Examples, two Sites

To illustrate the rapid growth of the ARV project, a short description is given of the fast developments at two sites, namely St. Joseph's Care and Support Centre at Sizanani Village in Bronkhorstspruit, and Nazareth House in Johannesburg.[22] The assumption of the SACBC AIDS Office that ARVs could be rolled out successfully in resource-poor settings proved to be right.

The home-based caregivers team of St. Joseph's Care and Support Centre at Sizanani mobilised at the first blood taking day at this facility in February 2004, the astonishing number of 80 patients who came to give their blood for a CD4 count test, whereas 20 patients were expected. The home-based care team had received a two days' drugs literacy training on top of their 69-day home-based care training, their practicals in the hospice for the terminally ill and their counselling training. Besides their practical experience in their townships as home-based caregivers, this made them the best and most committed tool in achieving a well-functioning ARV roll-out programme.

In October 2004, St. Joseph's Care Centre at Sizanani had 122 patients on ARVs (35 male adults, 78 female adults and 9 children < 14 years old), in April 2005, 315 patients had their ARVs (80 male adults, 216 female adults and 19 children < 14 years old) and in August 2005, 364 patients received there antiretroviral therapy (90 male adults, 254 female adults and 20 children < 14 years old). Adherence rates of more than 95% were reached.

Together with the rapidly growing number of patients on ARVs the number of patients dying in St. Joseph's Care Centre dropped significantly. In 2004, the admission rate in the hospice for the terminally ill dropped with 27%. Also the number of new AIDS orphans in our programme, which had been growing very fast between 2001 and 2004, came to a standstill and stabilised around 625 orphans.

Another effect of the ARV roll-out was a diminishing of the stigma attached to being HIV-positive. The support group for people living with AIDS with six members started in 2003 and grew into a whopping group of 60 HIV-positive members, which established nine small support groups in nine different locations with 70 members under the guidance of peer councellors trained in 2005. People living with AIDS witnessing openly about their status in front of factory workers, school pupils, farm workers, church members and colleagues became more and more common.

In Nazareth House the initial focus was to help the 35 HIV-positive children that live in this convent because their parents or other family members died or abandoned them or rejected them because of their status. The viral load in all these children was tested and 14 out of the 35 were put on ARVs. The ARV project in Nazareth House would never have become a success without the dedication of some female doctors who helped out on a part-time basis, some of them specialists in paediatric HIV.

After the initial phase which only included the children, Nazareth House ARV project started to link with two home-based care teams from outside, who agreed to prepare and follow up the outpatients. In Nazareth House in October 2004 we had 44 patients on ARVs of whom 14 were under 14 years old. In April 2005 we had 116 patients on ARVs of whom 16 under 14 years old and in September 2005, 163 patients on ARVs of whom 17 under 14 years old, mainly clients from the above mentioned home-based care teams.

The experiences in St. Joseph's Care Centre and Nazareth House were similar. Not only are ARVs 'miracle' drugs which can save people living with AIDS from the grave and which can change patients who are mere skeletons to healthy, normally functioning citizens, also the ARVs can totally change the atmosphere in the home-based care teams. Providing home-based care in a setting where ARVs are not available can be extremely strenuous, because all the time patients are dying under very painful circumstances. When ARVs are available, the home-based carers and their patients regain hope and that alone makes the work and life much easier.

## 7. Working Relationship of University and SACBC AIDS Office

End 2004, the SACBC AIDS Office and the Faculty of Social Sciences of Utrecht University, The Netherlands, agreed that Social Science students of Utrecht University would investigate the effect of ARVs on the social-emotional development of children at several points of service, beginning at St. Joseph's Care Centre and Nazareth House. In May 2005 the first investigation started in Sizanani. After four months of investigation, two new students took over in September 2005. They scaled up their investigation to more points of service besides St. Joseph's Care Centre and Nazareth House. Results and findings of the first investigation can be found in Chapter 15.

## 8. Way Forward

Both St. Joseph's Care Centre and Nazareth House are rapidly reaching the goals set for them by the SACBC AIDS Office. St. Joseph's Care Centre's task was to have 400 patients on ARVs before 1 April 2006. This goal has almost been reached already in October 2005. In the meantime St. Joseph's Care Centre has been informed by the SACBC AIDS Office that they are allowed to scale up to 550 patients on ARVs. Nazareth House was asked to have 200 patients on ARVs by 1 April 2006 and has also nearly attained this goal. In the meantime Nazareth House has been informed that it can scale up to 250 patients by the first of April 2006.

PEPFAR agreed to provide all patients in this programme with their ARVs for at least for 5 years. In the longer run, SACBC AIDS Office intends to hand over patients to government points of service, when the roll-out of the government would have been scaled up.

At the moment the SACBC AIDS Office is negotiating with Kwa-Mhlanga Hospital, circa 50 km from St. Joseph's Care Centre at Sizanani in the Mpumalanga province, about taking over stabilised patients on ARVs from that site. Kwa-Mhlanga Hospital has been recently accredited, but the roll-out there is still slow. The accredited site nearest to Nazareth House is Johannesburg General Hospital. This site has been accredited longer. This hospital would prefer Nazareth House to only hand out ARVs to the children on site and to refugees. Nevertheless, the pressure on Nazareth House to take patients living in the neighbouring areas of Berea, Yeoville and Hillbrow (very impoverished neighbourhoods in the old inner city of Johannesburg) is great, also because the Johannesburg General Hospital has a waiting list. Also patients prefer to be in the Nazareth House ARV programme, because the service in Johannesburg General Hospital is poorer and patients have to pay a fee to be admitted to the ARV programme, whereas the service in Nazareth House is free.

The whole ARV project of the SACBC AIDS Office now serves nationwide more than 4000 patients and after the government of South Africa, the SACBS AIDS Office is the largest single provider of ARVs in South Africa. This does not mean we can sit back and be happy about what has been achieved. The stark reality is that still the majority of South Africans who need ARVs are either in denial about their HIV status, or are mixed up and wrongly informed about how to survive with HIV, or simply cannot get ARVs. Therefore, there is still a lot of work to do!

# Acknowledgement

We would like to thank Sr. Alison Munro, director of the SACBC AIDS Office, for her review of the final version of this chapter.

## Notes

1.  *Mail & Guardian,* 3-9 October 2003, 'African's leader or its laggard? Mbeki must find the political will to fight AIDS or risk blotting his legacy', by Ferial Haffajee.
2.  *The Sunday Independent,* 5 October 2003, 'Replace Mbeki with man who cares about people', by Pieter-Dirk Uys, South Africa's most famous comedian.
3.  *Bangkok Post,* 16 July 2004, 'Mbeki should be here for forum', by 'Bewildered'.
4.  *Mail & Guardian,* 2 January 2005, 'The A to F of Mbeki's Cabinet'.
5.  *Sunday Times,* 29 May 2005, 'Manto pushes AIDS diet in hospitals', by Kerry Cullinan.
6.  *The Star,* 30 June 2005, 'Minister's advice "amounts to malpractice"', by Democratic Alliance opposition party Health spokesperson, Diane Kohler-Barnard.
7.  *The Sunday Independent,* 9 January 2005, 'The gentle child who opted for a private life', by Maureen Isaacson.
8.  *The Star,* 7 January 2005, 'Join Madiba and beat AIDS stigma: The disclosure of the reason for his son's death is a powerful blow against the disease's stigma', by Jovial Rantao.
9.  *Mail & Guardian,* 27 February 2004, 'Roll-out or cop-out? Implementation of the government's AIDS plan will be uneven over the provinces', by Nawaal Deane.
10. Search for project descriptions 'Medicines sans Frontières Kayelitsha' on the internet.
11. *Responsibility in a time of AIDS: A pastoral response by Catholic theologians and AIDS activists in Southern Africa,* edited by Stuart C. Bate, OMI, 2003, ISBN 0-620-30482-0. See also www.sacbc. org.za.
12. The South African Clinicians Society is an organisation of doctors and clinicians, initially meant to gather professionals in this health sector, which became more and more vocal against the foot-dragging AIDS policies of Dr. Manto Tshabalala-Msimang, when she refused to make nevirapine available in public health to prevent mother-to-child transmission of the HIV virus in 2002.
13. The Treatment Action Campaign (TAC) is the biggest organisation of AIDS activists in the world. Under their world famous leader Zackie Achmat (HIV-positive himself) they are continuously campaigning for access to treatment for all. They campaign for free ARVs in the public health sector for all infected South Africans, and for free nevirapine for HIV-positive mothers. Besides that, they have trained large numbers of unemployed, HIV-positive South Africans to be drugs literate and sent them out to help government hospitals and NGOs which hand out ARVs, but are lacking counsellors and staff. They have structures in all South African provinces. E-mail: info@-tac.org.za.
14. COSATU stands for Congress of South African Trade Unions. COSATU co-operates with the ANC (African National Congress) and the SACP (South African Communist Party), all supporting South Africa's ANC government. Under their leader, Vavi Zwelenzime, COSATU has become increasingly critical of the HIV/AIDS policy of the ANC government, which is characterised by a slow pace, broken promises and a lack of political will.
15. The CD4 count shows how the resistance of the body is affected by the HIV virus. A normally healthy person has a CD4 count of between 800-1500. The HIV virus starts to eat the cells that normally keep all infections outside our bodies. If a person has a CD4 count of 200 or less CD4 cells, this means that he/she has entered the AIDS stage and in principle can get all life-threatening infections like TB, pneumonia, meningitis, candida, carposi sancoma, etc. that will ultimately kill him/her.

16. Peer counsellors are PLWAs who take ARVs and are trained to counsel other PLWAs who have just started on ARVs about how to take these medicines, about the possible side effects and what lifestyle people who use ARVs should adopt.

17. Memisa/Cordaid in The Hague, The Netherlands, is one of the largest donor organisations in The Netherlands. Organisations like Memisa/Cordaid receive funds from the Dutch government to distribute among their partners in the Third World. Memisa/Cordaid uses its worldwide network of mainly Roman Catholic NGOs. Of all the work done worldwide in the fight against HIV/AIDS, circa 25% is done by Roman Catholic organisations (figures from Caritas Internationalis, Rome, Italy). Other important Dutch donor organisations are ICCO, HIVOS, NOVIB and PLAN Netherlands.

18. The first five ARV sites under the SACBC AIDS Office were: St. Joseph's Care and Support Centre at Sizanani in Bronkhorstspruit, Nazareth House in Johannesburg, St. Francis in Johannesburg, the project in Winterveld (all in the Gauteng province) and Marianhill in Durban, KwaZulu-Natal.

19. PEPFAR is an initiative of US President George W. Bush to fight AIDS worldwide. In 2004, the US Congress made 15 billion dollars available for the fight against HIV/AIDS over a period of five years. From this money, support is given to projects in fourteen different countries around the globe which are active in the fields of HIV prevention, home-based care, palliative and hospice care, handing out of ARVs and orphan care. Sometimes PEPFAR works through national governments but mainly through national organisations like the SACBC AIDS Office, the Hospice and Palliative Care Organisation in South Africa, etc. In prevention PEPFAR likes to emphasise to abstain and be faithful en tends not to support the supply of condoms.

20. Catholic Relief Service (CRS) is a large US donor organisation that has its own office in South Africa and can monitor the use of PEPFAR funds through its partners more effectively than the US Bush administration itself.

21. The infrastructure of the projects in Botswana and Swaziland is similar to other SACBC AIDS Office projects in South Africa, which means that a well-trained home-based care team is present and nurses and part-time doctors are sent for specific training on ARV implementation in Southern Africa.

22. At the two points of service the author has been appointed as a part-time coordinator since February 2004.

*Address for correspondence:*
Mr. Ricus Dullaert
St. Joseph's Care and Support Centre
Sizanani Village
P.O. Box 2016
Groblersdal Road (R 25)
1020 Bronkhorstspruit
South Africa
e-mail: ricusdullaert@gmx.net

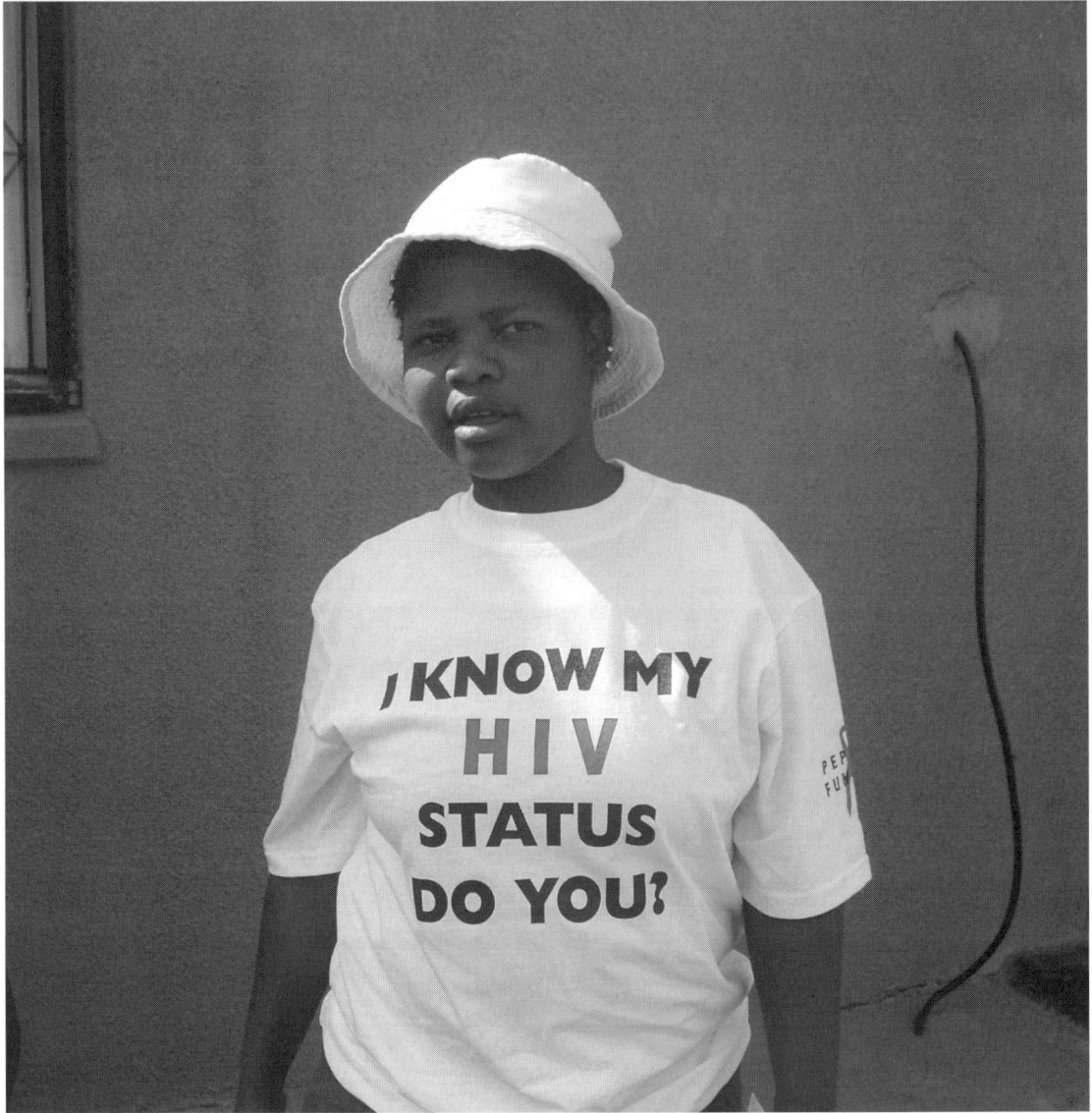

# Chapter 13

# Turning of the Tide: A Qualitative Study of ARV Treatment Programmes

*Maretha de Waal* [1,2]

[1] University of Pretoria, Pretoria, South Africa
[2M] Assisted by Sr. Ouma Nakedi, Southern African Catholic Bishops' Conference AIDS Office, Pretoria, South Africa

## Abstract

The Southern African Catholic Bishops' Conference (SACBC)-AIDS Office has been actively fostering the development of local community-driven initiatives in their response to the HIV/AIDS pandemic. More recently, the SACBC-AIDS Office has secured funding to coordinate the implementation of ARV programmes for people in its home-based care and hospice programmes. The ARV programme sites of the SACBC AIDS Office aim at complementing government programmes in areas where government-funded ARV treatment is not available, notably in resource-poor communities.

ARV programme implementation poses almost insurmountable challenges to programme managers, health care staff and human and financial resources. ARV centres face huge patient backlogs and growing demands for ARV treatment. Research into the social and organisational dynamics of ARV programmes in the initial phase of implementation is crucial to identify both positive and negative consequences of current processes and systems, with a view to sustaining and improving service delivery. This qualitative study explores the formal and informal institutions relevant to the implementation of SACBC's ARV programmes. Selected themes and cross-cutting issues were studied on an individual, institutional and community level. The study focused on the themes relevant to ARV programmes: social coherence and stigma tendencies, organisational dynamics, capacity, resources and service delivery, and individual responses to ARV treatment. Three cross-cutting issues were included in the study as these relate to social institutions impacting on HIV/AIDS prevention, treatment and care, namely gender, generation and social support structures.

The experience of the SACBC ARV treatment programme at the selected research sites yields several lessons for ARV programme implementation and 'scale-up. The needs and concerns raised by programme staff, as well as the narrative reports of patients on receiving ARV treatment, provide a valuable set of strategic issues that need to be considered by programme managers. These issues are critical as treatment programmes are expanded to reach larger numbers of people in more areas of South Africa. Programme maturation also brings its own set of strategic issues. The treatment and care of children pose particular challenges, and require specific attention of programme managers.

## 1. Introduction

Across the world, 60 million people are HIV-positive. More than six million people living with HIV and AIDS in the developing world need AIDS-inhibiting drugs to significantly extend their lives. Currently, an estimated number of 700,000 people receive such drugs. Initiatives are undertaken to raise this figure to three million people in low and middle income countries by the end of 2005 (UNAIDS, 2004).

The availability of ARV treatment has been documented to reduce the problem of HIV and AIDS to a manageable chronic disease. The availability and proper administration of AIDS inhibitors, together with facilities to treat opportunistic infections and conditions to lead a healthy lifestyle, have indeed been proved to play a key role in decreasing AIDS-related suffering and mortality.

In South Africa, the first signs of the HIV/AIDS pandemic began to be noticed when, in the early 1990s, annual antenatal surveys of women attending state clinics showed that close to 3% of them were HIV-positive. At the time, HIV/AIDS was still thought of as primarily a homosexual disease, and then the government was slow to respond to these statistics. Early responses by this government, whose legitimacy was questioned, had little impact. The AIDS plan of the government that came to power in 1994 focused on prevention and declined to accept AIDS-inhibiting drugs at reduced prices, and even at no cost, from pharmaceutical companies (MacFarlane, 2004).

One of the South African government's arguments for not accepting AIDS drugs has been that the health care infrastructure, especially in many communities, could not cope with the demand for the provision of treatment. Other arguments against public availability of AIDS inhibitors related to the dangerous side effects of these drugs. The South African government responded to the AIDS epidemic by formulating policies and setting up structures and programmes for the implementation of policies without making treatment publicly available. These included adopting a National AIDS Programme and STD (sexually transmitted diseases) management protocols, free access to male condoms, the training of thousands of secondary school teachers in HIV/AIDS to implement life skills programmes targeting the youth, the introduction of an annual HIV surveillance system, setting up an AIDS directorate in the Department of Health, and the adoption of an HIV/AIDS/STD Strategic Plan for South Africa 2000-2005 (Department of Health, 2000).

After several years of resistance and prevarication, the Constitutional Court ruled that the South African government had to provide nevirapine or 'equivalent treatments'. Government finally announced its support in principle for public sector provision of highly active antiretroviral therapy (HAART) in August 2003. Preparations for programme roll-out commenced at the beginning of 2004. The initial aim was to establish at least one accredited service point in each health district by the end of the first year of implementation. Furthermore, the plan stated that by the end of March 2004, 54,000 people would be on ARV treatment. That deadline has already been missed, and has been moved to March of 2005. MacFarlane (2004) suggests that this target is also impossible in view of the fact that by October 2004 only 19,500 people were on treatment through the government's ARV programme.

It has also been suggested that by far the majority of HIV-infected people will not be able to receive the life-prolonging drugs from the South African government. A report published by the Centre for Actuarial Research in 2003 estimated that about 1.6 million people are in need of ARV treatment or will soon need it (SAIRR, 2004). According to the report, approximately 6.5 million South Africans were HIV-positive, 75% of whom were in WHO stages 1 and 2 of the disease's progression, which meant that they had not yet developed any symptoms and possibly did not know their status. It also meant that they might be in need of ARV drugs in the near future.

The limitations of government's ARV programme roll-out have raised immense concern both locally and globally. Faith-based organisations in general and the Catholic Church specifically have become central role players in a range of activities to combat the pandemic. The SACBC opened its AIDS Office in January 2000 in order to coordinate the response of the Catholic Church to the HIV/AIDS pandemic in five Southern African countries. The SACBC AIDS Office has been actively fostering the development of local community-driven initiatives in their response to the HIV/AIDS pandemic, including provision of food aid, income generation/skills training, HIV/AIDS awareness, home-based palliative care, hospices and orphan support. In addition, the SACBC AIDS Office embarked on a process to secure funding and to coordinate the implementation of ARV programmes for people in its home-based care and hospice programmes. Plans for the implementation of ARV programmes through funding secured by the SACBC AIDS Office commenced in 2002, at a time when there was no commitment from the South African government to make ARV treatment available (see also Chapter 12).

## 2. Background to the SACBC's ARV Treatment Programmes

Using the John Snow international tool, 22 sites were selected and funding proposals submitted to international donors. These sites have been providing care and support for people affected by HIV/AIDS for many years and are committed for the long haul. With funding secured, the SACBC AIDS Office set up pilot projects in poor rural areas across South Africa where the government has not provided ARV treatment. Letters of agreement have been obtained from each provincial Department of Health. After the initial piloting of programmes in six sites in Gauteng and KwaZulu-Natal, and after securing additional funding, the SACBC pilot sites expanded their programmes from initial facilities that served a relatively small number of people to facilities that serve a significantly larger population (so-called 'scale-up'). The first blood samples were taken on 16 February 2004 and the first patients started medication on 5 March 2004. In each location, drugs are to be provided to 100 HIV-positive patients in the first year, 200 in the second year and 400 in the third year of the programme cycle.

The ARV programme sites of the SACBC aim at complementing government programmes in areas where government-funded ARV- treatment is not available, notably in resource-poor communities. All SACBC sites work with government referral sources and use the government's treatment protocols and treatment regimens. Staff are trained in government accredited programmes. It was agreed to also use the government's patient tracking forms, so that patients who move around may be able to continue treatment. In addition, SACBC ARV programmes also accept patients on long waiting lists at government hospitals and are open to both South African and non-South African citizens. Patient numbers are reported to government using the government format.

The programme operates along a continuum of prevention, care and treatment, involving all aspects of AIDS. ARV treatment is linked to prevention, in that people receive counselling about not becoming re-infected and not infecting other people. Treatment is also linked to holistic patient care, regardless of whether this takes place in the context of a hospital, hospice or clinic. Home-based care is the backbone of the treatment programmes.

Programme preparation commenced in February 2004 at the various sites, with staff recruitment and training as a first step. Each site employed a doctor, a professional nurse and a project coordinator. After the nurses and doctors had finished their training, accredited by the Foundation for Professional Development, so-called drug literacy courses were presented to home carers, the remaining medical staff and patients. Each site employs the same procedure designed to speed up the treatment process, avoid unnecessary delays in the delivering and administration of the AIDS-inhibiting drugs, personalise treatment and maximise adherence:

Home carers identify patients – who in their opinion meet a number of strict criteria – for a blood test at the ARV treatment centre. The doctor and nurse draw blood from patients on site, which is then sent by courier service to a laboratory in Johannesburg to be tested for CD4, viral load and full blood count (where necessary, liver function tests are also performed). The sites are informed of the results by e-mail. Adult patients with CD4 counts below 200 are put on treatment. Drugs are ordered electronically by the site doctor from a pharmaceutical company in Johannesburg. These are pre-packaged individually for each patient and delivered to the site, where they are given to the patients. Each patient has to undergo adherence training and treatment of opportunistic infections before commencing with treatment (Viljoen, 2004). Criteria for taking part in the SACBC's ARV treatment programme correspond with the patient selection criteria for ARV of the National Department of Health South Africa (2004):

– Adult patients must have fewer than 200 CD4 cells per 100 ml of blood (the point at which HIV develops into AIDS).
– Patients must live in an area where home carers are working and must agree to be supervised by one of these home carers.
– They must have informed the people they live with of their HIV status.
– They may not have taken AIDS inhibitors before and must be prepared to take them for the rest of their lives.
– They must keep a lifestyle suited to treatment with AIDS inhibitors (no alcohol addiction, safe sex, eating as healthily as possible).
– They must have followed a drug literacy course and must have a basic understanding of HIV/AIDS and AIDS inhibitors.

The first screening visit takes place two to four weeks before starting ARV therapy. The aim of this visit is to confirm the selection criteria, both clinical and laboratory, to treat any opportunistic infection, to complete patient information records, to meet with the multidisciplinary team for information sessions, to discuss treatment with the patient, to provide a 28-day supply of antibiotics, and to arrange a date of return.

The home-based care worker/treatment counsellor visits the patient at home to assess home circumstances, correctness of contact details and support structures, including disclosure and drug storage facilities. The second visit includes clinical assessment, an information and education session, pill count and adherence counselling to patient and patient advocate if available. The ARV commencement visit includes (for first-line and second-line treatment in adults) reassessment of patient's readiness, pill count, reinforcing of drug-dosing details and detailed discussion of drugs and adherence issues with the patient and his/her advocate. Thereafter, patients visit the ARV clinic monthly to collect medication and for the professional nurse to monitor drug tolerance, adverse events and adherence. Patients should be seen by the doctor at 4, 8 and 12 weeks and every three months thereafter, if well. If not well, patients should see the doctor more frequently. Safety blood tests are taken as per schedule.

CD4 counts and viral loads are done six-monthly while patients are on the regimen.

# 3. Problem Statement

ARV programme implementation poses almost insurmountable challenges to programme managers, health care staff and human and financial resources. ARV centres face huge patient backlogs and growing demands for ARV treatment. With growing numbers of HIV-infected people and people reaching WHO stages 3 and 4 of the disease before seeking ARV treatment, programme sustainability poses very serious challenges to both implementing agencies and patients receiving or awaiting ARV treatment. On an organisational and service delivery level, programme implementation poses serious challenges to implementing agencies, especially non-governmental service facilities, their resources, systems and focus. ARV programme implementation requires very intensive and holistic care and systemic linkages to other parts of the health care system. Can service providers secure the necessary resources, systems and focus to sustain quality prevention, treatment and care programmes (also in view of government's limited facilities for ART programmes)? Scaling up ARV treatment requires assured long-term political support and funding. Any lapse in support could result in collapsed ARV programmes, with resultant interruptions in treatment, giving HIV the opportunity to become drug resistant and render entire treatment programmes useless if drug-resistant strains of the virus start spreading (UNAIDS, 2004).

Health staffing is also crucial to the prospects of extending ARV access. According to the UNAIDS 2004 Report on the Global AIDS epidemic, many nurses and doctors seek better salaries, working conditions and opportunities in higher-income countries, 70% of doctors trained in South Africa currently live abroad. Can service providers secure the necessary multidisciplinary treatment teams to provide integrated treatment and patient care?

On an individual patient level, adherence to treatment, the effect thereof on the individual and the occurrence of opportunistic infections show great variation from one person to the next.

How do gender, age and family/community support affect an individual's response to treatment and the way in which individuals are stigmatised and ostracised, or integrated into their families and communities?

Faith-based organisations play a crucial role in the fight against HIV/AIDS. The involvement of faith-based organisations is multifaceted and includes organisational, spiritual, emotional, psychological and value-related issues. Faith leadership plays an important role in motivating people to become involved in HIV/AIDS-related work. Also, faith can be a source of comfort both for those infected and affected by HIV and AIDS. Faith underpins and propels the response of the Church as an institution to the HIV/AIDS epidemic. The morality of care and compassion obliges individuals and organisations to become involved in the prevention of the spread of HIV and to care for the sick or those whose lives are affected by the sickness or death of family members. On the other hand, faith and religion can also prevent HIV-infected people from accessing treatment, or encourage people to rely on witchcraft or traditional medicine which may interfere with ARV drugs.

Walker (2004) argues that social scientists have been slow to respond to the HIV/AIDS epidemic and that much work remains to be done on the social dynamics of HIV/AIDS. Research into the social and organisational dynamics of ART programmes in the initial phase of implementation is crucial to identify both positive and negative consequences of current processes and systems, with a view to sustaining and improving service delivery, and ultimately to save the lives of women and men, adults and children, in rural and in urban areas.

Despite a burgeoning amount of research in the area of HIV and AIDS over the past number of years, many questions remain unanswered. In addition, the bulk of the research up to date has been undertaken in a context where ARV treatment has not been publicly available. The context of HIV and AIDS prevention, treatment and care in South Africa has changed drastically since the implementation of government's ARV treatment programmes in the beginning of 2004, opening up a host of unanswered questions regarding the impact of ARV on service providers and on the recipients of ARV treatment: Does stigma disappear when people have the prospect of accessing treatment? Would women who have not been able to negotiate safe sex before be able to do this while they are on ARV treatment to prevent re-infection? Would families, where disclosure of HIV-positive status meant rejection and ostracisation, now embrace family members on ARV treatment and support their adherence to ARV medication? Would children who have suffered bereavement and traumatisation while family members were sick and died of AIDS in their presence, be able to pick up the pieces of their lives and continue to lead 'normal' lives? Would children who have been stunted due to AIDS and AIDS-related family resource depletion be able to catch up on their development milestones and become re-integrated into the family and community?

This study explores some of these questions, in an attempt to document 'lessons learned' in the initial phases of ARV programme implementation at selected SACBC-funded sites.

## 4. Focus, Aims and Scope of the Study

This study explores the formal and informal institutions relevant to the implementation of ARV programmes. Selected themes and cross-cutting issues were studied on three levels, namely an individual, institutional and community level. The study focused on the following themes relevant to ARV treatment programmes: social coherence and stigma tendencies, organisational dynamics, capacity, resources and service delivery, and individual responses to ARVs. Three cross-cutting issues were included in the study as these relate to social institutions impacting on HIV/AIDS prevention, treatment and care: gender, generation and social support structures. The table below summarises the focus and scope of the study.

| Levels | Themes | Cross-cutting issues |
|---|---|---|
| Community | Social coherence and stigma tendencies | Support structures |
| Institutional | Organisational dynamics, capacity, resources, service delivery in relation to ARV programming (incl. HIV prevention, positive living, orphaned and vulnerable children and voluntary counselling and testing) | Stigma |
| Individual | Individual responses to ARV programme implementation and patient treatment | Gender and generation |

Figure 1: Focus and scope of the study

The aims of this exploratory study are threefold:
1. Documenting experiences, expectations and perceptions regarding ARV treatment of health care workers at the various facilities involved in ARV implementation, and of patients (women, men, children) who receive ARV treatment.

2. Comparing programme implementation at the various kinds of implementing organisations, namely:
   a. home-based care facilities;
   b. facilities for children;
   c. hospital facilities;
   d. hospice facilities.
3. Developing a set of 'lessons learned' from the initial stages of ARV programme implementation at the seven pilot sites to inform programme scale-up and programme implementation at other sites, with a specific focus on the following:
   a. increasing social coherence in the community and decreasing stigma;
   b. supporting women as well as men - according to their different roles, needs and resources - in testing, treatment and care;
   c. increasing the effectiveness and efficiency of ARV programme implementation, but not at the cost of other services and programmes;
   d. improving sustainability of ARV programme implementation and coordination with other HIV and AIDS programmes (e.g. prevention);
   e. identifying possibilities of and opportunities for institutionalising emotional and spiritual support for caregivers, patients and their families and relatives.

The following questions were formulated to guide the research:
1. What is the role of ARV therapy in individuals' experiences, perceptions and expectations of *social coherence and stigma*?
2. What is the effect of ARV therapy on *women* in general and more specifically with regard to their *gendered positions and relations in households and public life*? What is the effect of ARV therapy on *men*?
3. What is the effect of introducing ARVs on the role, resources, capacity and service delivery of the *implementing organisation*?
4. What measures do implementing organisations take to enhance *sustainability* and *interconnectivity* of their ARV programmes to other health care programmes (including HIV/AIDS programmes)?
5. What is the role of *spirituality and faith* in the various aspects of service delivery in ARV programme implementation?
6. How do *children* experience their HIV-positive status and respond to treatment?
7. What are the *specific strategies and issues/constraints* pertaining to the various implementing programmes at hospitals, hospices, home-based care centres and centres dealing mainly with children?

## 5. Methods

### 5.1. Research Design

In general, the qualitative paradigm stems from an anti-positivistic, interpretative approach. It is ideographic and holistic in nature, and aims mainly to understand social life and the meaning that people attach to their everyday experiences. It is for this reason that the qualitative research paradigm was selected for the study. Qualitative research produces descriptive data in the participants' own words. It thus involves identifying the participants' beliefs and values that underlie the phenomenon. True to the nature of qualitative research, the researchers attempted to gain a first-hand, holistic understanding by means of a flexible strategy of problem formulation and data collection (Marshall & Rossman, 1999).

## 5.2. *Selection of sites*

Data for the main research project were collected at the following ARV treatment centres funded through the SACBC AIDS Office:
– home-based care centres: Sizanani (Bronkhorstspruit), Tapologo (Rustenburg) and Sinosizo (Stanger, KZN);
– children's centres: Nazareth House (Yeoville), St. Francis (Boksburg);
– hospital: St. Mary's Hospital (Marianhill, KZN);
– hospices: Holy Cross (Pretoria), St. Francis (Boksburg), Nazareth House (Yeoville).

Seven interviews were conducted in each of the seven sites (N=49). Respondents for interviews were identified from the following categories of members of the ARV team at each site:
– ARV project management and administration;
– medical practitioners;
– professional nurses;
– trainers;
– volunteer caregivers;
– adult male patients receiving ARVs;
– adult female patients receiving ARVs.

## 5.3. *Data Collection Techniques*

### *Observation*

The role of the researchers in the observation process entailed being objective observers to form a comprehensive and holistic view of the implementation of each of the programmes in each of the seven research sites. Field notes were kept and analysed in terms of the objectives of the research.

### *In-depth Interviews*

Two types of interviews were conducted:
1.  Interviews were conducted as *informal conversational interviews* with patients. This type of interview resembled a chat, during which participants sometimes forgot that they were being interviewed. Most questions asked flowed from the immediate context.
2.  *Standardised open-ended interviews* were conducted with professional and project staff at the various ARV facilities included in the study. A set of open-ended questions were set and arranged for the purpose of minimising variation in the questions posed to the participants. Main questions were supplemented by probes and follow-up questions to acquire sufficient detail and to pursue the implications of answers to the main questions.

Interviews were audio-recorded for the purpose of transcription, translation and analysis.

## 4.3. *Data Analysis*

Triangulation was used by seeking out secondary information resources such as annual reports and workshop proceedings that could provide insights about the social dynamics of ARV programme implementation. Natural meaning units were identified to explore categories and patterns in the data, which would ultimately assist in the interpretation of the data and the formulation of 'lessons learned'.

## 6. Description of Programme Sites

The seven ARV programme sites are:

### 6.1. *Holy Cross Home*

Holy Cross Home is situated to the west of Pretoria. Originally a hospital and maternity home serving Pretoria's former black township of Lady Selborne, Holy Cross became a frail centre after the implementation of the previous government's policy of forced removal of the black residents of the area. Five years ago, it also opened a hospice with ten beds. The home trains health carers and has an outreach and home-based care service in the nearby informal settlement of Plastic View, a reference to its residents living under sheets of plastic. Holy Cross Home has a reputation for its excellent quality care. In 2001, it was named in a survey by the *Pretoria News* as the institution providing best quality health care in the Pretoria area (Viljoen, 2004). In March 2004, Holy Cross started putting its patients on ARV treatment. The ARV team comprises 1 part-time doctor, 2 registered nurses, 5 auxiliary nurses, 2 lay counsellors and 1 voluntary care worker. Initially, 25 patients were selected for treatment.

Treating opportunistic infections to get patients well enough to commence in some instances required referral of patients to other treatment centres.

*Strategic issues and constraints:*
– Securing accurate and timely diagnosis and treatment – and continuation of ART – from hospitals to which patients have been referred in cases of opportunistic infections.
– Continuity of treatment in the case of referral to outside hospitals and adherence after discharge cannot be assumed; sustaining a system of care with all role players, including home-based care and referral hospitals is essential.
– The need to secure funding, build linkages with other groups and service providers, and build own capacity and support mechanisms to sustain integrated, holistic care of the patient as an individual. This goes beyond medical care, spiritual and emotional support, to tailor-made support based on an understanding of the context into which the patient will be discharged. Many patients are discharged to informal settlement areas where basic infrastructure is lacking. In many instances this requires support to access disability grants and education and spiritual guidance to change lifestyle.
– Patients who are flourishing after discharge could be powerful role models in the community to promote timely testing and HIV prevention

### 6.2. *Nazareth House*

Nazareth House is situated in Yeoville, serving the inner city of Johannesburg. Over the years the social needs of the community changed, so the Sisters of Nazareth House changed their focus to meet those needs. This area is renowned for its crime, substance abuse and prostitution, as well as its highly transient population (including a very high percentage of refugees and economic migrants from all over Africa). Nazareth House is home to mentally disabled people, frail old people and destitute, terminally ill people. It is also home to HIV-positive abandoned and orphaned babies and children (Viljoen, 2004). The Sisters and lay staff care for 35 HIV/AIDS orphans, 9 adult terminally ill AIDS patients, 78 frail aged and 18 mentally challenged women. Most of the residents of Nazareth House can no longer adequately care for themselves or be maintained by family or community. Nazareth House was one of the first sites where SACBC started its ARV roll-out. Initially, the orphans residing in the centre were tested. Out of a total of 35, 14 had CD4 counts below 200.

They were immediately put on treatment. About two months later, treatment was started for adults and outpatients The outpatient clinic operates every Friday afternoon for adult patients. The multidisciplinary team of staff consists of two part-time doctors (a general practitioner own support group and meet on a weekly basis to discuss their issues and concerns. One of the sisters works within the inner city settlement areas on an outreach programme, addressing the spiritual, emotional and social needs of infected and affected people in the community. She supports and provides specialised home-based care when required. The programme also gives food, clothing and support especially to grandparents and single parent families who care for orphaned children. Nazareth House works in partnership with government, business and the community. For example, the home-based volunteers are supervised, trained and supported by government health workers. Three schools assist the children with their homework. Local businesses donate food, including baby food and immune booster supplements. The HIV Clinicians Society provides a 24-hour telephone support service.

Nazareth House also works in close collaboration with the Johannesburg General Hospital and the United Nations High Commission for Refugees (UNHCR). The arrangement was made for Nazareth House to accept Johannesburg General Hospital patients (South African citizens) on its waiting list for ARV treatment onto its programme until they get appointments at the Hospital, after which they would become government patients. In addition, Nazareth House accepts the non-South African citizens who applied for treatment at Johannesburg General Hospital (but who are not eligible for government-funded treatment) on to its ARV programme with UNHCR financial support. UNHCR uses the services of French and Portuguese-speaking counsellors to facilitate the partnership. Also, in order to strengthen linkages and build linkage systems, health care workers attend lectures at Baragwanath Hospital once a month regarding HIV issues in children's homes and issues relating to coping with grief and loss.

*Strategic issues and constraints:*

– Responding to the various problems and needs of children affected by the AIDS epidemic is an immense task. As more children begin to thrive after commencing ARV treatment, the need to find suitable foster homes and to re-unify HIV-infected children with their families is increasing. The kind of care required is also changing, as the needs of children who are on treatment and whose health has improved drastically, are very different from those of sick children.
– The notion of confidentiality of a child's HIV status in all circumstances may in some instances, especially in the case of school going children, compromise the health and well-being of the child, friends and teachers. The child's willingness to disclose and

skills to deal with the social responses to disclosure may vary from one child to another, and may change as the child grows older. On the other hand, many children receive ARVs without their knowing or understanding why they are sick and why they have to take the medication. This raises concerns regarding the availability of counselling services specifically developed for children to deal with these and related issues.
— Medication alone is not sufficient to effectively impact on the AIDS pandemic. The impact of HIV/AIDS on health, living standards, morale and general well-being of people requires a more comprehensive response. Empowering people to take responsibility for their own lives is an essential aspect of this approach. Also, working in partnership with government enterprises is vital to the success of the programme.
— Maintaining the spirit of adherence to the ART programme in the future, with a focus on prevention strategy, education, development, collaboration, openness and dialogue.

## 6.3. Sinosizo

Sinosizo was established in 1995 as a programme of the Archdiocese of Durban. It provides home-based care, an orphan and vulnerable children (OVC) programme, training and ARV treatment services. Its standard of training has made it one of the foremost training organisations in South Africa, providing training on all aspects of HIV and AIDS. It also has a large network of caregivers, providing care to the terminally ill in all parts of Durban. In 2003, 17,226 home visits were made to people living with AIDS. It has eight home-based care staff, 11 OVC staff, eight training staff, 3 ART staff and 154 volunteers.

Sinosizo prepared to participate in the SACBC's ARV programme in February 2004. It identified the rural area of Groutville in Northern KwaZulu-Natal (outside Stanger) as the site where it was to provide ARV treatment to its patients (Viljoen, 2004).

Sinosizo is rather unique as an ARV site, in that it is not linked to a clinic, hospice or hospital. Patients with opportunistic infections, as well as paediatric cases and pregnant women are referred to Starnger Hospital. The Groutville centre is next to an independent VCT (voluntary counselling and testing) centre. The Groutville clinic as well as community members act as sources of referral to Sinosizo. It employs the services of a part-time clinic doctor, project manager, professional nurse, social worker, therapeutic counsellor and clinic counsellor. The Groutville centre works in close collaboration with the Department of Social Development, which sends an official on a weekly basis to assist with social grant applications. The ART programme connects to its other programmes in important ways, for example records of children who are referred to the paediatric section of Stanger Hospital, are kept and followed up by their OVC programme officers.

## Strategic issues and constraints:
— Improving linkages, networks and communication with other ARV treatment centres and health facilities via data sharing to ensure patient follow-up and adherence. This would entail more effective record keeping, preferably computerised, not only to relieve the administrative burden of programme officers, but also to provide a better service to patients.
— Implementing a programme in a rural area poses particular problems with regard to setting up of infrastructure to support the services rendered. In particular, in view of the remote areas serviced by the programme, transport needs of staff to conduct home

visits and for patients to pay regular visits to the ARV treatment centre, have definite financial implications.

## 6.4. St. Francis Care Centre

St. Francis is not only one of the oldest Catholic hospices in the country, but also the largest. Situated in Boksburg, a mining area 30 km east of Johannesburg, it serves an urban area with migrant mine and industrial workers. The hospice was started more than ten years ago by Fr. Stan Brennan, a Franciscan priest. It has a residential facility for AIDS orphans, where more than 30 reside. It also provides home-based care in two areas, Vosloorus (the former 'black' township of Boksburg) and Reiger Park (the former 'coloured' township of Boksburg) (Viljoen, 2004). Initially, St. Francis started providing ARV treatment to its resident orphans, functioning as a satellite of Nazareth House. Currently 12 children receive ARV treatment. With funding from other sources, an ARV clinic was recently opened up. Already before completion, St Francis was receiving enquiries from potential patients in the Boksburg-Vosloorus-Reiger Park area. With the new wing that opened last year, it currently provides palliative care to more than 30 patients. Staffing includes a paediatrician, a part-time doctor, a professional nurse, counsellors and a social worker. At the time of the research interviews, preparations were underway to start treating adult patients. Patients had been selected for treatment and had been receiving counselling and treatment for opportunistic infections.

*Strategic issues and constraints are:*
- Well-trained and motivated counsellors form an essential part of the ARV programme. One of their important tasks is to support patients to disclose their status and to find a person to assist them in adhering to their treatment.
- Children are particularly vulnerable and staff are often confronted by the harsh impact of stigmatisation of children living with HIV and AIDS, and discrimination against sick children in families and communities. Communicating the message of treatment and improved health remains a vital part of the ARV programme to counter stigmatisation and discrimination against especially children with HIV/AIDS.

## 6.5. St. Joseph Care Centre, Sizanani Village

St Joseph Care Centre, Sizanani, is situated at Bronkhorstspruit, about 60 km east of Pretoria. Sizanani Village, started in 1989, has provided focused AIDS programmes since 1999. It is a large centre, containing a home for physically disabled children, a conference centre, a crafts workshop, training centres and a palliative care hospice. The hospice was started by a former nun and professional nurse, in response to the plight of dying people who were dropped at Sizanani's doorstep by relatives from the surrounding rural villages who were unable to care for them.

St. Joseph is the basis for an extensive home-based care programme. It provides voluntary testing and counselling, as well as palliative care and runs a number of support groups for people in the surrounding communities. The centre operates a number of day care centres for AIDS orphans, providing them with food, clothing and medical care. The Department of Health recognised the excellence of St Joseph as one of the country's top five models of best practice for home-based care and palliative care.

In addition, Sizanani provides support to community-based organisations. It houses an ARV treatment programme. St. Joseph has been earmarked to have 200 patients on ARV treatment by the end of February 2005. Starting with 80 clients presenting themselves for

VCT, there are already 92 patients on treatment. With funding from other donors, it has erected a new treatment wing with consulting rooms and training facilities, as well as a storage space for medicines. Sizanani has so impressed Department of Health officials with the quality of its service that it was selected by JSI (the organisation developing the computerised patient tracking system for the government) as one of the sites where the proposed patient tracking system would be field-tested (Viljoen, 2004).

*Strategic issues and constraints:*
– As the programme begins to mature and as patient numbers and the demand for its services increase, so does the need for self-sufficiency, which include more sophisticated equipment, appointment of extra staff and a more efficient electronic record-keeping system.
– As the numbers of patients who are thriving because of the ARV treatment increase, they begin to form a valuable 'pool of resources' for the ARV treatment centre, as they often avail themselves as volunteers to support the programme in various ways.

## 6.6. St. Mary's Hospital

St Mary's Hospital is situated at Marianhill, on the western outskirts of Durban. It is one of only two remaining mission hospitals in South Africa and serves the 'Outer West' health district of metropolitan Durban – an area with a population of close to 750, 000, consisting chiefly of very poor, mostly unemployed people living in informal settlements. This is one of the areas with the highest HIV infection rates in the country. The hospital has been on the forefront of providing care to people with AIDS. It has been offering ARV treatment for a number of years at its iThemba clinic (in association with Harvard University). In addition, it recently offered a prevention of mother-to-child transmission (PMTCT) programme at its St. Anne's Clinic. Both of these programmes functioned vertically, and were housed in separate buildings outside of the hospital.

Despite the extraordinary success of the programmes, the hospital currently faces problems in sustaining these services. With the termination of the previous funding, iThemba patients have been transferred to the current SACBC ARV treatment programme since the middle of 2004. The hospital now faces challenges relating to the integration of the iThemba and St. Anne's programmes into its mainstream services.

At the end of August 2004 the hospital had 178 patients on ARVs. The intention is to reach a target of 750 by the end of February 2005. This means that an additional 100 patients must be enrolled every month. At present, the hospital is on target with regard to enrolment of new patients (Viljoen, 2004).

Staff comprises 2 full-time doctors, 1 professional nurse, 1 staff nurse, 1 HIV counsellor, 1 community outreach director, 11 therapeutic counsellors, and 1 clerk in training. The multi-disciplinary team has a daily 1-hour pre-clinic conference to discuss their patients and to discuss various HIV-related topics. One day per week is set aside for team-building, staff education, patient case review, sharing of clinical cases, invitation to guest speakers and sharing of patient support, methods and tools.

The therapeutic counsellors (TCs) provide an important link between the patient, the clinic and the community. They undertake home visits, provide counselling and support and are able to identify side effects and barriers to adherence before non-adherence begins. A patient support group meets on a weekly basis. HIV-positive basic health and treatment literacy workshops and talks are given during selected support group meetings. Also, a range of community-based activities is coordinated and supported by the therapeutic counsellors.

*Strategic issues and constraints:*
– Integrating the ARV programme with existing hospital infrastructure and systems has both advantages (such as sharing of limited human resources and equipment) and disadvantages (such as dealing with stigma). Mainstreaming of ARV programmes at public health facilities may alleviate many of the current concerns.
– Recruiting and training of programme staff to deal with increasing numbers of patients, strengthening community support groups, maintaining a database for patient tracking and reporting that will meet various criteria, takes up a considerable amount of time and resources of the small team of programmestaff, in addition to dealing with increasing patient loads.

## 6.7. Tapologo, Rustenburg

Rustenburg, the world's largest source of platinum, is currently the fastest growing town in South Africa due to the sustained high prices of platinum. Home to migrant labourers from various African countries, the mineworkers live in single-sex hostels close to the mineshafts.

Following in their wake, women have set up informal settlements close to the gates of the hostels, providing various income-earning services and networks to the mineworkers. Over time, retrenched workers have erected shacks in these settlements as well, hoping to find employment again on the mines. In this way, shack settlements have grown around the gates of the hostels, accommodating poor, desperate and uprooted people. All of these settlements are on Bafokeng tribal land. With the Bafokeng not wanting them there, local authorities are

unable to provide services to the area or to secure tenure (Viljoen, 2004). There is a high incidence of HIV infection in the area, due to the extreme poverty of its inhabitants, a lack of extended families and a lack of personal and community resources.

The Tapologo programme of the Diocese of Rustenburg serves the mining community stretching north-west to north-east of the town, through the Freedom Park clinic. Housed in converted shipping containers, the clinic provides curative services, home-based care, adult education and child day care facilities. Due to overwhelming demand, services have spread to all the surrounding squatter settlements. Currently Tapologo has a network of home-based caregivers running a programme that is financially supported by the platinum mines and that provides services to all these communities. Tapologo is currently constructing an administrative centre and a hospice on the grounds of St. Joseph's Mission in Rustenburg (Viljoen, 2004).

Tapologo started ARV roll-out in March 2004 as part of the SACBC-funded ARV programme. As at the end of August, Tapologo had 48 patients on treatment, with a view of scaling up to 300 patients by the end of February 2005. The ARV programme is strategically based in the community and linked to the other Tapologo programmes, including the Freedom Park clinic, the in-patient unit, the OVC programme, the psycho-social support programme and the outreach programme. For example, services offered through the Tapologo outreach programme include counselling and emotional support, HIV/AIDS education and awareness, positive living, support groups and ART adherence. The outreach programme staff comprises an outreach manager, 8 professional nurses and 96 community caregivers who provide care to approximately 2,700 patients. During 2003, the caregivers recorded 28,000 home visits, and enrolled 836 new patients.

*Strategic issues and constraints:*
- The main focus of the ARV treatment programme is the provision of ARVs. To be able to do this effectively, it required project staff to undertake multiple 'extra' tasks and roles, such as: dealing with stigma, illiteracy, and uninformed and/or misinformed communities and patients; addressing issues of poverty and malnutrition of patients, traditional values and beliefs, traditional medicine and healers; coordination with government programmes and actively promoting good relations and linkages; effective reporting and project evaluation.
- As the ARV treatment programme matures and expands, increasing resources for increased patient care are needed. Also, staff needs refresher training on medical protocols and procedures.

## 7. Results

### 7.1. *Narrated Experiences of ARV Treatment*
Information collected from staff and patients at the ARV treatment centres is presented in the following categories:
- Information collected from programme staff regarding ARV programme implementation, based on interviews with programme staff.
- Issues arising from information about programme implementation collected from programme staff.
- Information collected from patients receiving ARVs.

The information was also analysed in terms of cross-cutting issues (social institutions), namely gender, generation and social support, with a focus on the capabilities or strengths, as well as the vulnerabilities of the respondents.

Following the qualitative framework, the presentation of the information includes statements and views taken from the research interviews.

### *Adhering to the Principles of Quality and Holistic Health Care*
Commitment to personalised quality and holistic care offered at each of the sites is the key feature of the ARV programmes and by far the most outstanding and most commented upon aspect of the ARV centres in the study. This commitment is reflected in the one-on-one interaction of programme staff with patients, as well as in the way in which the programmes are managed to meet the set targets. One of the part-time doctors made the following observation: *'There are not many places that would take a dying person in and nurse him/her back to health... they give you hope'* and *'we are aiming for 100% adherence of patients to the treatment regimens'*. Care forms an integral part of the treatment: *'People with a CD4 count lower than 50 have a 20% chance of survival – and our patients are doing so well. It's the counseling, the care!'*

Holistic care involves quality clinical care, based on a treatment contract with the patient. Developing a treatment partnership with the patient has been a useful way of structuring and managing the relationship between treatment team and patient. The treatment partnership comprises a written agreement between the patient and the clinical team, which is time bound. The patient is made aware of the commitment of the team to provide AIDS treatment plus care for a minimum period of time - and what the patient needs to commit to in terms of adherence and contact with the treatment team. The underlying principle is succinctly described as follows: *'Treatment should be defined in the context of care and support. Treatment with medicines does not work in isolation.'* The notion of a 'contract' extends beyond the treatment period, to a 'commitment to life': *'ARVs cannot be isolated from a programme. You can't just give them out like this. It's a life contract.'*

Honouring this contract involves many aspects. The clinical team uses registers, time sheets, treatment plans and treatment cards to document, monitor and remind patients of their commitment to treatment, and to link the patient to community-based resources, support staff and support programmes. The commitment of the programme staff to this contract with their patients extends beyond clinical care of an individual patient, to reach families and communities as well: *'They [social workers] must be in the community. You cannot afford to miss one patient ... try to reach the couples... Go there. Don't stop here. Always be there, know what is happening.'*

Not only the treatment regimen, but also the care is individualised: *'For four weeks they carried her in here. For two weeks I did not put her on medication, I was afraid it might kill her. And now, when she comes in, she dances!'*

Faith plays an important role in the lives of many of the programme staff. Personal belief systems drive and sustain individuals and teams, without dominating the treatment and care programme: *'They say: Feed him, clothe him, heal him. And when he asks why, then you say: Jesus. That's the difference.'*

### Supporting Patient Self-Management

Programme staff members recognise the fact that the patient must understand and learn to manage her or his own condition due to HIV/AIDS. Although the clinical team and others at home and in the community can help (and will be there to provide support), patients need to learn to cope with the infection, to disclose to those they trust in order to get further help, to learn to practise prevention and positive living, and to understand and use prophylaxis and ARVs and other treatments. The results are overwhelming: *'Bedridden, sore, they don't want to die, and three months later they walk in here!'*

This implies, to a large extent, behaviour change through counselling, education and ongoing support, which gives patients the skills and motivation to self-manage AIDS and to sustain their adherence to the treatment programme: *'It is quite difficult to make sense to a patient. What you see is that patients often cannot come to the institution [for check-ups and Medicine], or they take the medication wrongly, or if they feel better they stop the medication, because there are a lot of myths around ARVs. It is very difficult to change human behaviour, like to use a condom, abstain... it's far-fetched. Your brain closes up and it tells you it is not for you, it's for someone else. Fear is not enough to change behaviour.'*

The responsibility remains with the patient. The programme team assists and empowers, if necessary, to promote self-management: *When you come to the house, you find people are sleeping. They are not sleeping because they are sick, but because they are hungry. There is no food. We ask what have you done yourself to overcome your poverty? What have you tried? Try to plant seeds. Try to restore your relationship with the extended family.'*

Successful self-management can only be possible when a person has been able to take charge of every aspect of his/her life and livelihood. The ARV team plays a key role in assisting patients to regain control over the various aspects of their lives as they nurse them back to health. In addition to the clinical care, patients are also assisted and counselled regarding, for instance, social and financial matters. This requires the inputs from a multi-disciplinary team of professionals and volunteers.

*Working as a Team*
The multi-disciplinary teams at the different ARV treatment centres are all differently composed, depending on the facilities, resources and focus of the various centres (for example hospice or hospital; adults or children). Teamwork takes place on different levels and in different contexts:
– Collaboration within the team to provide quality holistic care: *'Within our own team: if the patient has a complaint, the therapeutic counsellor phones the doctor, the doctor advises and the problem is solved, or the patient goes to see the doctor in person.'* The sense of trust and collaboration between professionals and volunteers is very important in this regard: *'Before the doctor comes, we weigh them, check blood pressure. We don't have a time to knock off, we have a time to come in... We enjoy it. Voluntary work is a very nice job. We are not qualified... We are helping each other with love and care. We are not expecting anything in return.'*
– Collaboration with other programmes offered by the ARV treatment centre in addition to ART, for example HIV prevention, peer programmes and children's programmes: *'We are one. Those who are referred, we keep their files. We monitor them; we work together. Once you open a file for home-based care, you open a card for the children so that you don't lose them.'*

Collaboration with other service providers and stakeholders outside of the ARV team forms an essential part of the holistic care given to the patients.

*Linking up with External Programmes and Stakeholders*
The ARV treatment centres do not operate in a vacuum. In fact, in the current ARV provision programmes they form a vital link with government, business and local communities. Similarly, they are also dependent on these external service providers. Setting up and sustaining linkages takes deliberate effort and commitment. These collaborative agreements cannot be assumed and taken for granted; they need to be negotiated and nurtured. Someone in the team needs to champion these collaborative agreements: *'We had met with local people and clinics - a shared kind of care...with stakeholders. People came to know us. The Department of Health's programme was also picking up steam. We are working hand in hand, not against them.'*
   Partnerships with stakeholders and networking with other programmes as service providers form essential interconnections with their own system of care and service: *'Good referral networks and procedures are required to sustain safe and effective treatment':*
– With business, for the provision of food parcels, and effective management of ARV programmes for employees: *'Trying to get funding for food parcels takes ages.'*
– With the Department of Social Development for social grants: *'The way the Department of Social Development helps us... they will be here... and process the grants. Within three weeks they will have it, because it is urgent.'*

– With local communities and non-governmental organisations: *'...for home-based care workers and to monitor adherence, to be able to extend services to more communities.'*
– With other programmes, especially peer education, positive living, HIV prevention and OVC programmes: *'We work with peer educators, and with other programmes, but we don't do peer counselling, because it is not our core business. Treatment and prevention are interlinked.'*
– Partnerships with other training providers: *'Lifeline for training of caregivers; the Church provides counselling...'*
– Collaboration with local government: *'... to be able to cover a greater area withoutduplication or overlap of services.'*

*Mainstreaming ARV Treatment in Public Health Facilities*
The lack of mainstreaming of ARV treatment programmes in the public health sector poses several challenges to the ARV treatment centres. Referral for the treatment of opportunistic infections is inevitable, in view of the current limited scope and resources of the ARV programme sites: *'We refer patients to bigger hospitals because we do not have specialist facilities to treat some of these opportunistic infections.'* Within this context, referral of patients for treatment of opportunistic infections has been reported to be particularly challenging: *'The fact that not every other hospital offers ARVs just says that people [receiving ARVs] will be sidelined.'* In severe cases, patients have simply been turned away:
*'Non-acceptance of AIDS patients in hospitals due to ignorance, fear.'* One doctor remarked: *'I have to battle to get them accepted at referral centres. Firstly because they tell you there are no beds, the beds are full. It is not a secret that most hospitals are overwhelmed by patients with HIV-linked diseases and you are looking at over 80% of beds... I have experienced resistance because of the stage of late presentation... maybe it's the prognosis...would rather give a non-HIV patient the resources...'*
In some instances, patients take the initiative to knock on the doors of these ARV treatment centres after being tested of treated at other facilities, for various reasons: *'ARV programmes presented elsewhere are often poorly managed and they come to our programme when they have problems.'* Also, patients seek a 'second opinion' after testing positively elsewhere, or after receiving contradictory test results: *Tested positive, then negative... then came to us.'*

*Dealing with Stigma, Myths and Misconceptions*
The provision of ARV treatment in a holistic and caring way involves a focus on the social phenomena associated with the infection, in addition to the clinical care. HIV/AIDS has shown itself capable of triggering responses of compassion, solidarity and support, bringing out the best in people, their families, caregivers and communities. But the disease is also associated with stigma, ostracism, repression and discrimination. Ignorance, lack of knowledge, fear and denial engender serious and tragic consequences, including undermining of ARV treatment.
The ARV team needs to counteract felt and enacted stigma on various levels of manifestation on a continuous base. This has been a particularly serious challenge in the initial stages of programme roll-out. However, over time, the presence of an ARV treatment centre in a community, together with its services and information campaigns and the fact that patients are disclosing their HIV status, has been reported to play a role in reducing stigma: *'Before we*

*started, stigma was higher. If I can put it on a scale of 1 to 10, I would say stigma was as high as 10 before we started, but now it is down to 6 or 7. It is coming down because of disclosure.'*

In some instances, the opportunity to receive treatment has been reported to overshadow the fear of stigmatisation as sick people come to the ARV treatement centres to join the queue for treatment. On this level and in this context, stigmatisation has clearly diminished: *'It has diminished in the closed circle of patients.'* Also, the availability of food parcels and the opportunity to be assisted in application for a social grant also seem to encourage disclosure and dealing with possible stigmatisation.

In the private domain of the family, responses to AIDS vary greatly. In some instances, ARV treatment has been a binding factor in a family: *'This is a private family matter. We have decided not to tell anyone outside of the family.'* Parents on treatment bring their children or other family members for testing and treatment. In this way, family members support one another in treatment adherence. On the other hand, stigmatisation and discrimination remain very real in the lives and homes of many people, even to the extent of locking up people with AIDS and preventing them from taking ARVs: *'... when the first daughter began to show the signs, the mother was in denial...she kept her locked up in her room.'* Experiences of stigmatisation and discrimination are abundant: *'I can see he is also sick, he is losing weight but now the way he is fighting with me! Whenever I say let's go for a test, he doesn't want to go ... he does not want to eat the food that I cook, because I am going to give him the disease; I must sleep outside; he does not want my kids now...'*

Stigmatisation also applies to the very people working on the ARV treatment programme: *'Before I started the programme I was scared to tell what kind of work I am doing... they were calling me names...but I know they will come...I was suffering before, not now.'*

Inevitably, patients on treatment have also died. This has given rise to all kinds of myths and misconceptions about treatment, in addition to already existing misinformation. The notion that "treatment kills" needs to be addressed continuously: *'The mother stood up and said "don't think it's the drugs that killed my child, she was just too sick".'*

The role of traditional medicine and the use thereof in conjunction with ARVs need special attention: *'We explain to them that it is not as if we are against traditional medicine, but we advise them that their cells are very weak now... we have to know which one is helping them... when she starts ARVs we must make sure that they do not use traditional medicine... traditional medicines are too strong, they die.'*

The fact that people's health and wellness visibly improve within a short period of time after commencement of ARV treatment undoubtedly contributes not only to destigmatisation of HIV-infected people, but also to a willingness to adhere to ARV treatment.

*Reaching Targets*

Different strategies are followed to reach target groups: numerically, geographically and demographically. The very purpose of establishing the SACBC ARV treatment centres has been to reach people who would otherwise 'fall through the system' of national ARV provision: *'Somebody decided to take the responsibility and said "we will do it", and not "why does government not do it?"'* The notion of 'reaching out' is very strong. The home-based care system is well suited to reaching the communities: *'We go out to the community, not vice versa.'* People are also referred from the VCT centres to the ARV centres. This implies understanding and addressing of the specific needs of specific communities, inter alia by means of local members of the community as home-based care (HBC) workers and through tailor-made training of HBC workers: 'It needs to be tailor-made for a particular area to be sensitive to culture, politics, etc., of the area.'

Reaching men is a particular focus of the ARV teams, as they have been recorded to face various gender-based barriers to access health services and to participate in programmes: 'Men, they are still in a stage of denial, but they are coming out now'. Despite possible initial reluctance to join the ART programme, men have been noted to become active programme participants: 'Men who have been with our programme for a while open up and talk'. Also, specific categories of men do not necessarily have the incentive or opportunity for testing, notably migrant workers and truck drivers: 'We have two truck drivers on treatment, and they are doing very well.'

There is a perception that it is easier for women to test and apply for treatment: 'More women come for testing and apply for treatment; it is "easier" for women to find another woman relative to disclose to.' On the other hand, testing positively and knowing your HIV status can also compromise a woman: 'Women are tested when they are pregnant. Or when their children are ill. Then the burden is upon the woman to tell the man... It is not easy if you are boyfriend and girlfriend, because if the woman tells the man she is positive, he will run away. How are you going to survive?'

With regard to the different generations, the ARV treatment centres have been able to reach every age group, from old to young, although children and young people often seem to be 'missing' at the centres: 'We see teenagers to those in their seventies. We don't see many children here. The hospital has a paediatric programme. There is a gap all right [with regard to small numbers of young school-going people on the programme]. It takes time to get sick after infection. As long as the symptoms are not showing, they are hiding it...'

The sad part is, however, those who could not be reached in time: '... I lost my sister to this... She was unfortunate; she did not get the treatment. So I am happy, those who are lucky are getting treatment. And I still have younger brothers and sisters. Maybe sometime they will be infected too...' A serious challenge to the programme is the fact that people apply for treatment only when AIDS has developed to an advanced stage. Ideally, patients should be identified before they reach this stage: '... the earlier one starts, the better...at the time when people are still borderline healthy.'

*Scale-up and Sustainability*
Specific measures are taken to extend services to geographic areas where ART programmes are not offered yet. This includes the recruitment and training of home-based care workers in these areas. All the centres have strategies for scale-up in place, and will be able to expand their services to reach the numerical targets set for 2005. Initial challenges regarding programme roll-out reportedly amounted mainly to issues of role allocation and the setting up of systems. Sustaining and scaling up of programmes will however be challenging, due to various factors. Respondents foresee the following problems:

'Problem of funding.'
'Problem of resistance to medication is always at the back of my mind – after six months you will see a response.'
'Staffing. We have two rooms now. In future we will need more space.'
'Getting more recruits as home care givers; takes time to train and keep them motivated.'
'Current patients who have been on the programme for six months will now come in once a month. We cannot cut down on monthly visits and HBC visits.'

*Experiences of Occupational Stress*

Programme staff invariably commented on the positive impact that ARV treatment had on their job satisfaction. Previously, they felt helpless and ineffective while caring for terminally ill patients. This has changed drastically since ARV treatment has given them hope, especially when they see their patients' radical improvement in a relatively short space of time. Many respondents commented on the emotional closeness that develops between caregiver and patient as well as between the members of the programme team.

However, staff also reported becoming seriously ill themselves after admission of a seriously ill patient and being stigmatised due to their participation in the ARV programme. Programme staff reported numerous sources of stress and frustration. In every research site, they mentioned the enormous emotional impact of the unexpected death of their patients: '*We all cried.*' Also, distress was reported due to the neglect of people with AIDS, especially children, in the care of relatives, who do not take proper care of the sick and leave them to suffer unnecessarily: '*I do not blame the family. I just want to get the message out to everyone – that they should not wait until it reaches this stage. Treatment is available. Do not let people suffer like this.*'

Following instances such as these, professional and volunteer staff reported their need for emotional and spiritual support. This is not always readily available and causes a great deal of distress among staff. Staff debriefing opportunities and the comfort and guidance received from colleagues have been noted to be very useful. Apart from the support they receive from their significant others, other coping mechanisms mentioned were 'internally' initiated on the part of the health care workers themselves, such as spirituality, or passive relaxation such as walking or gardening.

*Vulnerability of Children*

The issue of children with AIDS evokes highly emotional responses from ARV programme staff:

'*Children are not supposed to die; children are not supposed to have AIDS; children are not supposed to be raped or molested.*' Compounding to this, is the notion of the vulnerability of children affected and infected by AIDS: '*It happens all the time. As soon as the parents die, the children are all by themselves ... the children need an adult ... some take advantage of the situation. The children become their servants.*'

The availability of ARV treatment has changed the scenario regarding the care of children with AIDS drastically. In the past, children were supported to 'live positively and die peacefully'. This required a particular form of care and relationship with the children. As children receive treatment and get well, all kinds of issues arise, including disclosure (the children themselves often do not know that they are HIV-positive, or do not know what it means), adherence to treatment and reintegration into school and family life. Some of the children have been out of school for several months, even years, and have fallen behind with regard to the reaching of their developmental milestones vs. their chronological age. This poses particular challenges to the integration of children living with AIDS into mainstream schooling. Attempts are being made to address these issues in different ways: '*We have a good relationship with the school to take our children*', and '*we have students coming in to tutor the children.*'

Reintegration of children into family life is not easy either. Apart from the fact that many children have lost all their relatives to AIDS, some of the families of these children are so poor and under-resourced that it is just not possible for them to also care for these children with their special needs regarding nutrition and educational support: 'When the child comes back after a weekend at home, he is sick and we need to begin to build him up right from scratch.'

The following section comprises the reflections of the patients who receive ARVs as far as testing, treatment and care are concerned.

*Experiences of Diagnosis*

Recurrent themes in patients' accounts of their illness, testing and diagnosis seem to be notions of:
– not suspecting HIV infection;
– appreciation for support from health care workers during this time;
– confusion based on contradictory test results;
– taking other people, including children and partners, for testing; and
– rationalisation and blaming others for infection.

'I started getting sick in 2002. I was pregnant at the time. I got sicker after giving birth and was advised to go for tests. I didn't suspect that I had HIV; however I accepted the results and prayed. Health care workers were good and encouraging.'

'I started getting sick in October last year. I couldn't sleep most of the time and couldn't walk, but I didn't suspect that I had HIV. I tested in October. I was encouraged to do the test by the doctor who was very helpful and good to me. I felt bad about the results, but now I have accepted.'

'I got ill in 2000 but I didn't suspect it was HIV. I thought it would go away, but it didn't – the diarrhoea, discharge and vomiting... I got tested in 2000 because the hospital encouraged me and I was sick. The interaction with the health care workers was good, they were nice and they counselled me. The test came out positive and negative and then last year I tested positive. I didn't believe it at first, but then I had to test again when I fell pregnant. At three months it was positive and negative, and then at four months I tested again and it came out positive... the baby was born negative.'

'I started getting ill three months back. I did not suspect that I had HIV. I went for tests in July because I was sick and I didn't know what was wrong. Getting the results was very difficult and painful, but I accepted. The clinic staff was OK, they counselled me.'

'The health care workers were very good. I got the best love from the care workers. They are very good when it comes to working with people. They gave me support all the way until I delivered the babies.'

'I was so ill I went for the test. I did not know that I may turn out to be HIV positive. When the results came out I was shocked. I did not believe what I heard. I went for the second test, and I was again positive. I was tested by a special doctor. He counselled me first and told me about HIV/AIDS before he took my blood. He treated me right and explained everything from start to end.'

'I lost weight and had a headache. Sometimes I felt weak. I tried to use GrandPa, but it did not help. That is when I went to the clinic. As I was waiting to test for TB, I heard a nurse calling for people who have come to test their blood. Then I decided to go there. ...First I did not understand what the nurse was talking about. They asked me to bring my ID book in order to register for the grant. As a person you do not accept it at first. You think they are crazy because you know that you are well-behaved.'

'I never thought I was HIV positive. I thought I was bewitched.'

'I told my children. I wanted it to be a family matter. We do not tell anyone about it... I took my young child to do the test. She is HIV negative.'

'I used to love my wife even though she was mischievous. That is why I thought I got the disease from her... she worked in a restaurant... and she got out of hand.'

'I suffered from TB. I completed the treatment course. Then I began to lose weight. I went back again to the clinic for a blood test. That is when I was diagnosed as HIV positive. I thought the nurses were crazy because I respected myself and was never promiscuous. I did not go back to the clinic. I went to Tapologo...'

'Not suspecting' HIV infection and the tendency to 'blame others' for HIV infection are linked to the choices made regarding the timing and extent of disclosure.

## Experiences of dDisclosure, Stigma, Discrimination and Support

Disclosure is very personal, and varies from one context to the next. Decisions made regarding disclosure are linked to fears of rejection and stigmatisation on the one hand, and the need for support, on the other hand. The following narratives depict some of these variations in disclosure patterns: "I felt free. They did not say anything but kept quiet."

'I did not disclose immediately, only after a month ... to my husband and my mother, who told my father. I disclosed when I got too sick so that they would know what was going on and so that my husband can also go for tests. My mother was very supportive, but my husband was not supportive and he refused to go for tests ... I also disclosed to a distant female cousin who is also HIV-positive. My cousin was encouraging. My child, my other family members, the church, my friends and co-workers do not know that I have HIV. They just know that I am sick. Church members come to pray for me ... My husband's parents have not visited me at all.'

'I told my partner first on the day I got the results. She didn't react badly to the news. She also went for the tests and tested positive. Neighbours, relatives and the church do not know that I have HIV and at work they think it is TB. I am not sure if they know, but they treat me well. My supervisor used to remind me to drink my pills and also gave me time off when I got sick.'

'I did not disclose when I first found out. I only told the father of my child. His daughter disclosed my status to the community, who distanced themselves from us and chased us away from the place where we fetch water. Now we struggle to get water. It is painful to know that the community knows my status. People laugh at me and tell me I will die and won't survive six months... I visited a church one day and disclosed to the Pastor. He said he will pray for me and advised me to leave the father of my baby because we are not married. The next Sunday he preached about HIV and he said that people who are HIV get it from being sluts. That made me feel bad, because I know that I did not sleep around. I never went back to the church.'

'I disclosed to my mother because she may try to nurse me, only to find out later that she is also infected. She is supposed to take precautions such as wearing gloves when looking after me... She gave me love like she did when I was suffering from TB. She has not changed. She brings me money every month ... They are happy that I am better and beautiful. They love me so much.'

'I told my employer first, immediately after getting the results. He was shocked and heartbroken, but he accepted. After that I told my brother and then the rest of my family and relatives. They have all accepted and life is normal. They are happy that I am getting treatment and that I will be getting out of hospital. My colleagues and co-workers do not know what is wrong with me.'

These reports of disclosure and responses to disclosure are further analysed in the next section. The information collected in the research suggests that decisions regarding testing, disclosure, adherence and prevention are interlinked. Also, these decisions are related to the extent of the social support needed and received from family and community. An analysis of the capacities and vulnerabilities of people receiving ARV treatment was applied in this regard.

## 7.2. Capacities and Vulnerabilities of Adult Patients Receiving ART

The Capacities and Vulnerabilities Analysis (CVA) framework was designed to help plan aid in emergencies, in such a way that interventions meet immediate needs and at the same time (adapted from Anderson & Woodrow, 1989) build on the strengths of people and their efforts to achieve long-term social and economic development. The CVA is based on the central idea that people's existing strengths (or capacities) and weaknesses (or vulnerabilities) determine the impact that a crisis has on them, as well as the way they respond to the crisis. ARV treatment programmes should aim to increase people's capacities and to reduce their vulnerabilities.

Capacities refer to the existing strengths of individuals and social groups. They are related to people's material, physical and social resources, and to their beliefs and attitudes. Capacities are built over time and determine people's ability to cope with a crisis and recover from it.

Vulnerabilities refer to the long-term factors that weaken people's ability to cope with sudden or drawn-out crises. Vulnerabilities existed before the crisis arose, contribute to its severity, make the effectiveness of interventions harder and continue after the crisis or disaster.

Addressing vulnerabilities requires long-term strategic solutions, which are part of development work.

The following two cases illustrate the diverse life contexts of people receiving ARV treatment, and their diverse needs and concerns.

*Woman, aged 28*
**Previously:** Lived alone; involved in youth club; lived alone after father died and mother moved to another area; had a child, child stayed with grandmother; unemployed, supported by mother's social grant; tested positive when pregnant.
**Now:** Disclosed to husband and family friend; not to mother, relatives, church or community; got married, have twins; not working now; counsellor at ARV centre; receives grants for children; improved health.
**Dimensions Vulnerabilities Capacities:**
– Physical/material (resources, skills, hazards): Financial responsibilities towards three children and unemployed husband; has a home; trained as counsellor; receives social grants.
– Social/organisational (relationships, organisational structures): Lack of family support; father died; mother moved to another area; married; children.
– Motivational/attitudinal (ability to change and cope with change): HIV status not disclosed to mother, church, community; counsellor at ARV centre.

*Male, aged 38*
**Previously:** Not married; lived separately from his two children and their mothers; used to send them money; supported by his own mother, uncle, aunt; did piece work.
**Now:** Family and relatives have accepted him; supported by his mother; new girlfriend, also on ARVs; health has improved.
**Dimensions Vulnerabilities Capacities:**
– Physical/material (resources, skills, hazards): Previously income earning; now financially supported by his extended family.
– Social/organisational (relationships, organisational structures): Distant relation with children and previous partners; no direct responsibilities; own family has accepted his HIV status; new girlfriend.
– Motivational/attitudinal (ability to change and cope with change): Lives positively.

The focus on patients' strengths, assets, or resources and their vulnerabilities shed some light on the great variety of contexts and life situations of people receiving ARV treatment - with a view of understanding why some people may find it easier than others to disclose their status, to adhere to the treatment and to live a positive life. Whilst these case studies can by no means provide conclusive evidence, it seems as if a fair amount of family cohesion and resources constitute a context conducive to disclosure, adherence and positive living. It also seems as if women who have small children could be more vulnerable than other categories of women – they seem to experience insufficient social support and have insufficient resources, insecure living arrangements and more responsibilities, which put them at a disadvantage in terms of stress, positive lifestyle and nutrition.

## 9. Conclusions

An effective HIV/AIDS treatment programme is defined by its capacity to quickly and effectively treat a substantial number of people living with HIV/AIDS (WHO, 2003). The experience of the SACBC ARV treatment programme at the selected research sites yields several lessons in this regard. Although individual contexts may necessitate adaptations in view of available resources and location, an effective ARV treatment programme can be achieved when the following conditions are met:
1. Integration of AIDS treatment activities into the basic package of holistic care, including voluntary counselling and testing, prophylaxis of opportunistic infections, HIV prevention and psychosocial support.
2. Decentralisation of treatment services down to the primary care level to ensure wide coverage of geographic areas and community involvement in care and referral.
3. Setting up of simple regimens with standardised clinical guidelines to sequence the use of drugs and manage adverse events, encouraging ease of adherence for the patient and follow-up for the healthcare professionals.
4. Availability of reliable suppliers of antiretroviral drugs and laboratory services at a manageable cost.
5. Establishment of multidisciplinary teams, including home-based care with an emphasis on psychosocial support.
6. Adoption of a comprehensive approach to adherence, including counsellors, support groups and significant treatment literacy.

7.  Provision of specialist services, for example for referral of children to paediatric pro-
    grammes and effective treatment of opportunistic infections and emergencies.
8.  Addressing the specific challenges of long-term adherence to ARV treatment.

## 10. Recommendations

The recommended strategy aims at broadly expanding access to ARV treatment and providing ongoing adherence monitoring and support, while making certain that the unique requirements of HIV/AIDS treatment are met. While acknowledging the fact that scale-up can
happen in different ways, the following generic considerations are important:
– constraints in early phases differ from those in later phases;
– constraints may vary in different settings;
– information systems may help relieve constraints;
– local service delivery sites may not have control over / may not have the capacity to
  influence all elements. The scale-up should clearly identify cross-cutting support
  issues, activities and systems.

The following pointers may be considered in the scale-up of SACBC ARV programmes:
– Provide dynamic leadership and advocacy for effective action on the epidemic and the
  need for ARV programmes across the country.
– Mobilise and empower public, private and civil society partnerships and community
  engagement.
– Strengthen the management and dissemination of strategic information to guide efforts of programme partners.
– Build capacities to track, monitor and evaluate SACBC ARV site responses to the epidemic; also build capacities to identify resource gaps, costing and budgeting of programmes and strategic allocation of resources.
– Facilitate access to and efficient use of financial and technical resources, including integration and mainstreaming of HIV/AIDS programmes into relevant health care systems and programmes.

Further research is required with regard to children receiving and thriving on ARVs. The
impact of their new energy and zest for life pose new challenges and concerns regarding
their vulnerability, such as disclosure of children's HIV-positive status, facilities for schooling
and reintegration into family and community life (see Chapter 14).

## Acknowledgements

The researchers hereby acknowledge the Centre for the Study of AIDS of Pretoria University
for their role in the facilitation of collaborative research with the SACBC AIDS Office. We
also acknowledge the work done by Vanessa Barolsky in developing the original research
proposal.

# References

Anderson, M. & Woodrow, P. (1989). *Rising from the Ashes: Development Strategies in Times of Disaster.* Boulder and San Francisco: Westview Press,

Department of Health (2000). *HIV/AIDS/STD Strategic Plan for South Africa 2000-2005.* Pretoria.

MacFarlane, M. (2004). *Passing by on the other side. Fast Facts.* South African Institute of Race Relations No.12, December.

Marshall, C. & Rossman, G.B. (1999). *Designing Qualitative Research* (3rd ed.). Thousand Oaks: Sage Publications.

National Department of Health South Africa (2004). *National Antiretroviral Treatment Guidelines.* Pretoria.

South African Institute of Race Relations (2004). *South Africa Survey 2003/2004.* Johannesburg: SAIIR, 2004.

UNAIDS (2004). *UNAIDS at country level. Progress Report.* UNAIDS/04.35E.

Viljoen, J. (2004). *The SACBC's ARV roll-out: a narrative report.* 2 September 2004. Unpublished report. Pretoria: SACBC.

Walker, L., Reid, G. & Cornell, M. (2004). *Waiting to happen.* Cape Town: Juta.

World Health Organisation (2003). *Antiretroviral Therapy in Primary Health Care: Experience of the Khayelitsha Programme in South Africa.* Capetown: WHO.

*Address for correspondence:*
Dr. M. de Waal
Southern African Catholic Bishops' Conference AIDS Office
P.O. Box 941
Pretoria 0001
South Africa

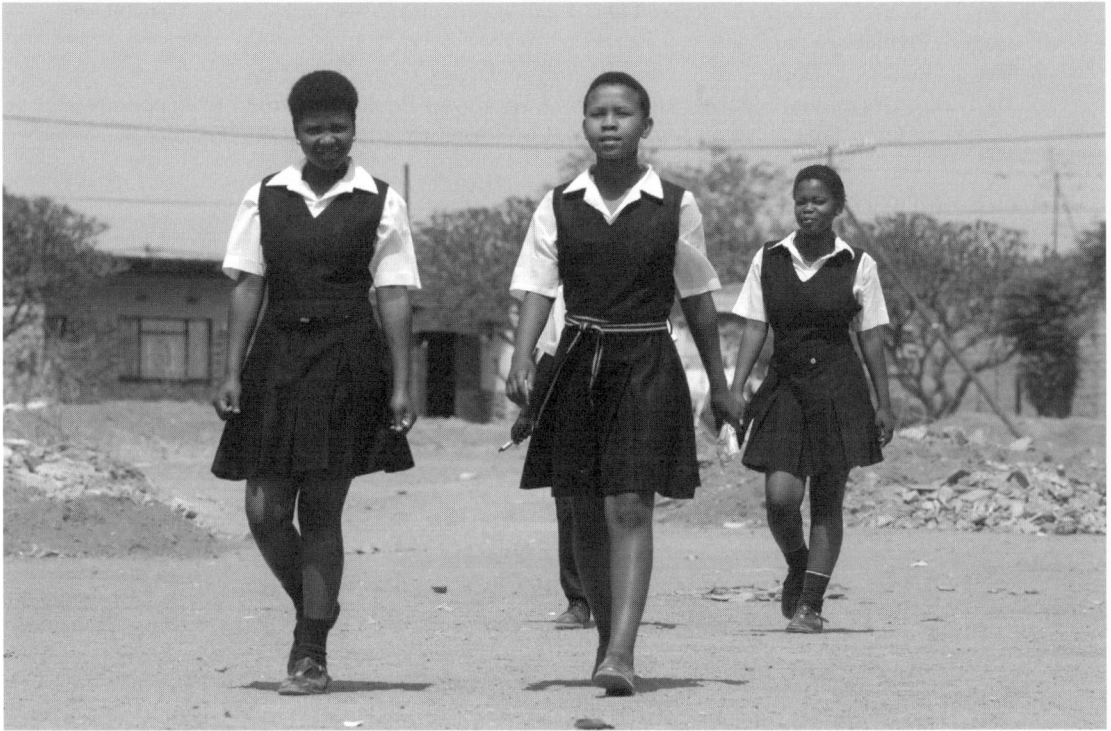

# Chapter 14

# To Live a Decent Life: Bridging the Gaps

*Tessa Marcus* [1]

[1] National Research Foundation, Pretoria, South Africa

*Love, Enterprise and Hope - Vukile's Story in 2004*
My name is Vukile. I am 15 years old.
Every day I wake up, brush my teeth and wash my face. I then fetch water from the well. I wash dishes. I go to the shops at 3pm to buy bread. Usually, I play with my friends, but I only play for three hours. Then I come back home and help granny light the fire and cook. We sleep at 10pm.
*The project first came in 1999-2000 when they heard about my mother's death. They came to comfort us and my granny. They brought food with them. Things changed when my mother died ….[ he stops talking].*
The hardest thing now is that there is no money at home. [Is there anything you can do about it?] Yes, my drawing and painting, I sell them. Also my gum boot dance group brings money. When I started the gum boot dance group I asked granny for boots and she helped me with that. My grandmother is the first person I go to [for help], but also Mrs Willeminah, our neighbour. She is granny's friend. I just feel alright, because my granny is around for us. I am doing well, especially with my dance group. Although, I was worried when you came. I thought you were the police, because my group is accused of stealing.
*[If you had three wishes?] I want to get my grandmother her pension here in Taung. I want to be a lawyer if only I am successful. And I want to get my granny better help so that she can take care of us.*

## Abstract

HIV/AIDS transforms the lives of everyone who is touched by the disease and epidemic. This paper reports the findings of a study of the Southern African Catholic Bishops Conference's efforts to bridge the gaps that AIDS-related illness and death generate for children, their families and their communities in South Africa and Swaziland. It reveals the importance of grass-roots initiatives to the lives of people marginalised by poverty and disease. These efforts are influenced and directed by the presence or otherwise of government policy and would be greatly enhanced by systemic interventions. In looking at the SACBC initiatives, the study foregrounds the importance of children as the kernel of a response system that will help them and society survive the epidemic.

## 1. Introduction

This is a study of Southern African Catholic Bishops' Conference-supported AIDS initiatives in South Africa and Swaziland. It was commissioned by the SACBC in order to understand the programmatic responses to and impact on children, and the context in which they are occurring.

When you sit at the bottom of the pile and seek to attend to the needs of the millions of children, women and men who, through life's circumstances, find themselves in a wretched place, you can't help but ask yourself what it is that can, must and should be done to make a difference? Of course, posing such a question at the personal level will yield a multitude of responses that follow familiar patterns of reasoning and explanation. Yet, each of us knows or needs to know that taking responsibility for the world that we live in is the precondition of securing our humanity. This is a lesson of history and experience that is particularly relevant in Africa in the 21st century, where the HIV/AIDS pandemic threatens the physical and social existence of millions of people – as individuals and in their various collectivities as families, communities and societies. This study provides a small insight into the ravages of the pandemic and the conscious responses that people are making, through the SACBC, to weather the tide of AIDS destruction and destitution.

## 2. The context

The study framing document defines context in terms of the national, regional and local setting in which the SACBC interventions are operating. There is a vast literature on this subject which – nationally, regionally and at times locally – elaborates variously on:
1.  the extent of HIV infection, AIDS illness and AIDS-related deaths;
2.  the age dimensions of the epidemic especially in respect of the children and the aged;
3.  the gender dimensions of HIV and AIDS impacts;
4.  the extent and nature of poverty and inequality and its interface with HIV and AIDS;
5.  the medium and long-term economic and social impacts of HIV and AIDS;
6.  the political and social responses from key institutions and organisations of society – be they governance, business, service, faith and civic society structures that claim to represent, act for and protect individual and collective interests.

Some key notions and facts include the following:
1.  South Africa and Swaziland are in the eye of generalised HIV and AIDS epidemics that are amongst the worst in the world. At the end of 2003 South Africa and Swaziland had HIV prevalence rates of 21.5% and 38.8% respectively, which translated in numbers terms into 5.3 million and 220,000 HIV-positive adults and children (2004 Update South Africa; 2004 Update Swaziland UNAIDS/UNICEF/ WHO). These epidemics are creating chronic illness and untimely death for successive generations of young and middle-aged adults that can be expected to persist for much of the rest of this decade, if not beyond. The AIDS epidemic was already visible by the year 2000 and continues to mount as the natural history of the disease sees people progress to full-blown AIDS and death in ever increasing numbers. In 2003 alone, AIDS deaths reached some 17,000 AIDS in Swaziland and 370,000 in South Africa (ibid.) with an estimated half a million people who are AIDS sick.
2.  The HIV and AIDS epidemics render up an unprecedented number of children without adult protection and care. In 2003 there were an estimated 1.1 million AIDS orphans in South Africa and 65,000 in Swaziland (2004 Update South Africa; 2004 Update Swaziland UNAIDS/UNICEF/WHO). It is presently estimated that approxi-

mately 23% of Swazi and 16% of South African children will be orphaned by 2010 (Africa's Orphan Generations 2004 UNICEF). Within the decade as many as 30% of 15-17 year olds will be orphaned.

3. The epidemic is shifting the burden of child and family care upwards to the aged, outwards to relatives, friends, neighbours or even strangers and downwards, to children themselves. In the process, the family, the traditional institution of care and support for children, is being incapacitated as it strains to attend to even a modicum of the reproductive and productive needs that are demanded of it.

4. Women bear the biggest brunt of the disease. They are disproportionately infected at an earlier age than men. In South Africa in the age group 15-24, prevalence rates among men were just under 5% compared to over 15% for women in 2003 (UNAIDS 2004). Women also carry the lion's share of coping with epidemics' consequences. 71% of households with orphans in South Africa and 50% of those in Swaziland are female-headed (Africa's Orphan Generation UNICEF 2004). They carry this burden on fewer resources because women are economically disadvantaged in both societies.

5. The social and economic effects of HIV and AIDS are long term and myriad – impacting negatively on nearly every aspect of local and national life. HIV/AIDS is not a disease of poverty, but it creates poverty and aggravates inequality. At the household level the economic impacts of HIV/AIDS on families are felt up to eighteen months prior to adult death and for years thereafter. It is estimated that Gross Domestic Product declines by 1% per annum where 15% of the adult population is HIV-positive (UNFPA State of World Population 2004 Report). Cumulatively the worst case scenario prepared for the World Bank predicts that in three generations there could be complete economic collapse (SA Reserve Bank October 2003 'Labour Markets and Social Frontiers'). Generally, it can be expected that poverty and inequality will grow in both absolute and relative terms, and the core institutions of society will become increasingly dysfunctional.

6. The economic, social, political and psychological consequences of large scale young adult HIV infection, chronic illness and early death as well as widespread orphanhood will resonate through both societies for decades to come. Their desire to create democratic, knowledge-based, socially stable environments that can compete in the contemporary global order will be difficult to achieve. Certainly, they already find it difficult to provide conditions that allow the majority of their citizens to meet their basic needs.

7. There is a need for multiple and various interventions at all levels of society to help South Africa and Swaziland see their way through these epidemics. There has been an unprecedented response from millions of ordinary people, in particular, those who have been directly touched by the disease syndrome and the epidemic. This response has been matched (although not always equally or adequately) by non-governmental and faith-based organisations. Both governments have created national oversight and technical bodies to coordinate and manage the national response. And both have set aside resources – the South African government set aside R1.3 billion for the 2003/4 financial year, while the Swazi government has secured US $2.2million. While South Africa has yet to actually cost the real financial needs, the estimated resources needed to tackle the epidemic in Swaziland is put at US$62 mil-

lion over five years – 30 times the present funding (UNAIDS National Response Brief South Africa; Swaziland 2004). Presently, everyone's best efforts reflect a struggle for survival and they are critical. However, they are unlikely to make significant inroads into the disease and its consequences without a clear and unequivocal commitment from the respective governments that is purposively translated into practical and meaningful interventions on a significantly different scale.

These and other ideas provide the wealth of knowledge and understanding about the epidemic and the disease that underpins SACBC programmatic and project initiatives.

## 3. Methods

### 3.1. The projects
Briefly, the 29 projects in this study reflect SACBC orphan-related initiatives in seven of South Africa's nine provinces and in one province in Swaziland. While some of the initiatives spring from the Catholic Church's care for children and adults in need that dates as far back as the 19the century, the focus on HIV and AIDS is relatively new. Ten projects began working on HIV and AIDS in the early to middle 1990s. They are pioneers in the field and can be expected to have a wealth of experience. The remainder were initiated in the five years 1999-2003, with the exception of two which began in the year of the study (2004). This means that although the majority are fairly new they too have already accumulated several years of experience in a field that changes rapidly.

Projects range in scope, scale and impact. Some concentrate on emergency needs, others try to address both immediate and longer-term issues of child care, while others seek to address challenges of HIV/AIDS and child care in a more holistic way. All the projects focus, in the first instance, on delivering their programmes to communities and individuals in their locality (losely understood). In this sense, they are both local and community-based, operating in especially poor communities and working with marginalised people. They also all seem to have adopted more or less similar principles in their approach to children's needs and the epidemic.

### 3.2. Respondents
The field work for this study was carried out in the period June –July 2004. A total of 29 projects and programmes located in seven South African provinces and one Swaziland province were visited. Each visit yielded interviews with between two and three respondents – ideally a project representative, a caregiver and a child or group of children. Face-to-face interviews were conducted with 41 project representatives, 24 caregivers and 38 children. The responses of these 93 study participants provide the basis for the findings presented here.

None of the findings are representative of the class of people or the projects concerned as this would have required systematic sampling and more extensive interviewing. However, collectively the data provide the SACBC and other partners with an insight into the larger undertaking that they have embarked upon. Their work is clearly filled with both promise and challenge and it is hoped that this study will provide some insights into the work that they are involved with as well as ideas for programme focus and refinement.

In presenting the findings, respondents are quoted directly without making reference to their names or the projects they are working on. They are distinguished rather by their role in the initiative and, where appropriate, by their age.

# 4. Results

## 4.1. Project Representatives

### Educational Background, Responsibility and Experience

Who project representatives are and how they have come to AIDS work arguably is as important to the interventions as the context in which the programmes are operating.

There were 24 women and 17 men interviewed as project representatives.

Generally projects are led or are staffed by women and men who have completed matric or tertiary education. Of respondents whose level of education was reported (N=24) all but one person have completed matric. 62% (N=15) have tertiary education – specifically degrees in nursing, social work or teaching.

Project representatives all hold some level of management or supervisory function, with most describing their position as manager or coordinator of the project or a division of the project. 62% (N=15) had been appointed into their present position on joining their respective organisations. The remainder entered their organisations at a different level and had been with them anywhere between one and 25 years.

Most have been working in their present position for three years or less. Of those whose year of appointment is reported (N=25) only one had been in her current position for more than ten years. The rest took up their present responsibilities in or after 2000. Twelve had between two and three years experience in their present jobs, six had a year (more or less) and seven were only appointed in 2004.

### Education, Training and Experience of Working with Children

The extent of education and training or experience with children that project representatives have is instructive. All but one report some form of formal training and a similar number report personal experience with children. While the kind of formal training received was not always stated, that which was specified seems to be a mix of workshops and short courses with fewer mentioning modules within more systematic, formal higher education.

Education and training mentioned includes running holiday camps, children's rights and entitlements, orphans and vulnerable children, mother craft, AIDS and babies, student and lecturer placements in schools, trauma debriefing, play therapy, educare, memory work, HIV care, counselling, sexual abuse, children with disabilities, early childhood learning, children's voices, as well as formal teaching and training degrees.

Respondents experiential background with children is somewhat less defined, but nevertheless important. Apart from the three who say they have no or not much experience in this regard, most describe their personal exposure to children as part of their working life experience. In this sense they have learnt how to engage with and manage children's issues on the job.

> 'I have worked with orphaned children and have had to deal with the developmental needs of young people, as well as children's issues regarding foster families. Children's issues are mainly emotional and therefore, they have to be helped to learn to cope with their emotional development. This is not always easy as there are varieties of issues affecting different children.'

The few who mention adopting or fostering children themselves have crossed the divide between their personal and working lives.

*How come HIV/AIDS?*

Like many other people who work with people infected or affected by the pandemic, for the most part working in AIDS came to project representatives rather than it being a career choice that they had envisaged or planned. The details of each person's experience are always specific.

> *The suffering and neglect of children pushed me to ask myself how I could help; I met P(eople)L (iving)W(ith)A(IDS)s when I worked at the clinic; I saw the need and wanted to work in the community; There were many deaths in the community, meeting women at church I listened to their needs; Young people are dying and they can't speak for themselves; I saw many orphans and the work I was doing encouraged me to take this job; I was retired, I agreed to look after four children living with AIDS, I saw the rate the disease was killing families.'*

Some respondents saw it as a calling or in fact, it was something they were specifically asked to do.

> *'It's God's calling; The bishop asked me to become involved.'*

A few project representatives chose AIDS work. Some came into it as a direct consequence of their exposure to HIV/AIDS personally or within their families.

> *'I was sick and I felt that it would be better if I came out and talked about it; A close family member died and I wanted to overcome fear and care for children; My brother died of AIDS, there was strong family denial, even rejection. [This experience] made me want to work with marginalised people.'*

For others it was where their sense of mission directed them.

> *'I wanted to work and educate people to live positively with AIDS; I wanted to conscientise people, to assist the church and the community where I live; This is the biggest human crisis, you've got to be there, you can't miss it, it is the church's responsibility to the world.'*

And for a few, it was what they had been trained for.

> *'Working with orphans and vulnerable children is part of social work; It comes with working for child relief.'*

*HIV/AIDS: Knowledge, Education and Training*

Given the way most project representatives have come into working with the pandemic, like their knowledge of children's issues, their exposure to HIV and AIDS appears to be largely work-derived. When it comes to HIV and AIDS, all say they know the basics about the disease, while a handful (N=4) describe themselves as experts.

Most project representatives have been educated in this field through workshops, short courses or modules. One respondent describes herself as being exposed to the issues through her adopted children and to have no AIDS training. The remainder have done one or more courses covering various aspects of the disease syndrome. Amongst others these include: home-based care, counselling, HIV/AIDS basics, behaviour change, AIDS and medication, prevention, disclosure, voluntary counselling and testing, signs and symptoms, ARV administration and monitoring, palliative care, teachers' response to HIV/AIDS, advanced counselling, grief counselling, proposal writing, project management, lifeline courses, support systems.

Several respondents describe having done a long list of courses whilst others only mention one or two. Whatever the case, it would seem that beyond basics, knowledge levels are uneven and there does not seem to be systemic, formal continuous education and training on the rapidly changing, multiple dimensions of HIV and AIDS across the programmes. There are some individuals who do have vast formal knowledge and/or experience, but they are the exception, rather than the rule.

Perhaps of greatest importance to the projects and their representatives is that most report limited systematic formal child-focused AIDS education or training. Six respondents (of 24) say that none of their training covered issues relating to children. One person remarked that the issue only arose out of a debate in the group but it wasn't in the course outline.

With one exception, the remainder report being exposed to more limited and sporadic child-focused components in their training. Amongst others, topics mentioned include mother-to-child transmission, bereavement counselling for children, disclosure, awareness and identification of children infected and affected by HIV/AIDS, children's rights, discrimination and poverty. There is only one report of a respondent completing a medical short course on paediatric ARV and drug management. However, as this is a new area of learning it is to be expected that it will become an area for broader, rapid knowledge and skills development.

Given that most project representatives are exposed only to intermittent formal education and training in the course of their work, they need to and do draw on other resources for ideas. A few simply base their practices on experience. However, these are the exception. It is particularly noteworthy that most actively seek out information and new knowledge from various sources. Most respondents report getting ideas and information for their work from relevant literature (be they popular, official and scientific literature), the media, networking with other organisations, people (especially fellow staff, professionals, church leaders, and friends) and workshops (which combine information and knowledge sharing with networking and interacting with people in the same or similar fields).

HIV/AIDS is transforming. Everyone who is exposed to it gets to see the world through a different lens. Their understanding of their places in life and their roles and responsibilities are profoundly changed. Project respondents are no exception.

Direct exposure to the disease and the epidemic in the course of their daily work, coupled with their growth in knowledge and understanding through training, education and networking generally has deepened respondents' individual involvement with and commitment to the issues and challenges that are thrown at them. As they put it:

*'I have become more involved, there is a greater sense of urgency. At first I knew nothing, now every day people die; I've got better and better – when I think of quitting, I just see the children around me; With every new bit of information I become more involved, but it is depressing; I am gaining knowledge and hope, it gives me a positive outlook and makes me feel optimistic; I see much more of a need to work with children and AIDS; I have become attached to the reality side, less to the theory; It's about focusing on needs; I understand the disease a bit better and I am becoming more passionate; I used to feel at the periphery, now I feel at the centre; I have become*

*deeply involved with the disease as it brings out many issues; As we witness most deaths, children take us as part of their families, they confide in us.'*

Others have changed their role in the organisation and in the field:

*'Initially I ran the project, now the community is more involved. I will be replaced; less hands on, more at a national policy level where the impact is broader; numbers are big, involvement has increased and have become involved with the affected not only infected. Workshops have generated new ideas.'*

Equally, just as the lives of respondents are being transformed, the disease syndrome and the epidemic are also transforming individual and collective life in the communities where they work. Perhaps the most significant change that many respondents observe is the growing acceptance of HIV and AIDS:

*'There is lots of acceptance by the families and communities. People are no longer afraid to talk about it; People are beginning to realise that AIDS is like any other disease; before people were hiding, now they are coming out, accepting their status; There has been a change from blame to acceptance. It is no longer a sin. AIDS is manageable and care is part of it. It's become our problem – we have to have a positive goal and outreach; People no longer discriminate, more people are coming out and there is less fear; People are beginning to wake up. Prevention is being used more.'*

## 4.2. Caregivers and Children

The caregivers and children who participated in this study shed some light on who in the community is responding to initiatives to deliver community-based care needs and who they are caring for, without in any way being representative of these groups.

Caregivers interviewed tend to be young adults or elderly rather than middle-aged. In this study the average age of those whose ages are known (N=24) was 37 years old, with a range in age from between 19 to 70 years. However, with the exception of three, all are below 45 and most (N=19) are in their twenties and early thirties.

Also, all but three are women.

The educational profile of caregivers interviewed looks very different from that of project representatives. Nearly all caregivers (N=19) have matric or less, with only four reporting a post school diploma (N=2) or a degree (N=2).

Most caregivers in the study are unemployed. In terms of income, they therefore depend on others - individuals and systems - to survive themselves. Three have no source of income. Eleven depend on mostly old age pensions and other state grants, their own or others. Nine depend on incentives from projects in the SACBC programmes. And three depend on relatives (husband and children) in formal employment.

*'We are five in the house, my grandparents receive pensions; I am unemployed, there are 10 in the house; I depend on my mother's pension- there are 10 in the family; This job – I am the only earner at home; I work as a care giver; I get income from the day care centre run by my family; None. We are orphans, I have three siblings to look after.'*

The 21 caregivers who provided information about household income live on between R50 and R6,500 a month, with most (N=14) having incomes of R1,000 or less. They are all poor and, for the most part, in search of sustainable livelihoods.

Between them they look after or look out for 367 children. The story of the children in their care can be told in many ways. Table 1 below, depicting the barest details of only 1% of the children looked after by the caregivers in the study, captures these children's circumstances most starkly. The children range in ages from babies to teenagers. It shows that their parents are deceased or their whereabouts are unknown. In their present care arrangements sometimes they live with siblings and other relatives, at other times they live with other children who are not related. All have been or are in the care of someone other than their parents for varying but substantial parts of their young lives.

**Table 1: Characteristics of some of the caregivers and 'their' children**

| Caregiver | Thebe | Gladys | Helen | Beatrice |
|---|---|---|---|---|
| Age | 28 | 35 | 40 | 29 |
| Sex | Male | Female | Female | Female |
| *Child One* | | | | |
| Name | Vuyani | Venolia | Gontse Tl. | Mbali M. |
| Age | 15 | 13 | 4 | 3 |
| Parent name | Mmabatho | Mokgadi | Sinah | don't know |
| Mother Where | deceased | deceased | deceased | deceased |
| Father where | don't know | deceased | don't know | don't know |
| In your care | 5 years | 2 years | 2 years | 2 years |
| School grade | 10 | 8 | not at school | Crèche |
| *Child Two* | | | | |
| Name | Rethabile | Clement | Biotemelo Tl. | Lucky R. |
| Age | 12 | 15 | 10 | 7 |
| Parent name | Pauline | Mosina | Sinah | don't know |
| Mother where | deceased | deceased | deceased | deceased |
| Father where | don't know | don't know | don't know | don't know |
| In your care | 1 year | 2 years | 2 years | 6 years |
| School grade | 7 | 9 | 6 | 2 |
| *Child Three* | | | | |
| Name | | Nkele | Kenneth Tl. | Fezile B. |
| Age | | 9 | 15 | 9 |
| Parent Name | | Maria | Sinah | Mantombi |
| Mother where | | deceased | deceased | dead |
| Father Where | | don't know | don't know | don't know |
| In your care | | 6 months | 2 years | 6 years |
| School grade | | 5 | 8 | 3 |

The children map their world somewhat differently – articulating the bonds that bind, the relationships they miss, the ones they are building and the ones that they find hard to establish (Figure 1).

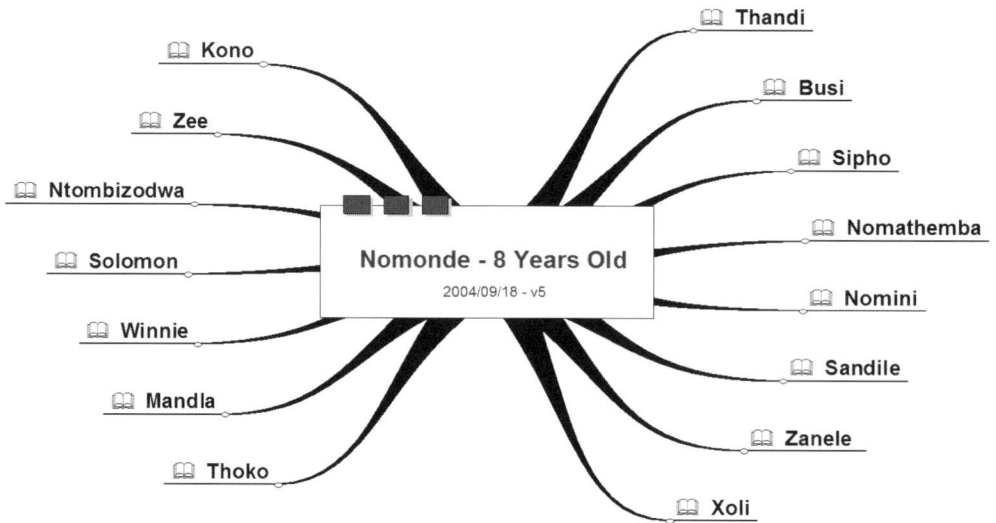

Figure 1: Bonds of a single girl

**Thandi** - My mother, she passed away

**Busi** - My cousin in Dobsonville. She is at crèche. She likes to play. I enjoy playing with her.

**Sipho** - My cousin in Dobsonville.

**Nomathemba** - My sister, she stays in Zola. She goes to school.

**Nomini** - Grandmother on my father's side. She is not working. She likes to send us around when we were staying at her place.

**Sandile** - My cousin, she is in Zola, Soweto. She is not working. I can't remember much about her.

**Zanele** - My aunt, she went to work. She works in town and stays in Zola. She likes to cook for us when we visit her place.

**Xoli** - My uncle, he went to work. He works in town and stays with us here. He likes to watch soccer on TV. I like watching TV with him. He prepares lunch boxes for me before he goes to work. I go to the shops and buy him things that he has sent me for.

**Thoko** - My grandmother on my mother's side. She is around the house. She likes to go to church. She also likes to tell us stories about my mother- like how she grew up and what she was doing. I like to talk to her. For example, we talk about school and what I want to become when I grow up. She washes our uniforms and she cooks for us when our aunts are not around. I make tea for her when I come back from school.

**Mandla** - My uncle, he is around. He is not working. He likes to move around the location with his friends. He gives us money to buy sweets sometimes.

**Winnie** - My aunt, she stays in Zola in our house where we used to stay with my parents. She likes to take us to town when we visit her. I like to be around her.

**Solomon** - My father, he passed away.

**Ntombizodwa** - My sister, she is in the house. She goes to the school which I attend as well. She likes to be on her own. I like to play games with her. She helps me to wash the dishes every evening. I help her wash dishes and accompany her to the spaza whenever our uncles send her.

**Zee** - My aunt who stays with us. She goes to high school. She likes to sing for us in the house. I like to help her when she is cleaning my grandmother's house.

**Kono** - My aunt, she stays with us here. She is not working. She likes to send us to bring things for her. I don't want to be around her. She washes our uniforms when my grandmother is not around. I help her to wash our clothes.

Both descriptions tell a difficult story filled with challenges for the children, in the first place, and for everyone interested in their and society's well-being in the second.

## 4.3. Children's Needs

A generalised HIV and AIDS epidemic significantly impacts on the shape and scale of need of children. This is especially the case when they live in resource-poor contexts where there are huge material and social demands on the adult women, and to a lesser extent men, who are their primary protectors and caregivers. Project respondents variously describe children as being robbed of their families, their childhood and their futures. They also consider the epidemic to be disempowering. For some, the enormity of this is summed up in their status. Simply put, in the words of a project representative: *'AIDS creates orphans.'*

Generally, children and those trying to care for them are confronted by a myriad of problems, often all at the same time. There is the trauma of children watching a parent who is in their care, die in front of them.

> *'Children are traumatised watching their parents die, becoming orphans; Home visits are the most painful, when children have to face seeing their sick parents; To lose a mother is an unbearable experience.'* (Project representatives)
>
> *'Three girls - Nelisiwe (6), Precious (4) and baby Ramona (10 months) - were found by a family friend in a small farm outhouse with the corpse of their mother. They had been alone with her for an unknown time. Nelisiwe had been taking care of the younger girls.'* (Caregiver – Love of Christ Ministries TLC)
>
> *'They ask lots of questions, they lose sense of their family and belonging. They wonder 'will my life ever be normal?'* (Project representative)
>
> In their own ways, the children express a great sense of loss and of missing.
>
> *'I used to stay with my mom but now I have to make friends. ...Whenever I begin to talk about it, it hurts a lot.'* (Boy aged 9)
>
> *'I feel sad because I miss my parents everyday.'* (Boy aged 5)
>
> *'The hardest thing is the fact that I can't forget about my mother's death.'* (Girl aged 13)

Then there are the issues of food and shelter, which often become more acute on the death of the parent.

> *'When their parents die, children are often left without care or food. Sometimes their land and property is stolen by relatives.'* (Project representative)
>
> *'We did not eat last night and our shack was too cold.'* (Boy aged 5)

Some are simply abandoned. Then they become the carers and breadwinners.

> *'A child of nine takes care of dying parents, then she is forced to become a prostitute as she becomes the breadwinner and head of the house; They become adults before their time; They are subject to abuse and vulnerable to prostitution; A four- year-old "mother" was found looking after her two-year-old brother, because the mother abandoned them. The two-year-old called her mom.*" (Project representatives)
>
> *'T is a young girl of 11 and is in grade 6. She is the first born of six children. She is taking care of her five siblings ranging between the ages of 5 and 10 years old. They are staying in a two-roomed house. Each room is about 2 meters. There is very little space for them to move around in the house. Her mother passed away during the first week of April 2004 and her father passed away three weeks after the death of her mother. They both died of AIDS-related diseases. When their parents were sick these children had to take care of them. They were taking turns to clean and*

*feed their parents until they passed away. T is now playing a role of mother and father. She is responsible for her siblings. She cooks for them and makes sure they go to school.'* (Field worker – Research notes)

Sometimes, dying mothers approach projects for help.

*'When they are very sick, mothers bring them to us because there are no relatives; There are children from far away places. These parents spoke to the social workers to place their child safely because they were sick – she was also HIV-positive. They got better but never came back to check on her.'* (Project representatives)

Others become dependent on family members after losing parents.

*'Their food and education become insecure; They find themselves poor, lonely and uncared for. They lose their sense of security, safety and parental care.'* (Project representatives)

Conditions in the homes of relatives and caregivers vary. There are always difficulties, even where children are well cared for.

*'Sometimes the adults who raise them don't tell them about their parents; There are children who have uncles and aunts who take good care of them; Things are fine for some as long as they are being fed and going to school, but when they might want something else, then it becomes a problem.'* (Project representatives)
*'My uncle buys for me and helps with educational tours.'* (Boy aged 15)

Equally, their circumstances can become harder whether they live in their own homes, with relatives, with caregivers in the community or in children's homes. In the words of the children themselves:

*'I always have to go to our neighbours and ask for the wheelbarrow so that I can go and fetch water on my own. ... It is too heavy for me. ... My grandmother always scolds me if I say I am afraid to go to our neighbours in the night to return their wheelbarrow.'* (Boy aged 5)
*'Things have changed a lot. We no longer stay at our house ... Everyday before we go to school my sister and I have to clean the house and (we) wash the dishes in the evening.'* (Girl aged 8)
*'My grandmother no longer treats us the way she did when my mother was alive. She treats us harshly.'* (Boy aged 16)
*'Sometimes I go to school without something to eat and now I have to do the cleaning, which I never did when my mother was still alive. I want to live in my own house because the people I stay with do not provide food or take care of me.'* (Girl aged 10)
*'In the evening I have to go outside and pump water and I am very scared. Every evening I have to go to lock classrooms on my own ... I should not have to go outside at night on my own. Someone should accompany me.'* (Boy aged 11)

Children are disoriented by losing their place in the world and especially, when they are separated from their siblings.

*'I no longer have parents, I no longer live at my own home, but where I'm adopted.'* (Girl, 17 years)

*'I feel bad most of the time- because of my mother's death, because there are no relatives, also being separated from my sisters.'* (Girl aged 17)

For many, whether they live on their own, in the home of relatives or even caregivers, schooling and education becomes problematic.

*'They are forced out of school because of no money; School performance drops; HIV/AIDS affects learning and children's opportunities to develop, dream, go to school and lead a normal life.'* (Project representatives)

*'After my father died things changed. Even school, I stayed for some time, not attending.'* (Boy aged 15)

*'The children miss their parents and they don't cope well with school.'* (Female caregiver)

*'I want to go to school. I have been out of school for three years. School is too far and I have to walk a long distance. It is not nice as I left my friends behind.'* (Girl aged 17)

Caregivers especially point to the problems facing children who are beyond the age of entitlement to child care support and of those who have left or finished school.

*'They don't get grants because they are over the assistance age. Some are really destitute but they need love, security as well as food. They loiter on the streets. They need to get educated even beyond school.'* (Female caregiver for 65 children)

*'How long am I going to keep these children in this shack. They will be teenagers and they will ask me lots of questions. What will happen to them when they are bigger? Will I be able to stay with them if they are over age? Will they be well educated?'* (Female caregiver for six children)

The situation for infected children is often made worse because their own health is often quite fragile.

*'AIDS is traumatic. The symptoms are vast. Everyday life is a bonus. The children suffer; Some go into isolations wards to protect them from infection; Children living with HIV can't play sports like others.'* (Project representatives)

*'I've been living here for seven years. When I first came I was sick, unhappy and crying. My family brought me because I was sick and they couldn't look after me. The hardest thing for me is not to see my family.'* (Girl aged 13)

All the children experience profound emotional hurt that manifests in many different ways.

*'SC is a 5-year-old who attends crèche in Orange Farm. He was tearful. He had lost his mother a few days before. He was in the care of his step-grandmother, who, on that same day, had thrown him out of the house. He had been sent to his father's grandmother whom he did not know at all. SC could not concentrate. Most of the time he does not seem to hear when he is spoken to. He does not participate in any activities. And he often just bursts into tears.'* (Field researcher – Notes from interview)

Several children are fearful, express a loss of trust in adults, and are guarded about what they feel they can ask for or expect.

> 'It is difficult to trust anyone; I don't have trust in them; I worry about things like clothing because I am afraid to ask them. It will be as if I am pushing my luck; I am afraid that they are going to hit.' (Children – various ages)

The fears they have are drawn from their experiences and insecurities, some of which derive from the role that adults, and men in general play in their lives.

> 'Most children are afraid of me. I am the only male.' (Caregiver responsible for five children)

The impact of HIV and AIDS on affected or infected children is overwhelmingly negative. The disease and the epidemic have far-reaching physical, material and emotional consequences for them. Generally, project respondents suggest that:

> 'There is apathy among these children. They have no sense of future, especially among teenagers; Children feel lost and angry; Some resort to alcohol and drugs because of frustration; Others are unruly and very difficult to deal with. You ask them what they want and they tell you straight that relatives "don't want me so I don't know what to do"; The psychological effects are great, even for those children who seem to lead a normal life.' (Project representatives)

By their own account AIDS-affected and infected children find themselves in a variety of circumstances. This differentiation is widely recognised by project representatives. As one respondent expressed it: 'you always have to be careful about categorising (them).' Equally, there is a common thread that runs through the experiences of all children - the loss of a parent and the disruption that comes with adult death.

Generally, the trauma of AIDS for children is multiple, massive and long-term. In such a context, it is necessary to ask how appropriate are notions of need hierarchies? There might be things that seem to take precedence in time, that seem to need immediate attention because they threaten the very physical survival of individual children – and therefore require priority – but generally, the context is more often one of multiple insults. Because of this complex reality, most project representatives articulate the need for a systematic, holistic response, even when their programmes are only able to respond partially to this need.

Just as working with HIV and AIDS deepens their understanding of the disease and the epidemic, so working with children influences project representatives' perceptions and understanding of children and the problems they face. Project representatives and caregivers express a general concern about the loss of childhood and all that this loss implies for their present.

> 'Their childhood is lost. They are given big responsibilities at an early age; They are placed at the level of adults in society, as heading families; Normality is taken away from them. Some become sexually active.' (Project representatives)

The children express this loss with worldliness beyond their years as this account clearly shows:

*'I stay with other children in the same house. Sisi Sinah is taking care of us as if we are her children. She prepares us every day if we have to go to crèche or to the clinic every Wednesday. Sisi Sinah wakes me up and bathes me first while the other children are still sleeping. She gives me soft porridge and tea …Here I sleep on a bed. Where I was staying with my parents I did not have my own bed. Sisi Sinah cooks well for us. Each time I get sick and Sisi Sinah takes me to Doctor. I have lots of sores all over my body. I came here last year. …Sisi Sinah came to the shack where I was staying with my parents. That time my mother was sick and my father had passed away.'* (Girl aged 5)

A related concern that project representatives and caregivers have, centres on the vulnerability that comes with being orphaned.

*'Children are very vulnerable; There is greater dependence; Children are helpless; Their safety is not guaranteed. They are vulnerable to abuse; They have to deal with abnormal behaviour. They are taught one thing and experience something else; A lot of children suffer; Children are ranked very low by society.'* (Project representatives)
*'It's difficult. Their guardians physically abuse them. One child came badly burnt – she was made to clean the house and she was only 9.'* (Female caregiver responsible for 20 children)
*'They stay with grandparents or uncles who abuse them or chase them out.'* (Female caregiver responsible for five children)
*'I don't trust my relatives. They could not help me when my mother beat me.'* (Girl aged 17)

Project representatives and caregivers also observe changes in their own feelings and behaviours as well as what they see in others.

*'People destroy children. We tend to judge them … The root of the problem is not the child but our insensitivities to their needs…; Children must be loved; I feel more compassion, I see them as a valuable asset; It has increased my love but I also get stressed and depressed by what I can't do; I worry for my own child.'* (Project representatives)
*'They don't wash. They don't have food. I really cry but as a man I don't show people around me that I am crying; We are devoted to these children. We become a family. It makes you sad when you see these children die.'* (Caregivers)

Certainly, several project representatives are far more aware of the need to talk to children about issues that previously, they might have considered inappropriate.

*'It is very painful when a baby dies. I sit down and talk to the children; We need to deal more effectively with children rather than focus on dying. Children are traumatised; I educate them about sex from 11 years, whereas in the past I would have done this at about 18.'* (Project representatives)

In general, respondents see AIDS as laying the seeds for future inequality and social instability.

*'They are being poorly equipped; The gap between children is widening; They will be discriminated against by society; They will become angry adults; I am not optimistic about (these) children's future.'* (Project representatives)

This astute insight into the future implications of the crisis of childhood unleashed by AIDS is perhaps the baseline against which programmatic interventions should be benchmarked.

## 4.4. Programmatic Responses

The overarching objective of all the SACBC programmes can be summed up simply - to create a decent life and a dignified death for children and adults who are infected with or affected by HIV/AIDS.

> 'Our objective is to bring life to these children so that they can live like other children; We aim to give children hope, love, a chance to play, and to interact without discrimination; The objective is to make the lives of orphans and vulnerable children a fulfilling and enjoyable experience; We focus on rescuing abandoned babies, giving them quality of life, and finding adoptive parents; We want to alleviate hunger and the need for care; Our objective is to look after the well-being of the whole child – spiritually, emotionally and psycho-socially; We want to restore children's dignity, humanity and trust and help them continue with their education; We care for HIV-positive people and their families; We work with people living with AIDS and orphans and vulnerable children to bring quality of life, to remove the focus on death and to help them turn to life; Our objective is to provide professional and holistic care for the homeless and destitute in the Johannesburg inner city.' (Project representatives)

### Interventions

How programmes set about realising their objectives varies in focus and detail. The greatest concentration of effort seems to be around providing food relief to children in need, either through food parcels that are given to them in their homes as part of home-based care, through feeding schemes that are run in the community, in schools and sometimes in shelters or children's homes and to a small degree through school and home garden projects. Invariably, most projects have to access this food - from government, through donations from the private sector or the community and also through direct purchase and they have to distribute it, unprepared or unprepared.

Caregivers comment that while this food is welcome, there are shortcomings. These include a lack of some essential items, a lack of variety, insufficient quantities and problems with periodicity.

> 'The children get food during the week but not at the weekend. On weekends we bring food from our homes; There is not enough food; I don't have enough food for new intakes. The food parcel has maize, samp, beans, peas, salt, fish oil peanut butter and powder milk - no paraffin, sugar, or tea.' (Caregivers)

Caregivers also point out that focusing on food does not accommodate other needs.

> 'They need clothes and toiletries and sanitary pads. I end up giving them mine; We need soap and money for clothes.' (Caregivers)

Many programmes support children's education. They focus variously on getting children into and keeping them in school and supporting their performance. The work here is wide-ranging. It includes negotiating over fees and space at local schools, providing fees, school uniforms and books, and helping children with their homework, in their homes, or at after-care facilities which they run.

A third area of activity in South Africa centres on securing children their statutory entitlements. This work includes getting relevant identification documentation, helping caregivers secure child support grants, supporting child placements in foster care or through full adoption and monitoring and preventing abuse by parents or guardians, helping them access primary health care and education and ensuring prevention of mother-to-child transmission.

A few projects directly work through and many actively include recreation as part of their programmatic support for children. Activities include play, arts, drama, dance, sports of various kinds, picnics and other kinds of outings. Recreation is regarded as both a learning as well as a physical and emotional therapeutic medium that makes a very important contribution to children's quality of life.

Several programmes include the provision of shelter for children in their initiatives – envisaged as temporary places of safety, or as permanent homes. Holistic care is usually provided in these homes, with several making considerable effort to integrate children in these institutions into life in the larger community.

Part of the care that programmes offer – whether they are delivered in institutions or through outreach home-based care in the communities – focus on child and adult health. Several projects provide medications for people living with AIDS, some provide respite and hospice care, one attends to the health of street children, and several attend to children's primary health care needs. The counselling services provided through numerous projects also seek to address the mental and emotional well-being of both children and adults. In this work the focus ranges from HIV/AIDS- related worries - testing, living with HIV, living with AIDS, death and dying - through to bereavement as well as trauma counselling. Counselling and support is also provided for caregivers.

Since caregivers and volunteers also live and work in extremely stressful and distressing environments, several programmes try to provide them with structured emotional and spiritual support. Usually termed 'caring for the carers', it is an essential part of ensuring that people stay with the programmes and are able to respond to the needs and deliver the services expected of them.

All projects do HIV/AIDS awareness work, mostly to try and stem the spread of HIV. Sometimes awareness extends to raising community understanding of children's and adults rights and to encouraging people to become actively involved in community-based care. Several projects reinforce their awareness efforts by actively developing the capacity of volunteers, peers and caregivers. Some go even further into development work – setting up or supporting and monitoring community-based organisations that generate income (e.g. gardening, spaza, bead making, sewing, bricklaying) or attend to children's needs (e.g. crèches, sports clubs, after school care).

Most of the projects are involved in multiple activities, since the needs of the children and the communities in which they work are many and broad-ranging. At the same time and without exception, they all make choices in their priorities and foci. One choice that they make relates to who they will support. Several focus on children: babies, young children, boys initially and now boys and girls, homeless children, HIV/AIDS-affected children, orphans, vulnerable children, infected children etc. Others focus on people living with AIDS and their families.

Thematically, many adopt a needs-based approach. They focus on what they describe as 'the basics': food, blankets, sometimes clothes, health and education. These are the needs that they consider to be urgent - understood as requiring immediate attention, and essential - understood in physiological development terms. Others offer specialised services like the securing of identification documents, the provision of primary health care or adolescent sexual health services which draw upon the set of specific professional skills. Because they have to make choices they all are aware that there are issues that they have to overlook or find other ways of dealing with. Several actively try to refer the needs that they overlook to other governmental or non-governmental organisations, while others just hope that these will be picked up.

There are project representatives, however, who identify and develop their interventions within a framework of holistic care. By definition, this approach countermands the idea that the needs of AIDS-affected children (or people) can be or are ordered in some sort of rigid hierarchy. Since their human and financial resources are inevitably limited, most of these programmes do not try to provide directly for all human needs and requirements. Rather, they choose to attend directly to some aspects of the health and care needs of the children or adults they support, while they also actively network with other organisations to provide for the areas that they can not address.

Several factors shape these intervention choices and decisions. As already indicated, they are influenced by the paradigmatic framework that guides the programme, be it needs-based or holistic.

Another factor that influences interventions is locality. Working in the inner city is very different from rural community-based work. It is also different from suburban, township life where settled and new migrant populations intermingle.

The presence or absence of other organisations - government and NGOs - working in the field of AIDS and children in the areas where they operate also shapes the kind of work they do. Some organisations are forced to take on a multitude of activities because there is little alternative organisational response and the communities where they work are weakly connected. Others are able to be more selective because there are greater levels of organisational support and higher levels of social organisation in their areas.

Programme activities are visibly influenced by government policy. Swaziland and South Africa differ in child care policy. The Swaziland government does not have a social security system. However, in the face of a state-declared HIV/AIDS national crisis, draft policy on children, including those who are vulnerable or orphaned has been formulated (2003). At present the social security needs of children are provided by the extended family, which by all accounts is overstretched as HIV/AIDS, combined with endemic poverty, social inequality and drought, has led to a deterioration in the circumstances of the majority of the population. Approximately 40% of children under five show signs of chronic malnutrition and 60% of the total population are food poor.

The South African government provides for statutory entitlements through the Child Care Act for poor children up to the age of 11 (the child care grant = R170 per month in 2004) and a special needs grant (R530 per month in 2004) to caregivers who look after orphaned children up to the age of 18 (the foster care grant). The Constitution and in it, the Bill of Rights provides for children's rights to shelter, education, protection from harm and appropriate care. As a consequence, a lot of effort goes into securing orphans and vulnerable children their statutory entitlements as South African citizens, as well as trying to fill the gaps where these are delayed or unmet. There are also some efforts to help secure them their human rights as children.

The choices that are made around interventions are also dictated by the availability of resources, both financial and human. Many project representatives recognise that their interventions are constrained by limits in infrastructure, money and skills, at times with far-reaching consequences. Transport could be described as the Achilles' heel of community-based family care. It is costly and intermittent, if not absent (especially at night). As a consequence, it is often hard to provide sufficient skilled routine care and support to families in their homes; it is difficult or impossible for adults or children to get the timeous attention they need when they become sick; and it inhibits the participation of children in educare and other initiatives, when they stay beyond a safe walking distance.

Equally, as several respondents point out, the challenges of delivering programmes through the voluntary labour of young and old people who themselves live in poverty and are in need of livelihood, constrains and even negatively impacts on the kinds of care and the systems of support that are necessary to make community-based family care work. It also contributes to the perverse uses of the system.

Lastly, programmes are influenced by assumptions about children, family and community, assumptions that will be looked at in some detail below.

### The Role of Children

For the most part, children have played little or no part in determining the foci of the programmes in the study. This is not unusual. In fact it is in keeping with societal notions of children's competencies, entitlements and responsibilities.

This said, because most programmes involve children in their practice, the content of what they do is influenced by the children they work with, to varying degrees. At one end of the spectrum, there are programmes with no or very little involvement from children, mostly because they deal with babies and infants and rightly regard such children as being too young.

> 'The children are not involved much. The children we deal with are too young; None, sadly so. They are too young; None.' (Project representatives)

However, there are some which have not thought of involving children or doubt the reliability of children's information.

> 'We go door-to-door interviewing parents about their children's needs; We listen to the children's needs, share their worries and difficulties, but mostly go to their homes to get the real information. It is difficult to listen to a child coming to tell you that they need grants.' (Project representatives)

For the majority of programmes the involvement of children occurs through specific activities. In several instances, however, what they learn from the children is more of a by-product of the activity that they are focusing on and is regarded as incidental rather than integral to shaping their activities and interventions.

> 'We involve the children in the food garden project, each has a patch. Life skills have helped them understand their status. There is an improvement in their lives. They feel a sense of belonging and ownership; We took the children to the car park at Spar and to do door-to-door campaigning. We wanted the community to learn more about AIDS and about being an orphan. It gave

*the children a chance to express themselves; We normally have a session with children to talk about HIV/AIDS. We engage them around the issues of sex; We call them to the parish once a month. We organise activities and find out about their needs; We do drama with the children when we go camping. They communicate their feelings and problems.'* (Project representatives)

In other programmes, children's responses - what they say and what they do - and their involvement is regarded as critical information and feedback to the success of activities or even the programme as a whole.

*'We ask them what they need. This way children help with assessing viability, responsibility and sustainability of the intervention or programme; We try to bring children in from school. They help us identify other orphans and they also express their needs; We involve children- choice is a tool for them. Making them drug literate helps them take their drugs on their own. It makes them independent. It gives them a sense of purpose and responsibility.'* (Project representatives)
*'Eight year old ZM does not come back if she is taken to school, so we have established a school in the home to safeguard those children who we are not sure of.'* (Project representative)
*'We ask them what they want, what they are happy with and then try to respond. I want these children to be happy since they have experienced pain; We study what the children say in the class room. Listening to the needs of children, observing them in classrooms has improved the methodology of teaching life skills.'* (Project representatives)

And then there are programmes where the involvement of children is such that it shapes, and even sometimes determines the direction and focus of programme activities.

*'We involve them in decision making, encourage them to develop their own projects, train them to handle problems; We try to get into children's shoes to understand their trauma and suffering; We have lots of discussions with street children and support groups. We run two information and education camps a year. Street children are difficult to keep track of, it places trust in them and helps them stay in touch with peers.'* (Project representatives)
*'We ask the children what they want to do, on the weekend for example. Based on their choices we decide how feasible that is. Older children have influenced us tremendously in forming sports teams and the sports committee. At the moment the Sports Committee is made up of two boys, three caregivers and a social worker. They can either invite schools or have other [children's] homes come and play with them.'* (Project representative)

Most programmes are very responsive to children's needs. At the same time, the potential value of children's involvement in programmes designed to assist and support them has yet to be fully realised across the organisations. As much as children themselves may have limitations of age and experience, assumptions about these limitations may themselves inhibit the kinds of contributions children can make to their own and others' lives.

Certainly, just asking children what they wish for reveals their immediate worries and concerns as well as their dreams and hopes. It also reveals just how much the epidemic has intruded on their well-being and sense of security. They talk about being cared for and caring for those who look after them. They also worry about their siblings and friends as well as other children who find themselves in similar circumstance. They want to help make sure they and others are looked after.

*'I wish to look after the family, to help people who are suffering; I want to get my grandmother better so she can take care of us.'* (Boy aged 15)

They talk about their homes, their wish to find comfort and to have everything they need. They wish for little things – a toy, a ball, a doll, a dress – that are personal and special, things that may be outside the realm of 'basic need' thinking.

*'I wish for a bicycle, toys and chips ...and some proper clothes, and that we have a big and proper house.'* (Boy aged 5)

All worry about their education – they want to stay in and finish school. This is not surprising since in both South Africa and Swaziland, schools and schooling are the social spaces specifically designated for children. These children also all wish for a 'normal' future, to become an adult, to work, to have a profession. They mention, amongst others, their desire to become a nurse, a doctor, a social worker, a business man, a mechanical or chemical engineer, a soccer star or just plain famous.

*'I wish to find a job and live a decent life.'* (Girl aged 14)

Most of the children hanker after a sense of certainty about their place in the world. They express this in their wishes to stop worrying and having to care so much, of wanting to be younger or older than they are – simply of just being able to be a child.

*'To stop thinking too much about my mother and my problems; I would love to change the way I live now; I would love to live free like any other children; I want to grow up; I want to be young; I wish that there weren't orphans in the world.'* (Children various ages)

Children need to be heard and responded to.

## Institutions, Family and Community

Programme activities are significantly shaped by ideas about family, community and institutions and the policies that inform them. By custom and law, parents are deemed to be the naturally and socially obliged protectors of children in the societies in which we live. Children who are orphaned, by definition, have lost the person or people who are their protectors. In such a context, the challenge for any society is to find a way of replacing the loss of a 'natural adult authority' with a guardian or system of protection that secures the rights, entitlements and needs of children affected in this way.

Historically, there have been two kinds of societal responses to the social crisis of being orphaned. Either adult kin - grandparents, aunts, uncles or older children - have been called upon to take up the responsibilities of parenting where their deceased relatives left off; or societies have created systems for surrogate parenting - through fostering and adoption to 'stranger' families or through the creation of institutions for collective child care - commonly known as children's homes (or formerly, orphanages).

Lessons of history, combined with contemporary economic thinking, and an idealised notion of both 'the family' and 'the community' greatly favour extended family absorption or in-community surrogate parenting for children affected or orphaned by AIDS. Generally there is a strong disinclination to support the creation of residential child care institutions.

As programmes in this study grapple with making the preferred model work, what comes through is a much more nuanced and subtle understanding of its limits and the challenges that this model poses to securing the well-being of children.

The statement that orphanages are not an option for HIV/AIDS orphans is rather categorical. Project respondents appear more or less evenly divided between those who agree and those who disagree with it. Yet on closer examination, the divide is far less clear cut. Many express a distinct preference for a community-based, surrogate family model because it keeps children socially and culturally connected and because they feel that institutions are inherently not good places for children to grow up in.

> 'Personally I don't think it is a good idea to put children in institutions. I promote community adoptions; Institutions should be the last option. I feel very strongly about community models, orphanages can't cope.' (Project representatives)

Equally, those who support the existence of institutional care, regard institutions as one of several options rather than as the model of preferred care. Their argument centres on the existing limits of family and community as well as the weaknesses of the state social work system, where it exists. While most would like children to remain with relatives or in surrogate families in their communities, the majority recognise that circumstances vary significantly and that, therefore, there will always be children needing institution-based care.

> 'Institutions should be seen as an option; There are not enough foster parents, and grandparents are dying; A lot of children are going to lack protection and care; Institutional care has a place, subject to changes in size and structure; I don't agree with government because it does not feel the difficulty we face in the community; We lack resources to support scattered orphans in the community.' (Project representatives)

While the preference is for children to be raised in a system of community-based, surrogate family care, all project respondents point to its challenges and limitations.

There is a common concern across South Africa about the child support grants provided by the state. These are often difficult to obtain, because children do not have birth certificates and they may live with grandparents, relatives or others who do not know or cannot remember when or where they were born. Equally the adults caring for them may not have documentation.

> 'When I began I thought it was an easy job. But it is difficult to get documents and therefore difficult to help.' (Project representative)

Also, care grants are differentially age prescribed. Presently, caregivers are eligible for child support grants for children of 11 years of age or younger, whereas foster care grants are awarded to caregivers until the children in their care are 18. As a consequence, children who are not in foster care - the majority of affected children - face an insecure future in their teen years.

And there is a problem of abuse of grants. Child support grants have stimulated a form of rack renting of children in many communities.

*'Families fight over adoption in order to get the grants; People are guardians of seven children. They get the grants but they abuse them and don't take care of the children; The grants are not used for the children's needs.'* (Project representatives)
*'When we start grant processing, new relatives come forward to claim the child. They were not there when the mother was sick.'* (Female caregiver responsible for six children)

It can be argued that such abuse is actively stimulated by the state, because while it is willing to put some child protection mechanisms in place, it has not responded similarly to generalised poverty, so that the care grants for children inevitably are conflated with poverty alleviation (Bouille & Meintjies, 2004).

The problem of poverty also influences the abuse of food parcels and other supports offered to children.

*'Some children live in overcrowded homes – we give them food parcels but they don't get to eat them; Families have their own burdens. You can anticipate hesitancy; Foster parents take children's belongings. The community-based care model can be abused by volunteers; Food parcels tempt those who are distributing them to steal as they are also hungry.'* (Project representatives)

Misuse of resources is not simply a matter of poverty. It is also about the challenges of neglect and abuse. One of the widely acknowledged problems of institutional child care is the absence of love and care and the risk of abuse. These are not simply institutional phenomena however, they are also typical of the family even before the crises of family life induced by AIDS. Simply put, children do and can find themselves neglected and abused in families.

*'Yes, children are in homes but what happens when they are neglected? We need to be concerned about their treatment at home. Children are not stimulated or loved.'* (Project representative)
*'The way they live at home. They smell bad. They don't wash when they wake up. They come with dirty clothes.'* (Male caregiver looking after five children)

Neglect can be both wilful or unintentional. The community-based home care model and the focus on family in itself, places an enormous burden on already overstretched women, and increasingly children who are the central pillars of everyday family life. It should not be surprising, therefore, that project respondents raise concerns about the burden of care that the model places on caregivers.

*'Caregivers are poorly trained, they lack supervision and direction. They become stressed and burdened and suffer from burnout; It relies entirely on volunteers; They can't cope with terminal illness, transportation and they are financially constrained.'* (Project representatives)

Given their own circumstances, where most caregivers mostly depend on state grants (especially the old age pensions of their parents or grandparents) or project-related incentives and activities, many wish that they could be paid or rewarded in some way for their caregiving.

*'You need to think of volunteers as people who need to eat; We need advice on how to use our volunteer skills to earn a living; I would appreciate it if we could be paid; We need incentives, we work very hard – we need something like R1000 a month, not just R500.'* (Project representative)

Concern about abuse of resources can itself lead to perverse responses. This is reflected in narrow interpretation of bureaucratic criteria, or even illegitimate withholding of entitlements. A caregiver who lives in the house her mother built reports that:

*'The social workers would not leave food parcels because they said my house was too big. This house was built by my mother. Should I break it down to get food parcels?'* (Female caregiver responsible for four children)

Listening to the children themselves, they talk about being loved and cared for:

*'I feel as if I have parents because I live a normal life again.'* (Boy aged 15)
*'I wish that Sisi Sinah will take care of me because my mother has passed away and I do not know any one this side.'* (Girl aged 5)

And they talk frankly when they find themselves in uncaring and unloving situations:

*'They are not good to us. They are not kind. They don't talk nicely. We eat bad food. They could try and be more caring. The sisters are cruel and they make us work too hard.'* (Girl aged 14)

Abuse arises out of the inequality of power between adults and children and, as is well known, it occurs in all contexts of child care.

Some people believe that the propensity to abuse increases in institutional settings, but there is no evidence of that. In fact, perhaps the opposite is the case. Children's homes often create safe places for children who are abused in their homes.

*'Perhaps as we speak my mother is drunk. My mother was selling me off to older men to sleep with me. She was always drunk and so she could not look after my younger sisters.'* (Girl aged 14)
*'My brothers and sisters are at home. My mother used to beat me up and say that I slept with her boyfriend. Later she asked other men to sleep with me.'* (Girl aged 17)

Although not intentional, the model of community-based home care creates dependency. On the one hand vulnerable families at times become dependent on caregivers. In the worst case scenario, for example:

*'They have a "patient" and they do nothing for her until the caregiver comes.'* (Project representative)

On the other hand, the caregivers themselves come to depend on the model to help them with livelihood. This is an inherently positive feature of community-based home care in so far as it provides for some income and resources relief, but like subsistence agriculture, it is presently simply a survival strategy that will do little to lift caregivers and their families out of poverty unless it is built into the functioning of the formal economy.

Project respondents point to family and community concerns that the system is intrusive and pries into their private lives.

*'They think that we come to their homes to spy on how they treat the elderly and abuse children. It takes time to motivate them.'* (Project representative)

And there are contexts where the model of community care just cannot work, because people live more as a collection of individuals than anything that might resemble notions of community.

*'Community care in the inner city is very limited. People move a lot, they are difficult to track, there is generally poor sanitation and there is a lot of crime, including trafficking in people. On the streets, you need small orphanages.'* (Project representative)

All this has a direct impact on the interface between institutional and community- based care. Children in institutional care are more likely to have their physical needs addressed at a higher level than if they were living in the homes of relatives, who themselves are invariably poorer.

*'In the orphanage they are all treated equally. Despite insufficient resources they are well maintained and catered for.'* (Project representative*)*

When the focus is on physical resources, not surprisingly children make comparisons between institutions as well as between the institutions they are in and the homes of relatives.

*'In cluster homes there is competition and children compare the facilities. This makes them less satisfied and they want to leave for the one with better resources; Children don't want to go back home as they feel that the lifestyle is different and there are inadequate resources. They are no longer used to a house with no electricity, hot water or TV. They also say that at home they don't eat food, such as macaroni, instead it's just puthu everyday; They feel that they are much better off than those staying in shacks.'* (Project representatives)

These differences make the task of encouraging children to keep contact with family and community much more difficult. Children also sometimes actively resist placement.

*'Finding families is always a challenge. Children become funny and uncontrollable when they are with families.'* (Project representatives)

Lastly there is the issue of children's sense of themselves and their place in society. Widely recognised to be a problem for children in institutional care, it is not generally acknowledged that many children face a similar challenge in community-based care. This, largely, is because of the assumption that self-esteem and identity issues will be addressed automatically in family settings. In reality this is not necessarily the case. There are many accounts of orphaned and vulnerable children who struggle for a place in their worlds.

*'A family member gets scared of the child whose parents died. They are usually not willing to take the child in; Families who were infected are marginalised by their extended family – they accuse each other of witchcraft.'* (Project representatives)

*Responding to the Challenges*

All respondents readily recognise that community-based home care for children is a model with many challenges. Programmes in this study are making efforts and have ideas about how to try address some of these weaknesses. The very need for institutional care is a positive and responsible alternative response where community- based family care fails. At the same time, project respondents working in institutionally based, child care programmes are possibly most conscious and proactive about their limitations both because of their disfavoured status in the larger scheme of things, and because ideally, they too support a system that keeps children closely linked to community.

> 'There are a variety of issues affecting different children, especially in this home. As a nurse and a nun, I have been fortunate to not only heal children physically, but to understand the need for children to be loved and cared for. This is what we try to do here.' (Project representative)
> 'We realise that we are not treating children in a way that is the norm in society. This usually creates problems of adjusting for children when they have to leave the home. So we now bring both boys and girls into the home. Children from the community attend classes in the home. We enrol them in early childhood development classes. We look after sick children. And we encourage visits to families and friends in the community.' (Project representative)
> 'Our motto is to care for children holistically as individuals and in groups.' (Project representative)

When it comes to community-based child care, which, succinctly put, requires 'ensur(ing) that children are safe in their homes, that they get responsible adult care and that the structures are in place to make it work', a variety of things need to occur in order to get it to work properly. According to project representatives these include:

– interventions with families – surrogate or kin – to provide them with the necessary support and guidance, and to raise their knowledge and understanding of the issues involved in fulfilling their undertaking to the children in their care;
– interventions with caregivers that capacitate, support and supervise them on an ongoing basis;
– active engagements with communities, to raise their awareness and understanding of community-based care for children;
– communication and networking strategies with all stakeholders including parish structures, crèches, ward counsellors and other non-governmental and governmental organisations;
– strategic interventions to get communities to take full responsibility for programmes and initiatives so that they are independent and self-sustaining;
– making inroads into the challenges of transport on which so much of the success of community-based care hinges;
– strategies to address the issues of livelihoods.

For the most part, programmes in this study have tried to address one or even several aspects of these concerns. For optimal realisation of the model, however, there is a need for structural and organisational changes to occur together. These need and can be catalysed and supported by the organisations involved in the care of vulnerable and orphaned children, but they have to be driven collectively by all parts of the system.

## 4.5. Impacts

The challenges of child care for orphans and vulnerable children, many of which have already been described, need to be read against the positive impacts of these programmes. These can be quantified in terms of the number of food parcels distributed, feeding schemes run, children placed in families or in institutions, child care and other grants secured, counselling sessions held, awareness campaigns run, school placements secured or paid for, uniforms and school materials bought; crèches run etc. These numbers matter and they are kept by many projects, often for accounting and monitoring purposes. They certainly can usefully be used for planning and strategic management decision making, although the extent to which they are used in this way was not explored in the study.

Equally, it is important to recognise that numbers only account for part of the impact of these programmes. The qualitative stories give us insight into how these numbers translate into individual, family and collective life. In many programmes qualitative information is collected informally rather than formally, which suggests that it is likely to be used in an ad hoc and unsystematic way, if at all.

Drawing from their responses to questions, respondents are generally very positive about the impacts these programmes are having on the children, families and communities they serve.

The emergency food relief schemes run by many programmes address the crisis of hunger that confronts children and adults affected by HIV and AIDS. Although these interventions especially target children, more often than not, they are channelled and supplied through families.

'The feeding scheme has meant that there is no more malnutrition, there is personal growth and children are opening up to us and each other. Feeding schemes are received very positively because old people no longer feel left out; We give them a decent meal, keep them off the streets, give them a sense of belonging; Children and family are integrated in a more holistic way – concern is shown for all [the family] not just the one who is lying [sick]; People are helped by us with food, counselling and education; They say they can survive because they have food.' (Project representatives)

'The project pays for my school fees and trips and they provide me and my younger brother and sisters with clothes.' (Girl aged 15)

'At crèche, they get healthy food. We cook fresh food and teach them to do it at weekends.' (Female caregiver)

Similarly, education-related interventions - be they payment or negotiation of school fees with local schools or the provision of uniforms, books or other materials - keeps children in school.

'Families are proud to say the child is theirs because they are able to send their children to school; We address their educational needs and help financially; Children and their families are going to bed with food and they can go to a place where they can be heard. Children can also go to school.' (Project representatives)

Helping families access child care grants has a similarly positive effect in respect of their food, educational and other needs in the short and medium term.

*'When they have kids, they get grants and these give them access to income and entitlements; I see happiness when they get the grant, they can buy food and go to school.'* (Project representatives)

The impacts of providing children with shelter and care, be it in institutions or in surrogate families, are also evidently positive.

*'We save the lives of about 400 babies each month; We have been able to give children a place to be themselves; Children are placed in closely monitored families. They are given space to love and to grow; We see an improved life style because they are cared for.'* (Project representatives)
*'They help us take care of these children, to give them love and protect them from bad people; Taking children from the streets and putting them with families gives them hope.'* (Caregivers)

Generally, project representatives talk of the relief that their programmes provide from the burden of care that poverty and AIDS impose as well as the hope and dignity that they are able to bring to affected individuals, families and communities.

*'We have been able to help unload the burden these families are experiencing; We are able to restore individual and family dignity; We give a lot of hope to children and families; We offer people a dignified way to die. (Recalling the words of a woman on her death bed) She said that it was the happiest day of her life because she had been treated with dignity.'* (Project representatives)

The notion of community is complex. It is used inter alia as a reference to people in a specific locality, to black people, to the Catholic Church, or to everyone outside the programme itself. Furthermore, most programmes do not have systematic ways of assessing and determining community responses to their initiatives. In the absence of a common definition as well as clear indicators and systems to assess these, they therefore rely on uptake and feedback from the people who use their services or who respond to their requests for assistance and support to understand community perceptions.

All project representatives believe that the communities they serve are positive and supportive of their programmes. This is reflected in the requests for and offers of help that they receive and in the responses of the children and caregivers who they interact with.

*'The community encourages and assists us; The community is coming in large numbers to ask for help, for food and clothes; People in the community send others to us. They are volunteering to work with us and more are disclosing their status; The larger community is waking up. There is interest, curiosity, offers of help, local churches bring clothes; The parish is supportive, schools make donations; They perceive the project as a place of sustenance even for the hungry. They also think that it is a place that can help protect their children and they are ready to drop off abandoned children at the home because they trust and believe in it. Mothers who cannot look after their children bring them to us.'* (Project representatives)

It is also reflected in the impacts that go beyond any specific interventions.

*'The community impact of this programme is wider "Education for Life" is sought after by the principal at the local school, and headmen encourage young people to attend behaviour change*

*courses; There is more of a coordinated effort. We are raising awareness.'* (Project representatives)
*'I was a client, now I am a caregiver. I have grown; If this) centre stops I will personally suffer. It alleviates my stress and I don't dwell on frustrations.'* (Caregivers)

There are significant livelihood dimensions of these programmes which project representatives but especially caregivers and volunteers recognise.

*'There has been livelihood created for the volunteers who feel that R400 is better than nothing for their families as there are no jobs.'* (Project representatives)
*'[If the programme stopped] I'd have no job; We would starve because there are no jobs out there; Who would help the children? Who would help our families?'* (Caregivers)

All impacts are not necessarily easily achieved, however. Several respondents talk of the difficulties of getting people to come forward as volunteers or caregivers, suggesting that responses have been slower than they anticipated. Several project respondents also suggest that at times, there have been negative responses from people in the communities, although none of these appear to have involved any kind of collective negative reaction from communities as a whole. These arise for various reasons, including fear, misunderstanding, unmet expectations, parochial jealousies, or bad personal experiences.

*'People associate Sizanani with the hospice, so they are afraid because they think of death; Some families don't want us to come to their homes because people will think that they are HIV-positive; the community believed that anyone who came to the project was living with AIDS; They complain that we don't cover all areas, but we are very few; There is jealousy but we try to educate people and show them that we mean business.'* (Project representatives)

Sometimes negative responses come from within institutions or care centres or from other groups.

*'There has been a negative response from older residents who feel children are not entitled to be here; the negative responses come from inside the care centre; other groups compete but we try to ignore them.'* (Project representatives)

Generally, such responses are to be expected. The critical point is that project respondents have actively worked to overcome negative responses as they have arisen or become aware of them or they have tried to ignore those that they felt to be petty or irrelevant to their programmatic objectives.

Project respondents readily acknowledge that a better understanding of the impact of their programmes would assist them with their work. They point to the need for:
– developing the skills sets needed by general staff and managers;
– guidance on how to develop a more systematic approach;
– regular stakeholder/user surveys;
– more information for caregivers;
– a review of the manual – in respect of content and language;
– monitoring and evaluation;
– more structure;

– more infrastructure (computers, physical space, transport).

## 5. Lessons from Experience

Project respondents, caregivers and children all provide us with valuable insights into programmatic efforts by SACBC partners to address the needs of orphaned and vulnerable children in resource-poor communities in South Africa and Swaziland. Child care in a complex context of poverty, inequality, family breakdown and a generalised HIV/ AIDS pandemic requires a spectrum of responses rather than an either/or approach. Across this spectrum, all approaches require strategic thinking followed by practical responses to make them work in the best interest of the children that they serve.

It needs to be reiterated that these programmes have developed because children find themselves unprotected and uncared for in society. They are, by definition, a response to system failure that is caused, especially in southern Africa, by the impact of HIV and AIDS on individuals and their families and therefore the communities in which they live. Programmes invariably seek to fill gaps and respond to needs in a way that addresses these immediately. However, many are also trying to find systemic solutions for the medium and longer term. A lot of what they can and want to do depends on the policy and social environment in which the programmes are operating.

The programmes in this study have numerous lessons to share based on their experiences of and engagement with the many challenges that face interventions to support children in need. To make sense of these, they have been grouped by what they have to say about the model and the who, what, where, when and how of intervention.

### 5.1. The Model

Community-based surrogate family care is the preferred model for intervening to care for orphaned and vulnerable children. There are real integrative and normalising benefits of attending to the needs of children through kin or surrogate family-based care. And it is an approach that can be sustained into the medium and long term.

This being said, the model has limitations, which include the potential for the abuse of children and the misuse of resources. These are serious issues that have to be planned for, not least of all because they already occur in families that are not surrogate. Programmes can anticipate them by having plans for their active management through  prevention and remedial action.

Community-based surrogate family care may also not be able to cope with the scale of orphanhood that AIDS is generating in South Africa and Swaziland. There already is a shortage of foster care placements and other forms of surrogate care may too become saturated. Also the model responds weakly to the needs of teenage children affected by AIDS or domestic disintegration. Both caregivers and children identify shelter as a large and desired need. There is a need to develop interventions that will respond to the specific concerns and requirements of the growing number of adolescent and teenage children who find themselves out of home and out of place.

The preference for community-based family care for orphaned and vulnerable children does and should not preclude institutional-based child care options, be they homes, shelters or hospices. Institutional-based care is an appropriate response to family-based care that fails, is absent or is unable to meet specialised needs, especially where children are chronically sick or severely disabled.

There is agreement that institutional care works best where it is contained in size, is physically and socially integrated into local community life, empowers children to become sociable, independent and responsible and is systematically monitored by organisations that are not involved in its routine daily functioning.

## 5.2. Who to serve

Thinking through who should or ought to be served by the intervention is critical. The general sentiment is that it is important to concentrate on all children be they orphaned, vulnerable, abused or disabled, rather than on orphans only. Inclusivity means that children are not identified by their problems but by their status as children. This approach works for some kinds of interventions like those that supplement food and clothing as well as school materials and school placements. However, it can be difficult to achieve in holistic programmes because it requires a complex skills set that can deal appropriately with the needs of children of various ages and statuses.

Surrogate family care in community presumes that many interventions to support children and their needs are mediated by adults. Several programmes recognise, therefore, that the best and most effective way of supporting children is to ensure that the adults who care for them get the necessary support. This means that interventions, by definition, need to include adult carers in their focus whether they are AIDS-sick parents or caregivers who have taken over the parenting of affected or infected children.

## 5.3. What to do

There is a need to make provision for children's special needs. South Africa already does this by law and Swaziland is in the process of creating a policy on children. However, where there is generalised poverty – as is the case in both countries in the communities served by these programmes and beyond – interventions to attend to the special needs of children inevitably conflate children's needs with efforts to relieve poverty, mostly because there is little in place to specifically address adult and child poverty. In designing interventions, therefore it is important to engage with the challenges of poverty and of policy in a way that does not countermand efforts to assist and support children in need.

Orphaned and vulnerable children have multiple needs and there is no formulaic answer that can meet these adequately and at all times. While some programmes are very focused in what they do, most argue for and some are able to offer more holistic care. Whatever service they deliver or need they attend to, all recognise that their effect is greatest when they actively network with other organisations.

Many programmes focus on alleviating immediate physical needs, especially where children are hungry and without adequate clothing to keep them warm. At the same time, there is widespread recognition that children who have been exposed to parental death, family disruption and looming or actual disintegration also need emotional support as they are often profoundly traumatised. Psychological and emotional interventions are not seen as being urgent in the same way as those responding to physical needs. Yet, by their accounts from experience, is this really the case? Can or should emotional trauma be seen as a second-order need that may or may not be attended to down the line? Or should it be something that is understood as integral to the experience of being affected by AIDS, and therefore integral to programmes that intervene to help children? Obviously, to adopt this approach requires professionally supported interventions so that volunteers and caregivers are equipped to address this need. But this requirement is no different from providing ARVs and other medications to HIV-positive people who progress to AIDS.

## 5.4. Approaches to Intervention

Experience shows that there are better and there are worse ways of conceptualising and developing programmes and interventions. Drawing from the knowledge gained in these programmes there are some critical ideas that need consideration. These are not presented in any order of priority.

### The role of Children

Various project respondents recognise that children can and do make very valuable inputs into both the conceptualisation of programmes and the implementation of interventions. In other words, they should not be treated merely as the end recipients of interventions but rather they should be involved as active participants in them, age and capacity considerations obviously withstanding. Children's experiences of interventions also provide valuable feedback that can assist programmes to effectively meet their own objectives.

### Community Involvement

Community-based child care, almost by definition, requires the active participation of community members as individuals and in their organisational capacity in order to take root. The strength and sustainability of programmes and interventions depends considerably on the extent to which the community is included in them, either by helping conceptualise them from the outset, or through their involvement in their implementation, or just by raising their understanding of the issues that the needs of orphan and vulnerable children raise. Community involvement creates opportunities for people, builds partnerships and creates spaces for others to respond to the inevitable gaps that arise. These all are critical to the sustainability of programmes or particular interventions. As programmes strengthen networks between people and organisations they also build citizenship, which in turn contributes to people's sense of belonging and responsibility towards each other.

### Financial Resourcing

Experience suggests that it is important to raise financial resources in advance and in a way that ensures consistency and continuity. This means that is important to have enough resources in place to start any imitative. And while all programmes can and do continuously seek donations to enhance their functioning, these should not be relied on to sustain them unless they have been regularised into long-term commitments.

### Sustainability

In addition to securing finance, two critical and related issues need to be addressed in order to ensure the sustainability of these programmes in resource-poor, livelihood constrained environments. The one relates to retaining and developing volunteer and caregiver capacity through some form of regularised incentive system. Not all programmes pay volunteers. To survive, volunteer carers are forced to look for ways of getting resources which often distract and reduce the kinds of inputs they are able or willing to make. The very success of creating supports services for a system of community-based family care for people living with and affected by AIDS demands reliability and consistency, especially as we enter into it an antiretroviral treatment phase. This, in turn, requires finding ways of linking livelihood security to volunteerism.

The second relates to embedding child care programmes in community life in ways that translate into livelihood generation activities other than through direct employment in the interventions themselves. With the right supports from government, faith-based organisations and relevant professional and non-governmental services, child care, aged care and care for the disabled and chronically ill are all potential services that can be developed at local community level. There are already some examples in operation in the form of crèches for pre-schoolers and aftercare centres for scholars in the communities. Such initiatives need to become integral to all dimensions of programme activity and in all geographical areas.

*Planning*

Planning is about conceptualising what the organisation or initiative wants to do - setting goals and objectives - and then developing a clear set of activities and processes that will make them realisable. Planning makes it possible to identify the resources needed, financial, personnel, infrastructure etc. It makes it clear to others - be they implementing partners or intended beneficiaries - where the focus of activity will be and therefore what can and cannot be expected from the programme or intervention. And it makes clear the parameters of engagement to the organisation itself.

Creating and implementing plans require information. There is a wealth of data already in the programmes that presently either is unused or poorly used by them. Equally, there is information that is needed by programmes that is missing because it is not collected systematically. These are present weaknesses that need to be addressed since both strategic planning and operational management of these programmes need to be informed by quantitative and qualitative data. If they are collected systematically and used purposively, they will help these initiatives achieve their specific programmatic objectives, engage in the larger issues of policy and resourcing and assist with practical day-to-day management.

*Personnel*

The level of education of project respondents interviewed is high. They also bring to their work considerable experience and especially a desire to learn and grow. This is evidenced by the fact that most of their learning about children and HIV/AIDS interventions has been 'on the job'. This is a huge resource in the SACBC programmes that needs to be tapped and channelled effectively.

The knowledge required to work in AIDS is both vast and fast moving. It is inappropriate to imagine or expect that any one individual will have all the requisite skills or be up to date in information and practices in all aspects in the field. This means that expertise has to be built continuously and it has to be complemented through team work. Furthermore, and perhaps most critical to these programmes, dealing as they do with children in complex adult and community contexts, there is a need to grow and deepen the organisational and management skills of all personnel.

This means that in addition to the need for staff to be properly selected it really is important that programmes build continuous education and training into their plans and practices for personnel.

Equally, ongoing education and training need to be integral to their intervention strategy with volunteer caregivers and children since they are key implementing partners and beneficiaries respectively. Everyone needs to be brought into a continuous learning framework.

258

*The Role of the Southern African Catholic Bishops' Conference AIDS Office*
While this study has not looked at the SACBC directly in terms of its objectives and functioning, from the programmes' perspective, it is seen as a coordinating and integrating partner that has a key role to play in the development and ultimate success of church-driven initiatives to support orphans and vulnerable children. Especially it is felt that it should concentrate on:

1. procurement or assistance with the provision of funding to help projects meet their objectives;
2. education and training in order to develop project and stakeholder capacity and skills in the areas of their work;
3. networking to encourage sharing of experiences and resources;
4. information provision and sharing in order to ensure that projects and programmes keep up to date with developments in their specific areas as well as in the larger policy environment;
5. creating a platform for innovative thinking and strategic planning.

## 6. Conclusion

HIV/AIDS transforms the lives of everyone who is touched by the disease and epidemic. Sparked by the evident and ongoing crisis of care for children caused by AIDS-related deaths, the programmes in this study show just how important grass-roots initiatives are to the lives of people marginalised by poverty and disease. They are the kernel of a response system to this epidemic that will help present and future generations survive the epidemic. With the right support and commitment from governments and other partners, they have the potential to give millions of children the chance to live a decent life and to create a decent future.

## References

Boulle, A & Meintjies H., Income Grant Can Support AIDS Care. *Mail and Guardian,* August 27-September 2 2004:37

Marcus, T. (2002). *Wo! Zaphele Izingane: Death and Dying with AIDS* (Johannesburg). CINDI, British High Commission, Sida – Embassy of Sweden

Marcus, T. (2005). *Beginning at the End: An HIV/AIDS Reader for Senior Phase.* Johannesburg: Heinemann.

Marcus, T. (2005). *Promise and Possibility: An HIV/AIDS Reader for Senior Phase.* Johannesburg: Heinemann.

Marcus, T. (2005). *Change and Chance: An HIV/AIDS Reader for Senior Phase.* Johannesburg: Heinemann.

Marcus, T. (forthcoming). *The Paradoxes of AIDS: Poverty, Globalisation and Sustainable Development.* Pietermaritzburg: UKZN University Press

SA Reserve Bank (October 2003). *Labour Markets and Social Frontiers.* Pretoria: Reserve Bank

UNAIDS (2004). *National Response Brief South Africa.* (www.unaids.org)

UNAIDS (2004). *National Response Brief Swaziland* (www.unaids.org)

UNAIDS (2003). *Epidemic Update (annual).* (www.unaids.org)

UNAIDS (2003*). Follow-up to the 2001 UN General Assembly Response to the HIV/AIDS Epidemic.* (www.unaids.org)

UNICEF (2004). *Africa's Orphan Generations.* (www.unicef.org)

UNFPA (2004). *State of World Population 2004 Report.* (www.unfpa.org)

*Address for correspondence:*
Dr. T. Marcus
National Research Foundation
PO Box 2600
Pretoria 0001
South Africa
e-mail: tessa@nrf.ac.za

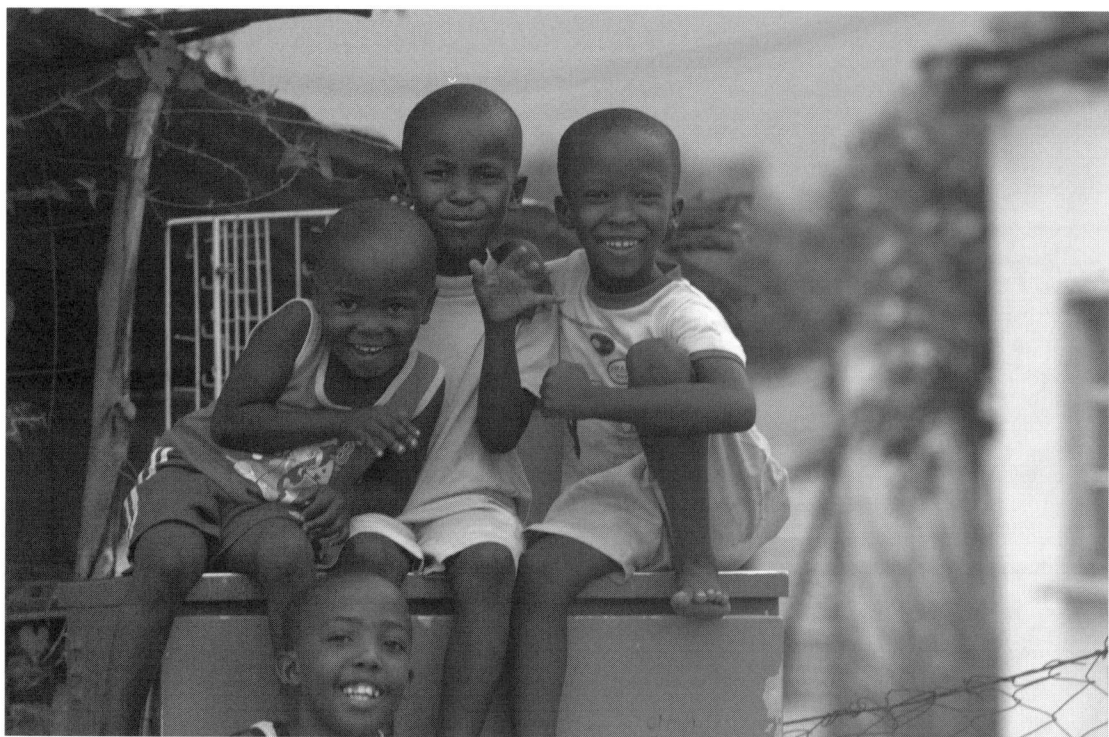

# Chapter 15

# The Quality of Life of Children with HIV/AIDS on ARV Treatment

*Anna Versteege[1], Leonie Korstjens[1], Marcel van Aken[1], Adri Vermeer[2]*

[1] Department of Psychology, Utrecht University, Utrecht, The Netherlands
[2] Department of Educational Sciences, Utrecht University, Utrecht, The Netherlands

## Abstract

There is not much information about the quality of life of children with HIV/AIDS in South Africa. Therefore, in this study the quality of life of children with HIV/AIDS on ARV treatment in South Africa has been investigated. ARV treatment will be a common treatment in the future and given the implication that more and more children with HIV/AIDS survive, it becomes relevant for their further development to investigate their quality. This information can be used in designing support programmes.

Using the 'Child Functioning Inventory – Junior Primary' (CFI-JPRIM) and the 'Child Functioning Inventory – Senior Primary' (CFI-SPRIM), several hypotheses have been tested with regard to the quality of life of children with and children without HIV/AIDS. The Child Functioning Inventory is designed to measure the quality of life by evaluating the present functioning of the child. Participants in this study were 13 children with HIV/AIDS on treatment and 13 children without HIV/AIDS. The children were living in a home or in a township in South Africa.

Results show that the quality of life of children with HIV/AIDS in South Africa is not different from the quality of life of children without HIV/AIDS. Results show also that boys with HIV/AIDS report a higher quality of life than girls and that children with HIV/AIDS living in a home report a higher quality of life than children without HIV/AIDS living in a home. No significant differences were found between the reported quality of life of children who are living in different conditions regardless whether they had HIV/AIDS or not.

Results seem to indicate that children with HIV/AIDS do not have a lower quality of life. It should be noted that all participants with HIV/AIDS are on ARV treatment, and it is discussed whether the lack of differences between children with and children without HIV/AIDS can be the effect of the ARV treatment.

## 1. Introduction

Sub-Saharan Africa accounts for nearly three quarters of the people in the world living with HIV or AIDS. By the end of 2002, there were over 29 million people with HIV/AIDS, 10 million of whom were young people (15–24) and 3 million were children under 15 years of age. In 2002 over 2 million adults died from AIDS. Eight out of every ten orphans in the world live in sub-Saharan Africa. The numbers of orphans will continue to rise throughout the next decade, reaching 40 million by 2010 (Foster & Williamson, 2000).

A large number of children in sub-Saharan Africa suffer from HIV/AIDS. They are in the final stage of infection with the human immunodeficiency virus (HIV). This is a retrovirus, which gradually impairs the immune system that is crucial for the suppression of infections, viruses and bacteria. As a result of the deteriorated functioning of the immune system patients may contract opportunistic infections and malignancies of which they, without therapy, ultimately die. HIV may also directly infect the nervous system causing morbidity and contributing to diminished survival. The impact of HIV and AIDS on affected or infected children is overwhelmingly negative. The disease and the epidemic have far-reaching physical, material and emotional consequences (Marcus, 2005). Fortunately, ARV therapy has a positive influence on the effects of HIV/AIDS (Geelen, 2002). It is said that the therapy improves the quality of life of those infected with HIV, especially of those who react positively to treatment. People with a positive reaction to treatment feel more hopeful, optimistic and relieved. They also feel less devastated, afraid and depressed than people with a negative reaction to treatment. (Catz, Kalichman, Benotsch, Miller & Suarez, 2001). A number of effective ARV drugs are now available in South Africa.

HIV/AIDS is a chronic illness. Chronic illnesses may be defined as any illness that persists for more than three months. It may be protracted but stable, or progressive and life threatening, or a non-fatal disabling condition, and it may profoundly affect a child's growth and development (Kibel & Wagstaff, 2001). It requires successful organisational and emotional adjustment of the child and the family. The way in which the child and the family adapt to the illness will affect their psychological well-being and their quality of life and in turn the clinical course of the illness itself.

Many cross-sectional studies have found that children and adolescents with chronic illnesses and disabilities are at increased risk of psychosocial problems. Chronically ill children and adolescents have been reported to have lower self-esteem, poorer body image and more problems in psychological well-being, behaviour, and social adjustment than those without chronic conditions (Huurre & Aro, 2002).

The quality of life regarding health-related issues, i.e. 'the individual's perception of problems in health status, combined with the affective responses to such problems' (Theunissen, 1999), consists of variables such as described above and is increasingly recognised to be an important issue in chronic diseases.

Two major correlates of the quality of life in adults are known to be self-esteem and a sense of primary control. Self-esteem is an evaluative component, that is, the individual's favourable or unfavourable assessment of oneself, and is an important facet of the self-concept. The attainment of a stable concept about oneself as an individual is an important stage in the cognitive development of children. By the age of 6 or 7 year, most children have definite ideas about themselves and their attributes as a person. For example, they know whether they are a boy or a girl, whether they are strong or weak, coordinated or clumsy, clever or not so clever, popular with other children or not, and so on. Throughout childhood and adolescence, self-concept changes in response to maturation and to environmental experiences. The effects of HIV/AIDS on the self-concept of children are largely unstudied.

The quality of life of children with HIV/AIDS is especially important, because the psychological impact in these children is enormous. In addition to possibly normal developmental problems, they also experience stigma and they suffer multiple bereavement through the loss of fathers, mothers, siblings, aunts and other relatives. In addition to direct losses caused by death, they also experience loss of familiar surroundings, friends and schooling, and can lose hope for the future due to consequent migration or a slide from poverty into destitution (Williamson & Hunter, 2000). It is also possible that children lose both their parents and become orphans. If there is an extended family, children can live with them and efforts must be made to support them for the sake of the well-being of the children. However, sometimes there is no extended family or it is not in the best interest of the children to live with them. Alternative care options should then be found (Desmond, Gow, Loening-Voysey, Wilson & Stirling, 2002). In South Africa there are different models of care but each situation is different so there are no guidelines in providing care (Desmond, et al., 2002).

For a variety of reasons, little attention has been paid to the situation of children affected by HIV/AIDS in Africa. Greater understanding of the impact of HIV/AIDS is important in the design and evaluation of programmes to support children living in difficult circumstances (Foster & Williamson, 2000). Because of this and of the fact that numbers of orphans will continue to rise throughout the next decade, the study of the quality of life in children with HIV/AIDS is important. The focus of this study will be on those children who are on ARV treatment, because it (hopefully) will be a common treatment in the future and because it is assumed that it improves the quality of life of those infected with HIV.

The following research questions will be addressed:
1. Does the quality of life of children with HIV/AIDS differ from the quality of life of children without HIV/AIDS?
2. Does the quality of life of boys with HIV/AIDS differ from girls with HIV/AIDS?
3a. Does the quality of life of children with HIV/AIDS living in a home differ from children without HIV/AIDS living in a home?
3b. Does the quality of life of children with HIV/AIDS living in a township differ from children without HIV/AIDS living in a township?
3c. Does the quality of life of children with HIV/AIDS living in a township differ from children with HIV/AIDS living in a home?

The expectation is that children without HIV/AIDS will have a better quality of life than children with HIV/AIDS, even when the latter are on ARV treatment. In view of the differences in living conditions there are no specific expectations, because it may depend on the quality of care. Normally it would be expected that living with a family is better than living in a home. But if the family has nothing to offer, a home can be better if there is intensive care and enough food.

## 2. Methods

### 2.1. Sample
The focus of this study was on children living with HIV/AIDS on ARV treatment between 7 and 13 years old. This age group was chosen because the acquiring of information could then take place with the children themselves. The aim was to include as many children as possible, regardless of their background or living conditions. It was difficult to find children in this age group who could participate, because for a lot of children ARV treatment came too late, so they died. Participants with HIV/AIDS were traced via the SACBC AIDS Office. Participants without HIV/AIDS were traced via social workers in Sizanani Village. In total there were 13 children with HIV/AIDS and 13 children without HIV/AIDS included in the study.

**Table 1: The age of the children with and without HIV/AIDS and of boys and girls**

| Age | 7 | 8 | 9 | 10 | 11 | 12 | 13 | Total |
|---|---|---|---|---|---|---|---|---|
| With HIV/AIDS | 2 | 3 | 1 | 2 | 4 | 0 | 1 | 13 |
| Without HIV/AIDS | 1 | 4 | 1 | 2 | 3 | 1 | 1 | 13 |
| Boys | 3 | 3 | 0 | 2 | 1 | 1 | 0 | 10 |
| Girls | 0 | 4 | 2 | 2 | 6 | 0 | 2 | 16 |

## 2.2. Instruments

To measure the quality of life two versions of the Child Functioning Inventory (CFI) were used:

- The Child Functioning Inventory - Junior Primary (CFI-JPRIM). This scale is specifically aimed at children between the ages of 6 and 9 (Appendix 1).
- The Child Functioning Inventory - Senior Primary (CFI-SPRIM). This scale is specifically aimed at children between the age of 10 and 13 (Appendix 2).

The CFI is designed to measure the quality of life by evaluating present functioning of the child. It contains four different scales:

- *Positive functioning areas:* perseverance, satisfaction, future perspective.
- *Self-perception:* anxiety, guilt feelings, lack of self-worth, isolation, responsible for others, lack of assertiveness.
- *Trauma dynamics:* memory loss, frustration, helplessness, attitude towards adults, mistrust, stigma, body image, personal boundaries, school problems (the CFI-SPRIM measured two extra items: alcohol use and drug use).
- *Relationships:* relationship with friends, mother, father, stepmother, stepfather, family.

All items items of the CFI-JPRIM (195) and of the CFI-SPRIM (209) are theses with three answering possibilities: 'no' (1), 'sometimes' (2) and 'yes' (3). A few examples of the theses are: *I work hard at school, I am afraid that things may go wrong, My body feels dirty* and *My caregiver and I do things together.*

Because most of the children that participated had lost their parents or had been abandoned, some of the items about relationships with mother, father, stepmother, stepfather and family were changed or deleted: items about the relationship with father, stepmother and stepfather were deleted and in items about the relationship with mother, the word 'mother' was replaced by the word 'caregiver'.

After collecting the data it showed that none of the children between 10 and 13 years old ever used drugs or alcohol. Therefore, the sub-scales about drugs and alcohol were not analysed. After these changes both questionnaires consisted of 163 items.

Because not all children were fluent in English, a student from the University of Pretoria made a translation of the questionnaire in Zutu and Zulu.

## 2.3. Procedure

It was not possible to have identical procedures for the different locations, because of their different living conditions and languages. As intended in advance, it was not always possible to play with the children and create a bond before questioning them. All children were told that the answers that they were giving were confidential. To thank the children they got some candy. The data were gathered on the following locations:

*Nazareth House (Johannesburg)*
This is a home for orphans with HIV/AIDS. All of them are on medication. Because HIV/AIDS is a difficult topic to talk about, the researchers first came a few times to play with the children and to create a bond. When the children answered the questionnaire they were sitting at one of the tables in the dining hall. The older children could fill in the questionnaire themselves. The researchers helped the smaller children; they read the questions to them so that the children only needed to tick the answer.

*Elandsdoorn (near Groblersdal)*
Children who live in the townships around Grobersdal were participating in the AIDS/HIV programme of the Ndlovu Medical Centre in Elandsdoorn and are all on ARV treatment. Parents had to bring the children to the clinic at an appointed time. The translator, somebody from the AIDS/HIV programme and an acquaintance of the children, read the questions to the children so they only needed to tick the answers. They where sitting in one of the rooms of the little hospital.

*Sizanani (Bronkhorstspruit)*
The children that lived around Sizanani participated in the AIDS/HIV programme in Sizanani and were all on medication. The researchers and a translator visited them at their homes in the townships. The translator, who was one of the social workers and an acquaintance of the children, read the questions to the children so that they only had to tick the answer.

*Germiston (Johannesburg)*
This is a home for children that have been abandoned, they are orphans or are difficult to handle. Most children are not infected. The researchers helped the younger children and read the questions to the children. The older children could do it by themselves.

*Schools in the townships of Zithobeni and Rethabiseng*
The children of the schools were not infected with HIV/AIDS. At Zithobeni the teacher read and translated the questions in class and they only needed to tick the answers. At Rethabiseng a few older children could answer the questionnaire by themselves. If they did not understand something they could ask the teacher or one of the researchers. The teacher was sitting next to the younger children and read the questions to them.

## 2.4. Statistics
To analyse the data, SPSS has been used. The items concern four different scales: Positive functioning areas, Relationships, Self-perception and Trauma Dynamics. The four scales were subdivided in different sub-scales. There were no missing values.

Because some of the items were measuring into different directions, they were changed with SPSS into the same direction for each scale. The quality of life is good when there is a high score on the scales 'Positive functioning areas' and 'Relationships' and a low score on the scales 'Self-perception' and 'Trauma Dynamics'.

266

Because of the small sample size, non-parametric tests were used to test the differences between the groups. To see if there was an interaction between gender and HIV/AIDS a two-way ANOVA was used.

## 5. Results

### 5.1. Does the Quality of Life of Children with HIV/AIDS differ from Children without HIV/AIDS?

No significant differences were found on the four main scales (see Table 2). Only a small significant difference was found in the sub-scale 'Lack of assertiveness'. On that sub-scale children without HIV/AIDS have a lower score, so their quality of life seems to be better in this domain than that of children with HIV/AIDS.

Table 2: Main scores of the quality of life of children with and without HIV/AIDS

|  | With HIV/AIDS Mean (n =13) | Without HIV/AIDS Mean (n=13) | Z-Value |
|---|---|---|---|
| Positive functioning areas | 11.85 | 15.15 | - 1.104 |
| Self-perception | 11.00 | 16.00 | - 1.667 |
| Trauma dynamics | 13.77 | 13.23 | - 0.179 |
| Relationships | 13.62 | 13.38 | - 0.077 |

* Significant difference between children with HIV/AIDS and children without HIV/AIDS (p<0.05)

### 5.2. Does the Quality of Life of Boys with HIV/AIDS differ from Girls with HIV/AIDS?

Significant differences are found on the scale 'Relationships' and the sub-scales 'Anxiety', 'Memory Loss', 'Stigma', 'Body Image', and 'Relationships with caregiver' (see Table 3). On those scales, the quality of life of boys seems to be better than that of girls. The two-way ANOVA showed that there was no interaction between gender and HIV/AIDS, meaning that the differences between boys and girls were the same in both groups.

Table 3: Main scores of the quality of life of boys and girls with HIV/AIDS

|  | Boys Mean (n =5) | Girls Mean (n=8) | Z-Value |
|---|---|---|---|
| Positive functioning areas | 6.80 | 7.13 | - 1.470 |
| Self-perception | 5.00 | 8.25 | - 1.464 |
| Trauma dynamics | 4.40 | 8.63 | - 1.903 |
| Relationships | 10.90 | 4.56 | - 2.895* |

* Significant difference between boys and Girls (p<0.05)

### 5.3a. Does the Quality of Children without HIV/AIDS living in a Home Differ from Children with HIV/AIDS living in a Home?

There are significant differences found on the scale 'Self Perception' and the sub-scales 'Guilt Feelings', 'Responsible for Others', 'Lack of Assertiveness' and 'Frustration' (see Table 4). Children with HIV/AIDS living in a home seem to have a better quality of life on these scales, than children without HIV/AIDS living in a home.

**Table 4: Main scores of the quality of life of children without HIV/AIDS living in a home and children with HIV/AIDS living in a home**

|  | With HIV/AIDS Mean (n =7) | Without HIV/AIDS Mean (n=7) | Z-Value |
|---|---|---|---|
| Positive functioning areas | 6.57 | 8.43 | - .8310 |
| Self-perception | 4.57 | 10.43 | - 2.619* |
| Trauma dynamics | 6.00 | 9.00 | - 1.342 |
| Relationships | 8.43 | 6.57 | - .8400 |

* Significant difference between children with HIV/AIDS living in a home and children without HIV/AIDS living in a home ($p<0.05$)

### 5.3b. Does the Quality of Life of Children with HIV/AIDS living in a Township differ from Children without HIV/AIDS living in a Township?

In the four scales and the sub-scales, no significant differences were found (see Table 5), indicating that the quality of life of children with HIV/AIDS living in a township did not differ from children without HIV/AIDS living in a township.

**Table 5: Main scores of the quality of life of children with HIV/AIDS living in a township and children without HIV/AIDS living in a township**

|  | With HIV/AIDS Township Mean (n =6) | Without HIV/AIDS Township Mean (n=6) | Z-Value |
|---|---|---|---|
| Positive functioning areas | 6.00 | 7.00 | - 0.484 |
| Self-perception | 6.50 | 6.50 | - 0.000 |
| Trauma dynamics | 8.17 | 4.83 | - 1.601 |
| Relationships | 5.58 | 7.42 | - 0.903 |

* Significant difference between children with HIV/AIDS living in a township and children without HIV/AIDS living in a township ($p<0.05$)

### 5.3c. Does the Quality of Life of Children with HIV/AIDS living in a Township differ from Children with HIV/AIDS living in a Home?

In the four scales and the sub-scales no significant differences were found (see Table 6), indicating that there are no differences between children with HIV/AIDS living in a township or living in a home.

**Table 6: Main scores of the quality of life of children with HIV/AIDS living in a township and children with HIV/AIDS living in a home**

|  | With HIV/AIDS Home Mean (n =7) | With HIV/AIDS Township Mean (n=6) | Z-Value |
|---|---|---|---|
| Positive functioning areas | 5.86 | 8.33 | - 1.144 |
| Self-perception | 6.00 | 8.17 | - 1.000 |
| Trauma dynamics | 7.57 | 6.33 | - 0.571 |
| Relationships | 5.86 | 8.33 | - 1.159 |

* Significant difference between children with HIV/AIDS living in a township and children with HIV/AIDS living in a home ($p<0.05$)

268

## 6. Conclusions

Our expectations have only partly been confirmed. There are no significant differences in reported quality of life between children with HIV/AIDS and children without HIV/AIDS. Children without HIV/AIDS do not report a better quality of life. This is not as expected, because children with HIV/AIDS experience stigma and suffer multiple bereavement (Williamson & Hunter, 2000). It was therefore expected that they would report a lower quality of life.

However, there are differences in reported quality of life between boys or girls. Boys report a better quality of life than girls. There are also significant differences between the reported quality of life of children without HIV/AIDS living in home and children with HIV/AIDS living in a home. Children with HIV/AIDS living in a home report a better quality of life. This is in contrast to what was expected because the living conditions are similar (both homes) and children with HIV/AIDS were expected to report a lower quality of life. It might be that the medical care (ARV treatment) and the extra concern for the children has a positive effect of their experienced quality of life.

In contrast, there are no significant differences between the quality of life of children with HIV/AIDS living in a township and children without HIV/AIDS living in a township. Because the living conditions are similar, children without HIV/AIDS living in a township were expected to report a better quality of life. There are also no significant differences in reported quality of life between children with HIV/AIDS living in a township and children with HIV/AIDS living in a home.

It can be concluded that the quality of life of children with HIV/AIDS on treatment in the locations of this research does not seem to differ from the quality of life of children without HIV/AIDS. However, it is known that children with HIV/AIDS suffer from physical, material and emotional consequences (Marcus, 2005). A reason for the fact that we did not find these differences, could actually be that ARV treatment improves the quality of life, and thus buffers against the negative effects the illness usually has. After all, earlier research showed that being on treatment gives people hope for the future. People on treatment also feel less afraid and more hopeful and optimistic (Catz, Kalichman, Benotsch, Miller & Suarez, 2001). It seems, therefore, that ARV treatment has a positive influence on the quality of life of children living with HIV/AIDS.

## 7. Discussion

It is not easy to do research in a country were stigma around HIV/AIDS is prevalent. One needs patience to be able to talk to people about HIV/AIDS. In this study there was enough time to build a bond, which was very helpful in executing the questionnaires.

Because ARV treatment has been publicly available in South Africa for just a short time, only a small number of children have been put on treatment yet. That is why it was very difficult to find participants for this study. Fortunately, there was enough time and the possibility to travel, so with help of the social workers in Sizanani Village it was possible to go to schools and visit children in the townships. But despite this help, the sample size remains quite small. For this reason, this study should be seen as a pilot study.

It should be kept in mind that the participants in this research who have HIV/AIDS, are all taking ARVs. Because there were no participants with HIV/AIDS without treatment, it is difficult to make a specific judgement about the effects of ARVs. It proved to be very difficult to include children with HIV/AIDS without treatment, because if children or their parents acknowledge their illness, they immediately get medicines. So, the participants who are known to have HIV/AIDS (and participated in this study), are always on treatment.

Because of the stigmatisation, however, it is possible that people do not know or do not want to know they have HIV/AIDS and are denying it. In this view, it is possible that the children living in Zithobeni and Rethabiseng that were involved in the control group of this study do have HIV/AIDS without knowing it. If this is true, the results might be influenced because they were supposed to be healthy.

The results can also be influenced by the language. Possibly not all children understood the question well enough and did not dare to say so. Also the use of translators and the different circumstances in which the children were questioned, might have influenced the results. Although there was a translated version of the questionnaire, it could be that the translators explained the questions in a different way than the researchers did. And in some of the circumstances the children had more opportunities to ask questions (because the groups were smaller) or were more or less distracted (or serious) than in other circumstances.

Another important aspect concerns the concept of 'quality of care'. It is our personal impression that the quality of care environment varies for the different locations. In Nazareth House there is a mother figure for the children. They live in a group, almost like a real family. In Germiston this was not the case. Children here are living in groups and do not have one mother figure. Children living in townships are sometimes living with their grandmother, but are living in poor circumstances. Because children with HIV/AIDS have the greatest needs for intensive care (which improves their quality of life; see Van der Eijk, Stockbrugger & Russel, 2000) and not every child receives the same quality of care, results may be influenced.

When time passes by, children who are on ARV treatment will be older, speak better English and there will be more children receiving medicines. This will make it easier to question them. For further research, it will also be interesting to look at the quality of care, as this can influence the reported quality of life.

Children with HIV/AIDS need special care. It is very important that they receive ARVs, so they will have a future again. HIV/AIDS has a great influence on the lives of everyone who is touched by the epidemic and the numbers of orphans will continue to rise. Therefore, children need help in creating a new future and living with direct losses caused by death and loss of familiar surroundings, friends and schooling. It must be clear that surviving HIV/AIDS and maintaining a high quality of life is only possible when children receive ARVs and special care.

# References

Catz, S.L., Kalichman, C., Benotsch, E.G., Miller, J. & Suarez, T. (2001). Anticipated psychological impact of receiving medical feedback about HIV treatment outcomes. *AIDS CARE, 13(5),* 631-635

Desmond, C., Gow, J., Loening-Voysey, H., Wilson, T. & Stirling, B. (2002). Approaches to caring, essential elements for a quality service and cost-effectiveness in South Africa. *Evaluation and Program Planning 25* (pp. 447-458). South Africa: Elsevier Science Ltd.

Eijk, van der, I., Stockbrugger, R, & Russel, M. (2000). *Influence of quality of care on quality of life in inflammatory bowel disease (IBD): literature review and studies planned.* Maastricht: Elsevier Science B.V. .

Evian, C. (2000). *Primary Aids Care: a practical care personnel in the clinical and supportive care of people with HIV/AIDS.* Houghton: Jacana Education.

Foster, G., & Williamson, J. (2000). *A review of current literature of the impact of HIV/AIDS on children in sub-Saharan Africa.* Zimbabwe: Lippincott Williamson & Wilkins.

Geelen, S.P.M., (2002). *HIV en AIDS bij kinderen en jongeren.* Eigen uitgave Wilhelmina Kinder Ziekenhuis, Universitair Medisch Centrum Utrecht, Utrecht.

Huurre & Aro, (2002). Long-term psychological effects of persistent chronic illness. *European Child & Adolescent Psychiatry, 11(2),* 85-91

Kibel, M.A., & Wagstaff, L.A. (2001). *Child Health for all. A manual for Southern Africa.* Cape Town: Oxford University Press

Marcus, T. (2005). *To live a decent life: Bridging the gaps.* Pretoria (RSA): National Research Foundation/Southern African Catholic Bishops' Conference AIDS Office.

Theunissen, N.C.M., (1999). *Health related quality of life in children.* Proefschrift. Leiden: Universiteit Leiden.

Williamson, J., & Hunter, S. (2000). *Children on the brink: Strategies to Support Children Isolated by HIV/AIDS.* South Africa: Health Technical Services Project USAID

*Address for correspondence:*
Prof. dr. A. Vermeer
Department of Educational Sciences
Utrecht University
Heidelberglaan 1
3584 CS Utrecht
The Netherlands
e-mail: a.vermeer@fss.uu.nl

# Epilogue

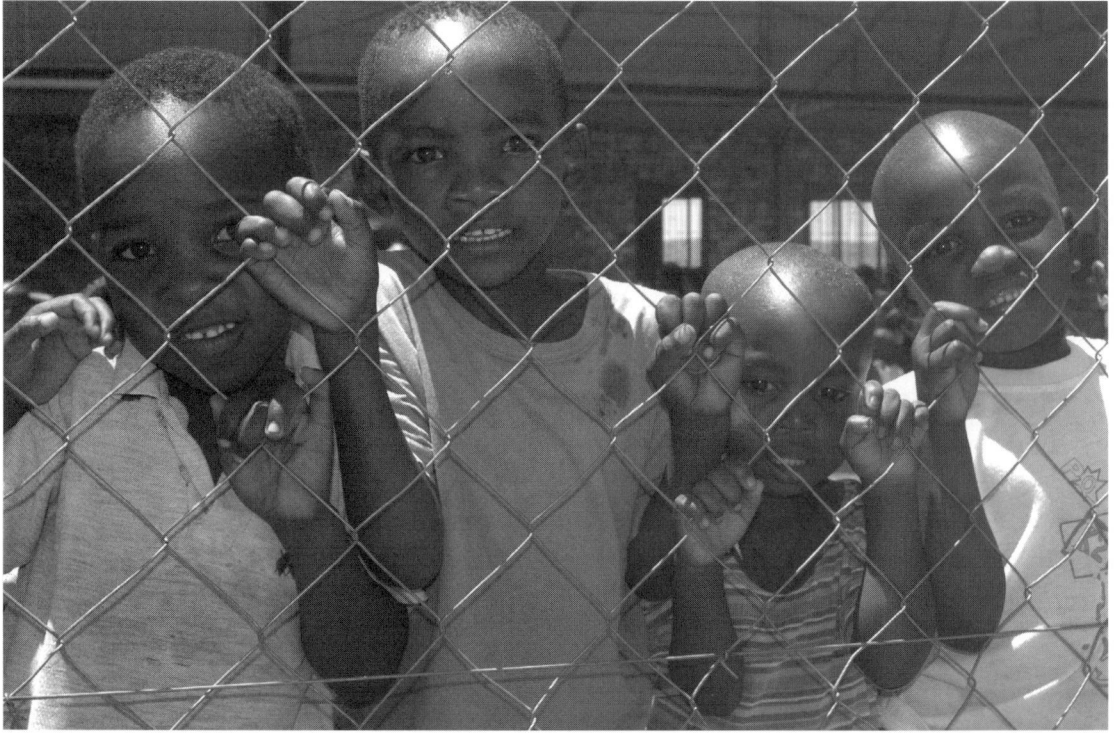

# Chapter 16

# Health, Knowledge and Society: In- and Exclusion

*Henk J. van Rinsum[1]*

[1] Utrecht School of Governance and Faculty of Social Sciences, Utrecht University, Utrecht, The Netherlands

## Abstract

This epilogue focuses on the intricate web of health, poverty, development and knowledge in Africa. Health and health care are seen as one of the resources in society. In Africa we see different concepts of health and illness which relate to an African worldview in which the seen and the unseen worldview are very closely related. At the same time it is argued that there are mechanisms of in- and exclusion relegating masses of people in Africa to a state of poverty. In the processes of improvement of health, health care and alleviation of poverty, knowledge is a crucial factor. The epilogue ends with a plea for joint activities in the field of health research.

## 1. Introduction

This closing chapter focuses on the intricate web of health, poverty, development and knowledge. Health and health care in a given society are determined by the availability of, and access to, different resources. The word 'resources' is used here in a very broad sense, referring to both material and immaterial resources. People, institutions at different levels and the resources together constitute a dynamic pattern of relationships.

## 2. Different Concepts of Health

When discussing the concept of health, it is imperative to differentiate between the different definitions of health that go hand in hand with the definition of their mirror image, i.e. illness. Perspectives on health and illness are part of a particular worldview in a particular cultural context (see e.g. the classical text by Helman, 2000). In the African worldview, health and illness form an integral part of a world that comprises both the world that we live in and the supernatural world. The African philosopher Godfrey Tangwa defined this worldview as an eco-bio-communitarian worldview stressing interdependence among human beings, animals, plants and inanimate objects and forces (Tangwa 2000; van Rinsum & Tangwa 2004). From this perspective, health relates to harmony, to the integral human being; a human being as integral part of humanity. Illness relates to disharmony and cannot be reduced to a strictly biophysical phenomenon, which can be cured (or even better prevented) by mainly biophysical means.

It is important to realise that plural societies use plural definitions of health and illness, a phenomenon that we see for example in countries in Africa. However, in the case of HIV/AIDS, we see different discourses of health and illness, that tragically lead to different but at the same time conflicting views on treatment (or prevention) of the disease. We will come back to this issue.

## 3. Economic Growth and Infrastructure

For health and health care, a certain level of economic growth and economic infrastructure is needed. This seems understandable as health and health care need 'to be paid for'. That means that there needs to be a minimum of income at household, regional and national level to enable people's access to resources that will positively affect their health or that will prevent them from falling ill.

Next to economic growth, health and health care are also determined by the functioning of an adequate infrastructure that facilitates the processes of knowledge development and knowledge transfer. Knowledge is more and more developing into a critical resource in the well-being of people. That means that access to knowledge-producing and knowledge-transferring organisations is a critical factor.

However, here again the concept of knowledge needs to be differentiated. Knowledge has to do with structured information, communication, learning and meaning. On the one end of the knowledge continuum we find scientific knowledge, produced according to global standards (although there is, of course, much discussion about these standards). This kind of knowledge is mostly produced within universities, research institutes and private firms and is dominated by the 'North'.

On the other end of the continuum we find what is labelled as indigenous, local knowledge, knowledge integrated in the cultural context, knowledge that enables people to give meaning to their own environment and their place in the world (which relates to both the seen and unseen world). This knowledge is mostly transferred along personal lines, within small-scale communities such as families.

These different knowledge systems are sometimes inclusive by nature but most of the time they appear to be exclusive, claiming dominance or even a monopolistic position.

## 4. Health and Development

It would be wrong, however, to suggest that health is only a dependent variable of other resources in society. Health is not only *resulting*, it is also *enabling*. Health and health care are essential prerequisites for the development of human dignity in a responsible and socially sustainable society. Here again there needs to be room for a pluralism of health concepts. And different health concepts will imply different systems of health care.

## 5. In- and Exclusion

It is not just the availability of resources that determines the level of health and health care. The available resources that people have access to, need to be relatively fairly distributed. And here we can discern an intricate relationship between the availability of, access to, and distribution of resources on the one hand, and processes of in- and exclusion on the other hand. If the distribution is uneven and society is characterised by inequality, more people will be excluded from the access to the basic resources such as health care. The result will be marginalisation and poverty. And this in turn, will negatively affect health.

In our global world we see mechanisms of distribution at work at different levels, which are reflected in mechanisms of in- and exclusion. At a global level, we talk about a 'North-South' divide, although this divide is increasingly differentiated by processes of mass migration that have taken place over the last decades. The North now sees the South in its backyard. One of the challenges for people in the North is to deal with people from the South in their midst. The other way around we see poor countries that have a powerful, relatively small, but very rich elite. The North-South divide and the mechanism of in- and exclusion represents itself increasingly in different guises. One of these guises can be found in South Africa today.

## 6. Paradigms of Inclusion

It is Thabo Mbeki, President of South Africa, himself who can assist us in formulating two paradigms of in- and exclusion. Thabo Mbeki made a statement in 1996 which has come to be known as the famous 'I am an African'-speech.[1] In very colourful and vibrant expressions he describes his roots back to the San, the Khoi, the European immigrants, the Malay slaves, the black slaves from Africa, etc. This speech resembles the rainbow concept as elaborated for example by Bishop Tutu. This *rainbow paradigm* is about a positive connotation of multiculturalism, about a colourful rainbow nation where people live together in harmony. It is about diversity of living creatures; it is about unity in diversity. It is a paradigm of a diversity of *inclusion*. People are included in the access to the resources that enable the development of human dignity. People are included in the health system.

## 7. Paradigms of Exclusion

However, Mbeki also formulated a different and opposite paradigm. He addressed the COSATU[2] 7th National Congress in 2000. In his speech he said:

> 'These masses want to see an end to racism. They want to see an end to the situation in which our country is divided into two nations, one well-off and white and the other poor and black. They want to see an end to the racism many people continue to suffer, including many farm workers. They want to see an end to sexism. They do not want black women in the rural areas for ever described as the poorest of the poor, with no education, no work, not enough food, no clean water, no electricity and no roads and difficult access to health services.'[3]

This paradigm is about inequality, about power relations, about racism, about living in townships or in luxurious resorts, about lack of basic needs. This two-nations paradigm is a paradigm of *exclusion* of resources. It is a paradigm of difference.

This two-nations paradigm of exclusion leads to a situation in which society, the South African society at large, has available the necessary economic infrastructure. The economic growth percentage may be up to or even exceeding international standard. At the same time, large portions of the population are excluded from the basic needs, including health and health care.

## 8. Health and Poverty

This two-nations paradigm is acutely present when we look at the HIV/AIDS situation in South Africa. The HIV/AIDS-catastrophe is unequalled. We can hardly assess the consequences of the figures regarding the rapid spread of HIV/AIDS. By the end of 2003, 5.3 million South Africans were infected with HIV. These figures are almost beyond imagination.

It was again Thabo Mbeki who made a curious contribution to the AIDS debate a few years ago, which was very controversial to many people as he disputed a direct connection between HIV and AIDS. In his statements about the non-connection between HIV and AIDS, Mbeki seemed to be transgressing the borders of his expertise. In fact, what he did, was questioning common scientific knowledge. He found support for this in the writings of some dissident Western academics.

At the same time, he also claimed that AIDS is a disease of poverty. And here he rightfully pointed at the intricate relationship between AIDS and poverty, between AIDS and exclusion. Des Martin, Head of the HIV/AIDS Clinicians Society, said in 2002 (Smetherham, 2002):

> 'I believe there will be no NEPAD [New Partnership for Africa's Development], no sustainable development and no African Renaissance [and, we could easily add, no Rainbow Nation, HvR] unless we deal with HIV/AIDS.'

Referring to this quotation, we argue that there can be no sustainable development - that implies inclusion of people in the basic resources - if we cannot deal with AIDS as an integral health problem in Africa. A scientifically based 'bio-medical' (Western?) strategy alone will not suffice. But, it should be added, neither will a 'garlic strategy'[4]. AIDS, poverty and malnutrition, poor sanitation etc. go hand in hand and require an integral strategy of poverty alleviation and supply of antiretroviral medicines (see also Cohen, 2001).

## 9. The Knowledge Factor

The relationship between health, health care and the access (or denial of access) to resources is a recurrent theme in this book. From different perspectives it presents the intricate relationships between health, food, sanitation and multiple processes of in- and exclusion of adults and children.

This shows that the 'knowledge factor' is crucial in different sectors that relate to health and society. Not only will knowledge help us understand the processes of marginalisation and of in- and exclusion, but knowledge is also a critical factor in intervention programmes. At the same time, however, we should be aware of the fact that knowledge - medical, economic, political, religious, cultural, global and local knowledge - is also part of the processes of in- and exclusion. The feminist philosopher Donna Haraway said that epistemology is about knowing the difference (quoted by Mary Crewe, 1997). It is fair to conclude that there is a political economy of knowledge in our world.

The development of knowledge takes place in different sectors. There is an academic world dominated by universities and research institutes. This academic world seems to be dominated by universities and institutes in the Western world. The thorny question to be answered is whether this dominance coincides with a dominant Eurocentric science model and how this dominance relates to universities and research institutes in Africa.

In any case, we have seen (and still see) a constant quest for the *African* university. The label 'African' seems to refer to two interrelated views on knowledge. One is to escape Western (i.e. colonial and neo-colonial) dominance. And the other is to re-evaluate and re-appropriate authentic, indigenous, local African knowledge. For many centuries, Africa has indeed been an old repository, storing precious local knowledge and wisdom which threatens to be marginalised by the 'cool rational' Western science. Can we 'reconcile' these different streams of knowledge? And if so, what should be our strategy?

## 10. The Knowledge Agenda

The 'knowledge agenda' should first of all presuppose the concept of inclusion. We should take different streams of knowledge really serious. And we should let people participate in the development of these different streams of knowledge. We should therefore open up our universities in the West to young people from Southern countries to study and be trained in the different disciplines. The dominant model of the internationalisation of universities is a flow of established researchers and young students to Southern countries. And the reverse is a flow of trained African PhDs that find a place in Western universities. Already some ten years ago the World Bank estimated that yearly about 23.000 qualified university teachers left Africa to find better working conditions at Western universities. We may safely conclude that since that estimate was made (many) more than 230,000 highly skilled persons have left the African continent!

The 'knowledge agenda' should encourage people in Africa to stay in their home universities in Africa by helping the universities and research institutes in Africa to develop a sound infrastructure. This should be the responsibility of Western universities, assisted by governments and donor organisations. Otherwise, we will see the further development of slums and townships in our global academic village, the rich and the poor, the haves and have-nots.

The 'knowledge agenda' presupposes the development of common research projects, projects that first of all reflect the needs of the people in the South. Dominance of the research agenda by Western academics (which seems to be a dominant trend) will ultimately fail. This book represents efforts from persons from both sides who have taken the responsibility to get to know each other, to work together in teams. This book provides good examples of a common research-agenda developed in a process of partnership.

## Notes

1. www.anc.org.za/ancdocs/history/mbeki/1996/sp960508.html
2. Congress of South African Trade Unions.
3. www.cosatu.org.za/congress/cong2000/tm000918.htm
4. I refer to some remarks made by the present South African Minister of Health, Manto Tshabalala-Msimang, who suggested that raw garlic and lemon can protect you from diseases. This is why some called her Dr. Garlic (see 'Aids groups condemn South Africa's "Dr Garlic"' by Sarah Boseley, Health Editor, May 6, 2005, *The Guardian*). Only recently, the UNAIDS envoy in South Africa, Stephen Lewis, accused the South African government of reluctance to provide sufficient supplies of antiretroviral treatment (*Mail & Guardian*, November 4, 2005).

278

# References

Cohen, D. (2001). Joint Epidemics Poverty and Aids in Sub-Saharan Africa. *Harvard International Review*, Fall 2001

Crewe, M. (1997). Commentary: How Marginal is a "Marginalised Group"? *Social science and Medicine, 45*(6), 967-970.

Helman, C.G. (2000). *Culture, Health and Illness*. Oxford: Butterworth-Heinemann (4th ed.).

Rinsum, H.J. & Tangwa, G.B. (2004). Colony of Genes, genes of the colony: diversity, difference and divide. *Third World Quarterly, 25* (6), 1031-1043.

Smetherham, J.A. (2002). Doctors' Plan to set up HIV-drug sites in all provinces; interview with Des Martin. *The Cape Times,* 3 September 2002.

Tangwa, G.B. (2000). The traditional African perception of a person: Some implications for Bioethics. *Hastings Center Report, 30* (5), 39-43.

*Address for correspondence:*
Dr. H.J. van Rinsum
Utrecht University
Faculty of Social Sciences
Heidelberglaan 1
3584 CS Utrecht
e-mail: h.vanrinsum@fss.uu.nl

# Contributors

Prof. M.A.G. van Aken, PhD
Utrecht University
Department of Developmental Psychology
Heidelberglaan 1
3584 CS Utrecht
The Netherlands

Mrs. A.V. van Dijk, Msc
Griftstraat 45bis
3572 GP Utrecht
The Netherlands

Mrs. J.B. van den Dries, MSc
Jutfaseweg 45
3522 HD Utrecht
The Netherlands

Mr. R. Dullaert
St. Joseph's Care and Support Centre
Sizanani Village
P.O. Box 2016
Bronkhorstspruit 1020
Republic of South Africa

Mrs. A.C. Gardeniers, MSc
Ndlovu Medical Centre
P.O. Box 1
Elandsdoorn 0485
Republic of South Africa

Mrs. G. Groenhuijzen, MSc
Koperslagerstraat 77
8043 EM Zwolle
The Netherlands

Mrs. E.E. Klop, MSc
Akkermans & Partners
Biltstraat 154
3572 BN Utrecht
The Netherlands

Mrs. L.A. Korstjens, MSc
Minervaplein 40
3581 XP Utrecht
The Netherlands

Mr. C.M.M.V. van der Lubbe, MSc
Ndlovu Medical Centre
P.O. Box 1447
Groblersdal 0470
Republic of South Africa

Mrs. Z. Magyarszeky, BA
St. Mary's Home
Sizanani Village
P.O. Box 1372
Bronkhorstspruit 1020
Republic of South Africa

Mrs. T. Marcus, PhD
National Research Foundation
P.O. Box 2600
Pretoria 0001
Republic of South Africa

Prof. dr. D. Martin
South African HIV Clinicians Society
Suite 233
PosNet Killarney
Private Bag X2600
Houghton 2041
Republic of South Africa

Mrs. M. Mbethe
St. Mary's Home
Sizanani Village
P.O. Box 1372
Bronkhorstspruit 1020
Republic of South Africa

Mrs. J. Okma, MSc
Dr. D. Herderschool
Singledwarsstraat WZ 22
3505 AB Utrecht
The Netherlands

Mr. H.J. van Rinsum, PhD
Utrecht University
Faculty of Social Sciences
Heidelberglaan 1
3584 CS Utrecht
The Netherlands

Mrs. M. Schinnij, Msc
Fluitekamp 49
3828 WD Hoogland
The Netherlands

Mrs. F. Stofmeel, MSc
Ferdinand Bolstraat 48
3583 AS Utrecht
The Netherlands

Mrs. T.C. Tamboer, MSc
Parc Spelderholt
P.O. Box 73
7360 AB  Beekbergen
The Netherlands

Mr. H.A. Tempelman, MD
Ndlovu Medical Centre
P.O. Box 1447
Groblersdal 0470
Republic of South Africa

Mrs. L. Tempelman
Ndlovu Medical Centre
P.O. Box 1447
Groblersdal 0470
Republic of South Africa
Mr. R. Valks, Tax Lawyer
Loyens & Loeff
P.O. Box 17
5600 AA Endhoven
The Netherlands

Mrs. J.N. Veenstra, MSc
Psychologische Praktijk Putten
Veldstraat 7a
3881 JM Putten
The Netherlands

Prof. A. Vermeer, PhD
Utrecht University
Department of Educational Sciences
Heidelberglaan 1
3584 CS Utrecht
The Netherlands

Mrs. A. Versteege, MSc
Pieter Nieuwlandstraat 104
3514 HL Utrecht
The Netherlands

Mrs. M. de Waal, PhD
Southern African Catholic Bischops'
Conference
P.O. Box 941
Pretoria 0001
Republic of South Africa

Mrs. F.E.M. Wehmeijer, MSc
Hanzenstraat 27-II
1053 SK Amsterdam
The Netherlands

Mrs. M.A.A. Westeneng, MSc
Utrecht University
Department of Methodology and Statistics
Heidelberglaan 1
3584 CS Utrecht
The Netherlands

Mr. L. Wijnroks, PhD
Utrecht University
Department of Educational Sciences
Heidelberglaan 1
3584 CS Utrecht